Advances in Specialist Hip Surgery

Wolf R. Drescher • Kyung-Hoi Koo
Russell E. Windsor
Editors

Advances in Specialist Hip Surgery

Springer

Editors
Wolf R. Drescher
Department of Orthopedics
RWTH Aachen University Hospital
Aachen, Germany

Orthopedic Surgery of the Lower Limb and Arthroplasty
Rummelsberg Hospital
Schwarzenbruck, Germany

Russell E. Windsor
Orthopaedic Surgery, Hip and Knee Replacement
Hospital of Special Surgery
New York, NY
USA

Kyung-Hoi Koo
Department of Orthopaedic Surgery
Seoul National University Bundang Hospital
Seongnam, South Korea

Department of Orthopedic Surgery
Seoul National University College of Medicine
Seoul, South Korea

ISBN 978-3-030-61829-2　　ISBN 978-3-030-61830-8 (eBook)
https://doi.org/10.1007/978-3-030-61830-8

This Springer imprint is published by the registered company Springer Nature Switzerland AG
The registered company address is: Gewerbestrasse 11, 6330 Cham, Switzerland

Foreword

Hip Replacement was successfully developed in Europe over 60 years ago and was quickly adopted throughout the world over the next decade. As the early success from total hip replacement was so encouraging, many other operations and treatment interventions around the hip including osteotomy and debridement were abandoned or greatly reduced. Fast forward to today we now recognize that both arthroplasty and non-arthroplasty procedures have a place in the armamentarium of the surgeon treating hip conditions. *Advances in Specialist Hip Surgery* is published at an opportune time in the present state of hip surgery. Just as surgeons in Europe and throughout the world specialized their practices to knee surgery several decades ago, somewhat corresponding to the success of knee arthroscopy, today more surgeons throughout the world have confirmed their practice to hip surgery, somewhat related to hip arthroscopy, the resurgence of hip osteotomy, and the development of biologic solutions for hip disease.

Wolf Drescher and his editors have assembled experts in every aspect of hip surgery throughout the world to compose *Advances in Specialist Hip Surgery*. The authors have comprehensively covered the gamut of treatment options for patients of all ages and all conditions of the hip. Preservation surgery is presented in three detailed sections. These include maturity disorders of the hip, arthroscopy of the hip, and two comprehensive sections on the treatment of osteonecrosis. The primary hip replacement section includes up-to-data information on all bearing surface options used in different proportions of cases throughout the world. An excellent example is the use of ceramic-on-ceramic bearings, which are uncommonly used in some countries and extensively used in others. Intraoperative strategies for accurate component placement are described in detail. In the revision hip section, new technologies in bone ingrowth enhancement and a comprehensive description of all the treatment options for femoral and acetabular bone loss are presented.

The editors should be applauded for developing a text with the toolbox of options available to these surgeons who confine their practice to hip surgery but also for any surgeon treating patients with hip disease whether it be in high or low volume practice. *Advances in Specialist Hip Surgery* will provide solutions for surgeons and their patients through this global perspective.

Iowa City, IA, USA John J. Callaghan

Preface

The idea for this book was developed by the underwriting editors during the Biannual meeting of the ARCO (Association Research Osseous Circulation) October 2017 in Berlin. The aim was first to present the current knowledge about femoral head necrosis to the broader international community of hip surgeons. Furthermore, the idea was to present the very current developments in the field of hip joint surgery.

This book describes current and emerging techniques in hip surgery, providing the essential, up-to-date knowledge that will be required by the orthopaedic surgeon who plans to become a specialist hip surgeon. The opening chapter offers a concise overview of the surgical anatomy, with particular attention to details relevant to the surgical techniques outlined in the book. The authors believe that a concise knowledge of the anatomy is key to successful surgery, and key to the advancement of existing surgical techniques as well as the development of new surgical approaches and techniques. The increasingly popular anterior minimally invasive approach to the hip and a microinvasive variation of this approach are then described. Subsequent chapters present surgical approaches to developmental disorders of the hip, including dysplasia and femoroacetabular impingement. Avascular necrosis of the hip is an often neglected but internationally relevant disease that can mutilate the hip in young patients. Therefore, this book contains one chapter on the state-of-the-art diagnostics and treatment of this disease. Finally, the latest techniques and implants for primary and revision hip arthroplasty are discussed in depth. The international author team consists of recognised leaders in the field, many of whom have developed the classifications presented and new surgical techniques.

The current knowledge in specialised hip joint surgery starting with joint preserving osteotomies in childhood and in the younger adult is presented in this book. Serving at a large orthopaedic hospital with several decades of tradition allows the surgeon to observe long-term results of procedures performed in childhood. For example, patients who were treated by Professor Heinz Wagner at Rummelsberg Hospital are today seen by one of the signing editors (W.D.). Wagner's techniques have shown to preserve hip joints for three or more decades before they now need hip joint replacement. This is very strong evidence and a strong argument to preserve and advance the knowledge about osteotomies, impingement surgery, cell therapy, and other preserving techniques for the coming generations of hip joint specialist surgeons.

Schwarzenbruck and Aachen, Germany Wolf R. Drescher
Seongnam, South Korea Kyung-Hoi Koo
New York, NY, USA Russell E. Windsor

Acknowledgements

At Springer, we would like to acknowledge

- Ms. Deepika Devan, Project Coordinator (Books)
- Mrs. Irmela Bohn, Ass. Editor and
- Mrs. Gabriele Schröder, Editorial Director, Clinical Medicine

for their continuous and professional support from start to finalising this international book.

Dr. Wolf R. Drescher

My Mentors

First, I would like to thank professor Cody E. Bünger, Dept. of Orthopaedics at Aarhus University Hospital, Denmark, for being my ever supporting supervisor during my experimental work on femoral head blood flow in the start of my career.

Second, I would like to thank professor Markus Tingart and professor emeritus Fritz U. Niethard, Dept. of Orthopedics at RWTH University Hospital, Aachen, Germany, for sharing their knowledge and teaching during my time at their department.

Also, I would like to thank Professor Thomas Pufe, Institute of Anatomy and Cell Biology at RWTH University, Aachen, Germany, for our friendship and research cooperation during more than 15 years now.

My Family

I would like to thank my wife Ana, my son Rudolf, and my parents for their loving support and patience.

Dr. Russell E. Windsor

My Mentors

I would like to thank Chitranjan Ranawat, Thomas Sculco, and Eduardo Salvati for teaching me about the art of total hip replacement at the Hospital for Special Surgery. I am particularly indebted to the late John Insall with him I did a year-long fellowship in Knee Reconstructive Surgery at the Hospital for Special Surgery. I also would like to thank Marvin Steinberg who taught me at the University of Pennsylvania and taught me much about the treatment of avascular necrosis of the hip.

My Family

I would sincerely like to thank my wife, Theresa and my children, Gillian, Russell and Eric for all their support for allowing me to work as an orthopaedic surgeon. They always are the bedrock that supports all that I do, and it would be impossible to surgeon I am without their love.

Dr. Kyung-Hoi Koo

My Mentors

I would like to thank my mentors: Drs Young-Min Kim, David S. Hungerford, John Paul Jones Jr., Yoich Sugioka and Gwo-Jaw Wang. I also thank members of ARCO (Association Research Circulation Osseous) and my fellow group.

My Family

I deeply appreciate my wife, In-Oak and my daughters: Kate, Jain, my son-in-law: James, and my lovely grand-daughter: Gia.

Contents

Part I

Anatomy of the Hip and Its Surgical Application

Surgical Anatomy of the Hip

1

Andreas Prescher and Wolf R. Drescher

"Not to know the normal anatomy is unexcusable and to confuse a point of abnormal anatomy can of course be disastrous"

Rush K. Aston

1.1 Surface Anatomy

The palpation of the hip joint and its structures is difficult, because the joint is covered by thick muscles and a variable amount of subcutaneous adipose tissue. Even in an obese patient the tendon of the adductor longus muscle is not covered by subcutaneous fatty tissue, so that it can be palpated at its origin [1]. On the posterior side the gluteal fold marks the inferior border of the buttock. The fold correlates with a condensed strip of the gluteal fascia, which is known as "Sitzhalfter." Topographically the gluteal line crosses horizontally the inferior part of the gluteus maximus at the level of the ischial tuberosity. The fold is the posterior flexure line of the hip joint. On the anterior side, somewhat caudally to the inguinal ligament, the fold of the groin crosses the femoral head. For orientation different lines and triangles had been defined in order to investigate the hip joint. Two important constructions should be mentioned: Roser-Nelaton's line and Bryant's triangle. Roser-Nelaton's line is connecting the anterior superior iliac spine and the ischial tuberosity. This line should pass the tip of the greater trochanter a bit proximally. Bryant's triangle is a rectangular isosceles figure, which is constructed by a horizontal line through the anterior superior iliac spine, a vertical line through the greater trochanter and a line connecting the anterior superior iliac spine with the tip of the greater trochanter. The vertical line through the trochanter is also called the "basal line" or "Bryant's line." An asymmetry of Bryant's line can be a hint to hip joint dislocation, fracture of femoral neck or coxa vara. Furthermore the pulsation of the femoral artery can be identified easily under the midpoint of the inguinal ligament, where the vessel is lying anterior to the femoral head, only the articular capsule and the iliopsoas tendon intervening [2]. The important palpable osseous landmarks are summarized in Table 1.1.

Table 1.1 Palpable osseous landmarks

• Anterior superior iliac spine
• Posterior superior iliac spine
• Iliac crest
• Ischial tuberosity
• Innominate tubercle
• Pubic tubercle

A. Prescher (✉)
Institute of Molecular and Cellular Anatomy, Prosektur, RWTH University Hospital, Aachen, Germany
e-mail: aprescher@ukaachen.de

W. R. Drescher
Department of Orthopedics, RWTH Aachen University Hospital, Aachen, Germany

Orthopedic Surgery of the Lower Limb and Arthroplasty, Rummelsberg Hospital, Schwarzenbruck, Germany
e-mail: wolf.drescher@sana.de

W. R. Drescher et al. (eds.), *Advances in Specialist Hip Surgery*,
https://doi.org/10.1007/978-3-030-61830-8_1

1.2 Proximal Part of the Femur

The proximal part of the femur is characterized by three essential structures: the head, the neck, and the trochanters. The spheroid or slightly ovoid femoral head presents at its medial area a rough pit, the fovea capitis femoris. In youth this fovea contains large and numerous nutrient foramina (Fig. 1.1a) for the vascularization of the proximal femoral epiphysis. After closure of the epiphyseal plate, the vessels of the ligamentum capitis femoris are no longer essential, so that they are partly diminishing (Fig. 1.1b). Between the femoral head and neck a subcapital sulcus can be recognized (Fig. 1.3a, b). This is important, because the neck measures only about three fourth of the equatorial diameter of the head. This anatomy enables a wide range of motion without an acetabular impingement. The femoral head is sitting on the collum femoris, which presents a somewhat flattened shape in the a.p.-direction and a greater diameter caudally than cranially (Fig. 1.2a). Furthermore, the strongest cortical lamella is also present at the caudal circumference. The femoral collum shows a slight posterior curvature of the femoral neck axis towards the head (Fig. 1.4d). Combined with the projection of the intertrochanteric crest, these conditions are responsible for a definite advantage of the lateral rotator muscles in movement of the hip joint, as it was outlined by Harty [3]. The posterior wall of the neck is a little bit concave in contrast to the anterior wall (Fig. 1.4d). The collum femoris and femoral shaft are forming the important collodiaphyseal angel. This term is a misnomer, because the collum femoris also belongs to the diaphysis. Therefore the designation as centrodiaphyseal angle would be a better term. Normally the angle presents values between 120 and 130°. A value greater than 130° signifies a coxa valga while an angle lower than 120° is called coxa vara. These conditions are important, because the load bearing area of the articulation differs, so that the loading is also different. In a normal hip joint the loading force is about 22 kp/cm^2. In a case of coxa valga the load-bearing area is smaller than in normal cases, so that a higher pressure of about 27.5 kp/cm^2 results. Therefore the coxa valga can be seen as prearthrotic deformity. But in cases with a well developed acetabular roof this can be compensated, because in such cases the loading can be normal, due to the enlarged area of the roof [4]. In case of a coxa vara the load-bearing area is enlarged, so that the load is diminishing to ~16.5 kp/cm^2. In these cases the greater lever of the femoral collum leads to a higher bending stress in the intertrochanteric region, so that the possibility of fracture is increasing [5]. Furthermore a serious limitation of the abduction can be caused by an impingement mechanism (Fig. 1.1d).

In addition to the centrodiaphyseal angle the torsion (declination) of the femur must be described. This declination is defined as the angle between the plane of the femoral condyles and the axis of the femoral neck. The torsion shows a wide range between coxa antetorta, the typical anteversion of 12–14°, and even retroversion.

Laterally we can recognize the greater trochanter. This large osseous mass is formed as a typical apophysis (Fig. 1.2a). The tip of the greater trochanter is bending medially over the trochanteric fossa. Furthermore the tip is covered by large muscular masses, so that it cannot be palpated. The lateral margin of the greater trochanter is V-shaped, because the superior part is bended medially and the inferior part extends from the inferomedial direction. According to this geometry a laterally protruding tubercle is formed at the lateral margin of the greater trochanter (Fig. 1.3b). Only this tubercle, called the innominate tubercle, is palpable and establishes an important landmark. Unfortunately the designation "innominate tubercle" is also used for the tubercle at the cranial end of the intertrochanteric line, so that confusion can occur. This tubercle is also known as "femoral tubercle" (Fig. 1.3a) and presents a useful landmark for osteotomies in anterior approaches [6]. The trochanteric fossa is the insertion point for the external obturator muscle. Normally this insertion is a more or less pronounced tray (Fig. 1.2b). But in some cases an irregular, osseous tubercle ("exostosis") can be seen in this region (Fig. 1.2c), which is considered by some authors as racial non-metric characteristic [7]. In contradiction to this view the first author is convinced that it is a simple fibroostosis of the tendon of the external obturator muscle

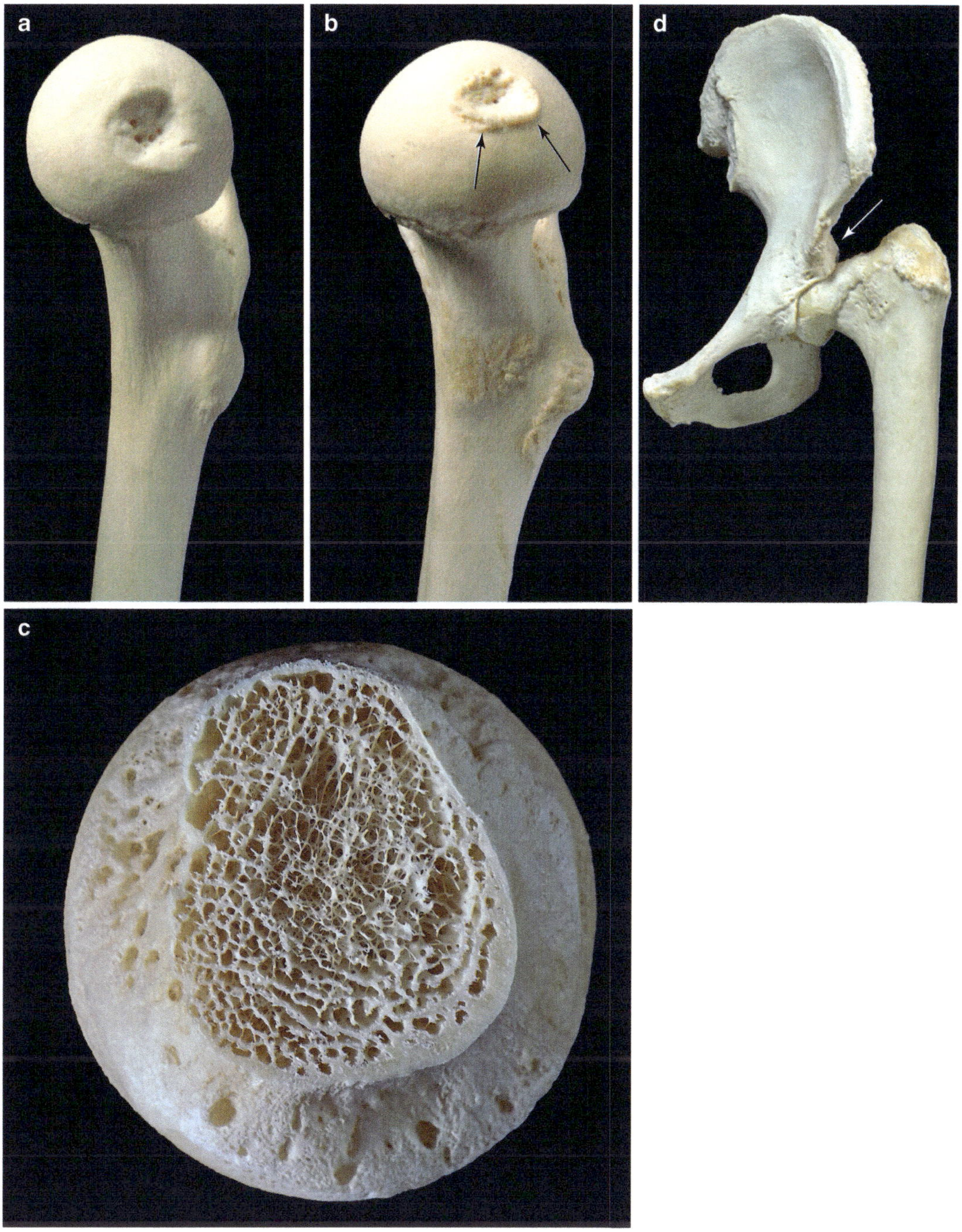

Fig. 1.1 (**a**) Caput femoris (20 year old male). Notice the fovea capitis femoris with numerous large nutrient foramina. (**b**) Caput femoris (71 year old male). Notice the perifoveolar osteophyte (arrows) as an early sign of arthrosis and the reduced number of nutrient foramina in the fovea capitis femoris. (**c**) Cross section of the femoral neck. Notice the different thickness of the cortical lamella and the geometry of the neck. (**d**) Severe coxa vara. Notice the blocked abduction (arrow)

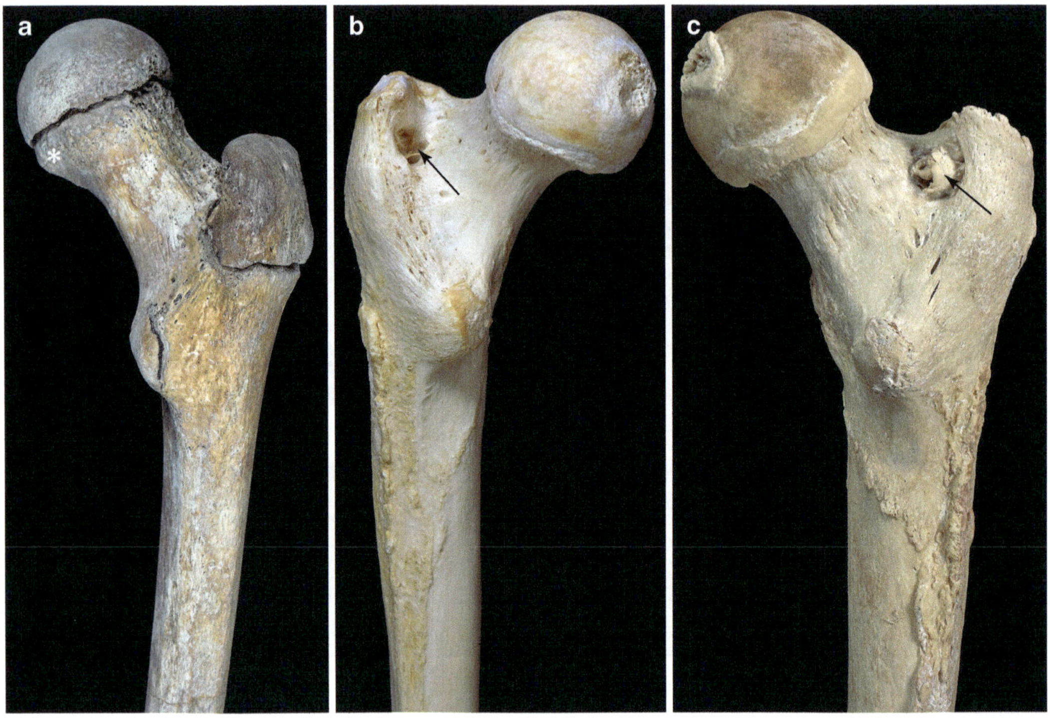

Fig. 1.2 (**a**) Proximal part of the femur (child, archaeological specimen). Notice the epiphyseal and apophyseal clefts which are separating the caput, the greater and lesser trochanter. Furthermore the balcony-like part of the collum (star) can be seen, which will be integrated into the femoral head in the further development. (**b**) Notice the deepening (arrow) in the region of the external obturator tendon insertion. (**c**) Notice the sturdy fibroostosis (arrow) of the external obturator tendon

and not an anatomical variation. Dorsomedially, at the inferior end of the intertrochanteric line, the not palpable lesser trochanter can be seen as a structure which presents a rough anterior surface and a smooth, polished posterior surface. This conical lesser trochanter, also an apophysis (Fig. 1.2a), is the insertion point for the iliopsoas tendon. Between the greater and lesser trochanter we see at the anterior surface the intertrochanteric line (Fig. 1.3a) and on the dorsal side the intertrochanteric crest (Fig. 1.3b). Nearly in the midpart of the intertrochanteric crest often a small osseous bump, the quadrate tubercle, can be observed, where the quadratus femoris muscle is inserting. At the intertrochanteric line the articular capsule is inserted, so that the whole anterior surface of the collum is an intraarticular structure. This is important, because the covering soft tissue of the anterior surface of the collum is not a real periosteum, as it was outlined by Schmorl [8]. Therefore this covering layer has no osteoblastic potential. During aging this leads to physiological bone loss at the inner surface, which is not compensated by appositional bone formation at the outer side. As a result of these processes a weakening of the femoral collum occurs, which is closely connected to the increasing danger of fracturing the femoral collum during aging. At the cranial end of the labium laterale of the linea aspera the rough gluteal tuberosity can be seen. In some cases this tuberosity is expressed as a third trochanter (trochanter tertius; Fig. 1.3c). The trochanter tertius is an anatomical variation without clinical interest but it is important for anthropology.

The inner part of the proximal femur shows a typical trabecular architecture. Normally we have to differentiate primary and secondary trabeculae [9]. Each group can be further subdivided into compression and tension trabeculae. Tension trabeculae are positioned in the lateral region and compression trajectories in the medial region (Fig. 1.3d). Between these two kinds of trajectories a weak area with a decreasing number of trajectories is visible (Figs. 1.3d and 1.4d).

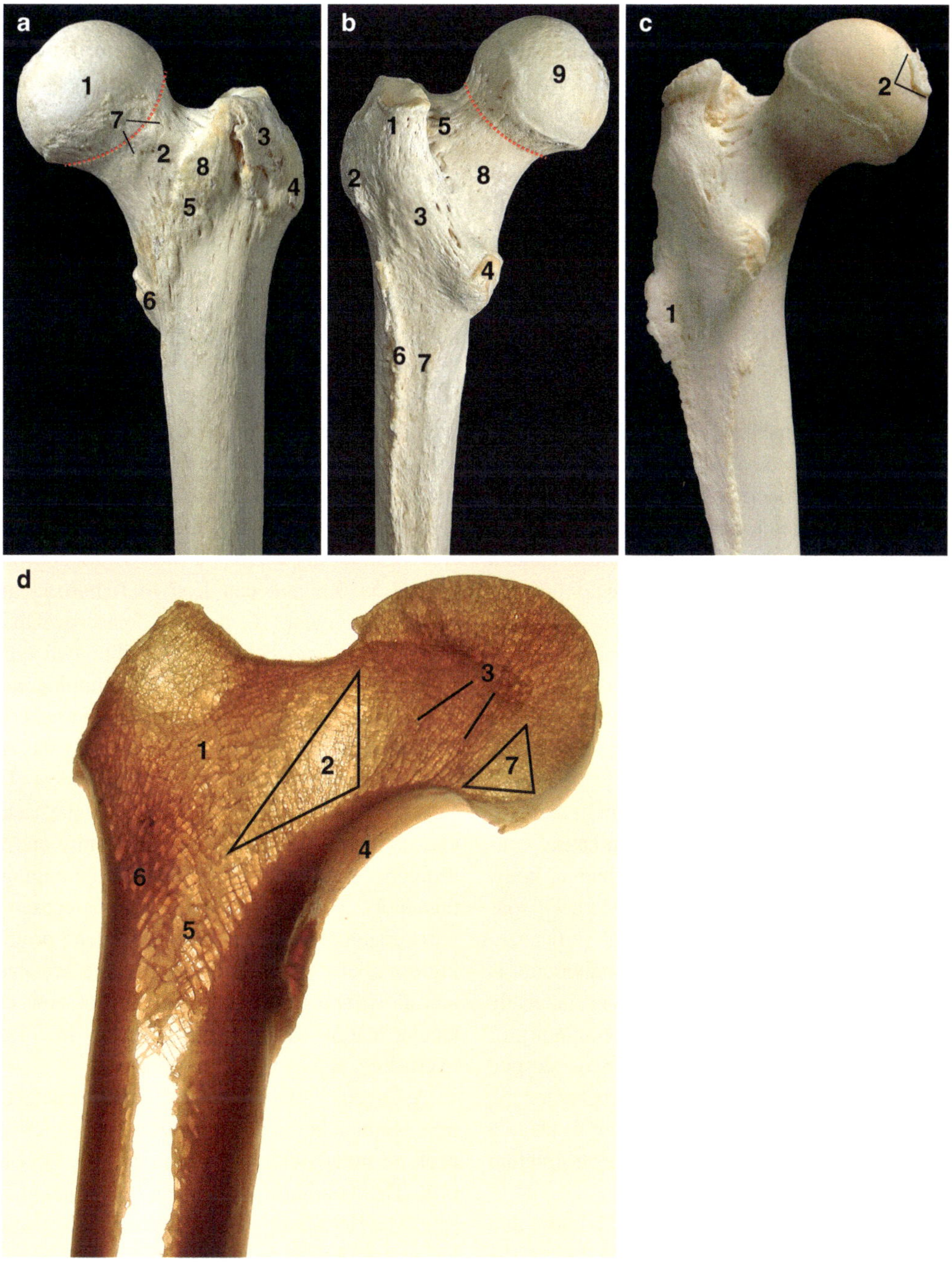

Fig. 1.3 (**a**) Anterior aspect of the proximal femur. **1**: Caput femoris, **2**: Collum femoris, **3**: Trochanter major. **4**: Tuberculum innominatum, **5**: Linea intertrochanterica, **6**: Trochanter minor, **7**: Walmsley's ridge, **8**: Tuberculum femorale. The slight line indicates the subcapital sulcus. (**b**) Posterior aspect of the proximal femur. **1**: Trochanter major, **2**: Tuberculum innominatum, **3**: Crista intertrochanterica, **4**: Trochanter minor, **5**: Fossa trochanterica, **6**: Tuberositas glutaea, **7**: Linea pectinea, **8**: Collum femoris, **9**: Tuberculum m. quadrati femoris. The slight line indicates the subcapital sulcus. (**c**) Posterior aspect of the proximal femur. **1**: Trochanter tertius, **2**: perifoveolar osteophyte as sign of a beginning arthrosis deformans. (**d**) Frontal section of the proximal femur in diaphanoscopy. **1**: Primary tension trabeculae, **2**: Ward's triangle, **3**: primary compression trabeculae, **4**: thickened medial cortical buttress, which is often misinterpreted as Calcar femorale, **5**: secondary compression trabeculae, **6**: secondary tension trabeculae, **7**: Babcock's triangle. Inset: explanation of the different kinds of trabeculae

This area is known as "triangle of Ward" [10]. In cases of coxa valga, Ward's triangle is diminishing, so that nearly only pressure trajectories are present. Another, smaller area with a decreased number of osseous trabeculae can be seen at the inferior region of the femoral head. This triangle is termed Babcock's triangle (Fig. 1.3d).

An additional, somewhat mysterious structure must also be mentioned: "Merkel's spur (Calcar femorale, Schenkelsporn) (Fig. 1.4a–d). Many authors (e.g. [11, 12]) confuse the spur with the thickened and condensed cortical buttress in the medial junction of femoral neck and shaft, as it was explicitly outlined by Harty [3]. This is also the situation in our days. Originally this structure was described by Friedrich Merkel in 1873 [13] but there are quite earlier descriptions and figures in the literature. The spur originates as a cortical lamella protruding from the dorsomedial region of the lesser trochanter into the spongious material of the proximal femoral end, fans out and points towards the greater trochanter (Fig. 1.4d). This orientation is important, because in cases of trochanteric fractures the spur acts as wedge and splits of the lesser trochanter and the intertrochanteric crest [3]. Merkel's spur is a structure which is only present in humans, so that it is hypothesized, that it is in causal connection to the verticalization of the human body. This is supported by the fact, that Merkel's spur appears ontogenetically in the time of verticalization and that it disappears, when an individuum is immobilized and horizontalized. Biomechanically Merkel's spur helps to preserve the continuity of the cylindrical femoral shaft into the neck, despite the backward projection of the lesser trochanter and the intertrochanteric crest. This anatomy leads to a reinforcement of the weak angulated bone structure in the proximal femoral region [3].

Merkel's spur can be seen in CT-scans and in classical X-rays, especially lateral and in the Lauenstein projections [3, 14].

In the region of the femoral neck different anatomical variations can be present. At the anterior surface, 1–1.5 cm laterally to the subcapital sulcus, a slight osseous ridge, orientated in a craniocaudal direction, can be seen in some cases. This ridge is known as "capsular ridge" or "Walmsley's ridge" (Fig. 1.3a). It must not be confused with the "Eminentia articularis colli femoris," described by Rudolf Fick [15]. This eminence extends horizontally from the cranial end of the intertrochanteric line to the femoral head. At the medial end of this femoral neck eminence a flat tray can be present, where the spongious material is often not covered by a cortical lamella. This region is termed "Empreinte iliaque Poirier" or "Allan's Fossa." Furthermore in some cases a superior extension of the articular surface on the femoral head towards the femoral neck can be seen, which is known as "Poirier's Facet."

A good description of all these entities was given by Walmsley [16], Odgers [17], and Angel [18].

In some cases the subcapital sulcus is not expressed in the superior circumference, so that the superior area of the femoral head is in continuity with the superior area of the femoral neck. This condition is known as "Pistol-Grip-Deformity" (Fig. 1.5a, b), and can lead to femoroacetabular impingement. Generally femoroacetabular impingement can be subdivided into two types: Cam and Pincer impingement. Cam impingement is characterized by an anterolateral, non-spherical osseous structure, which is pressed into the acetabulum during flexion or internal rotation. This causes an arthrotic degeneration only of the acetabular cartilage. The Pistol-Grip-Deformity and the different osseous bumps and lines are belonging to this entity. The Pincer impingement is caused by retroversion of the acetabulum or a lateral protruding acetabular roof. In these cases the acetabular labrum will be squeezed between the osseous acetabular margin and the femoral neck, which leads to crushing and tearing of the labrum.

As result of a chronic femoroacetabular impingement at the anterior surface of the femoral neck an intraosseous ganglion can be established [19]. This condition is known as "Herniation Pit" [20]. The Herniation Pit is characterized by a cystic lesion, surrounded by a sclerotic margin (important for radiologic diagnosis!) and a little opening at the anterior surface of the femoral neck (Fig. 1.5c, d).

1.3 Acetabulum

The acetabulum is formed by all three osseous components of the innominate bone by different amounts of material. 2/5 of the acetabulum are

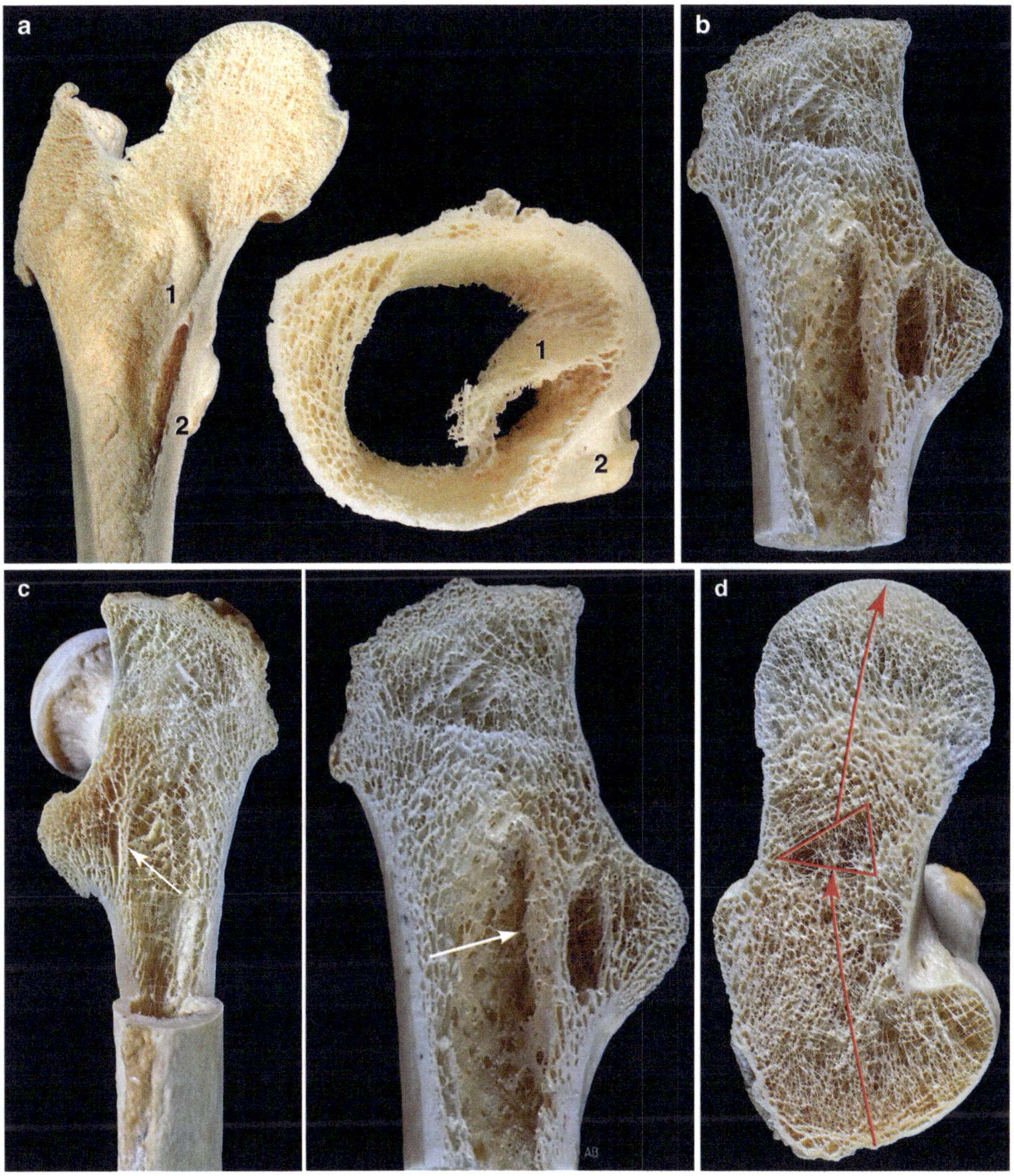

Fig. 1.4 (**a**) Frontal section of the proximal femur. **1**: Merkel's spur or calcar femorale. **2**: "calcar femorale": wrong designation for the medial thickened cortical buttress. (**b**) Horizontal section in the region of the lesser trochanter. **1**: Merkel's spur, **2**: Trochanter minor. (**c**) Sagittal section of the proximal femur. Merkel's spur (arrow). (**d**) Horizontal section of the femoral neck. The slight line indicates the anterior convex curvature of the femoral neck and the marked area indicates Ward's triangle

formed each by the os ilium and the ischial bone. The pubic bone contributes 1/5. These components are separated in young individuals by the triradiate cartilage, which presents an anterior, posterior, and vertical flange. In these young specimens a discrete protuberance towards the smaller pelvis can be seen on the medial aspect of the acetabulum. This protuberance is known as "physiological protrusion of the acetabulum" [21]. It should not be confused with a pathological protrusion (arthrokatadysis), which can be seen as accompanying feature of an osteomalacious process or a complication of a loosening endoprothesis. Furthermore primary acetabular

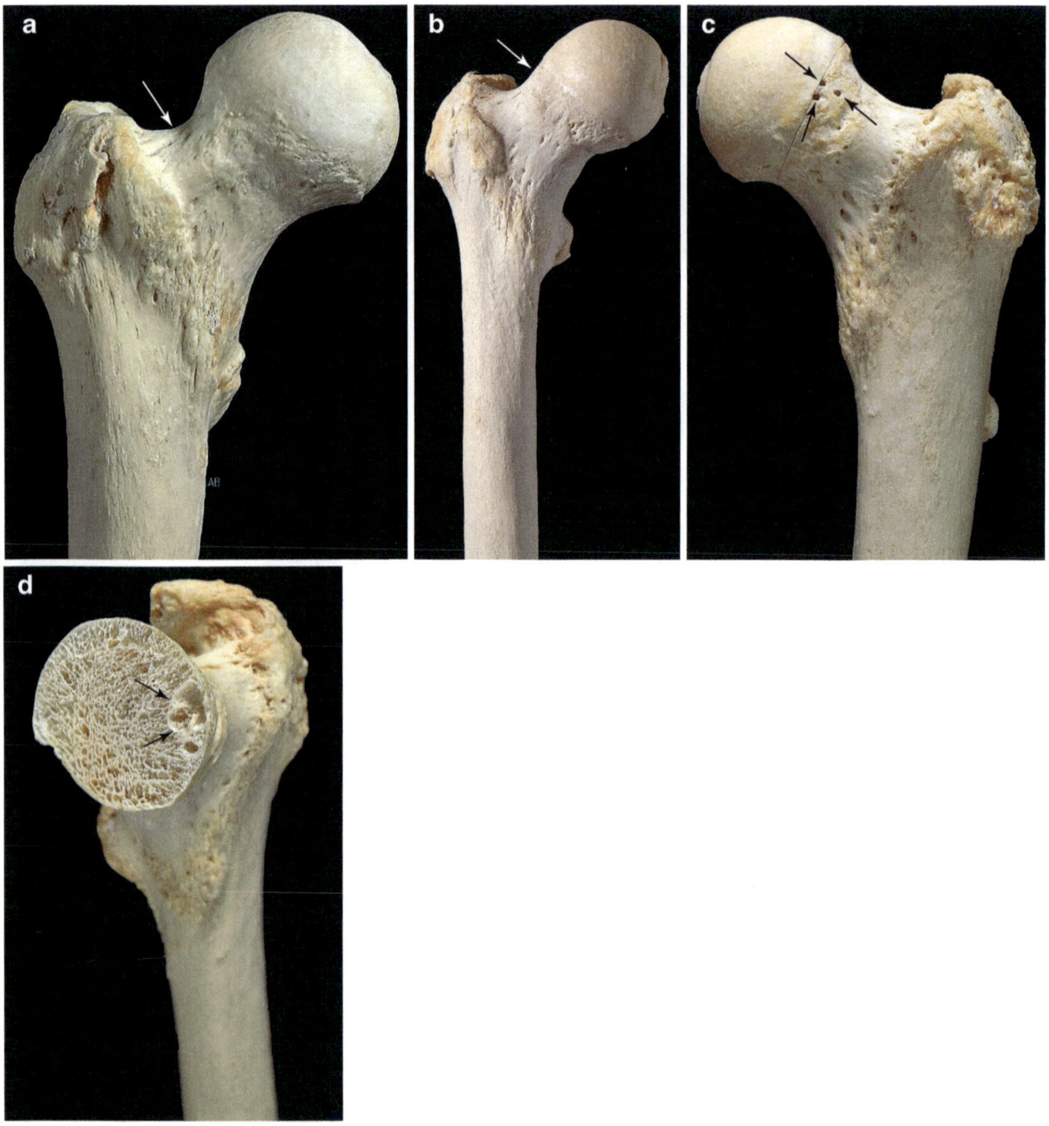

Fig. 1.5 (**a**) Anterior aspect of the proximal femur. The arrow indicates the regular waist-line of the femoral neck (subcapitular sulcus). (**b**) Anterior aspect of the proximal femur. The arrow indicates the lacking waist-line (subcapitular sulcus) of the femoral neck. The articular surface is in continuity with the superior area of the femoral neck. This morphology is known as "Pistol grip-deformity". (**c**) Herniation Pit. The arrows indicate three foramina, which are openings of an intraosseous cavity. (**d**) Herniation Pit: Cross section of the specimen of (**c**). The arrows indicate the osseous cavity, which is surrounded by a typical sclerotic wall

protrusion can be the result of an abnormal progression of the triradiate cartilage development [22]. If such a protrusion is affecting both hips, this condition is known as Otto-Chrobak-Pelvis. During ossification of the triradiate cartilage at first typical intercalated osseous islands are appearing within the cartilage. These ossicles represent the central epiphyses of the iliac, ischial, and pubic bone. The fusion of the triradiate complex commences around 11 years in females and 14 years in males and is completed at 15 years in females and 17 years in males [22].

The fully developed acetabulum is surrounded by an osseous ridge, the acetabular rim (Fig. 1.6a). This rim is not orientated in one plane. Especially in the dorsocaudal region the rim deviates medi-

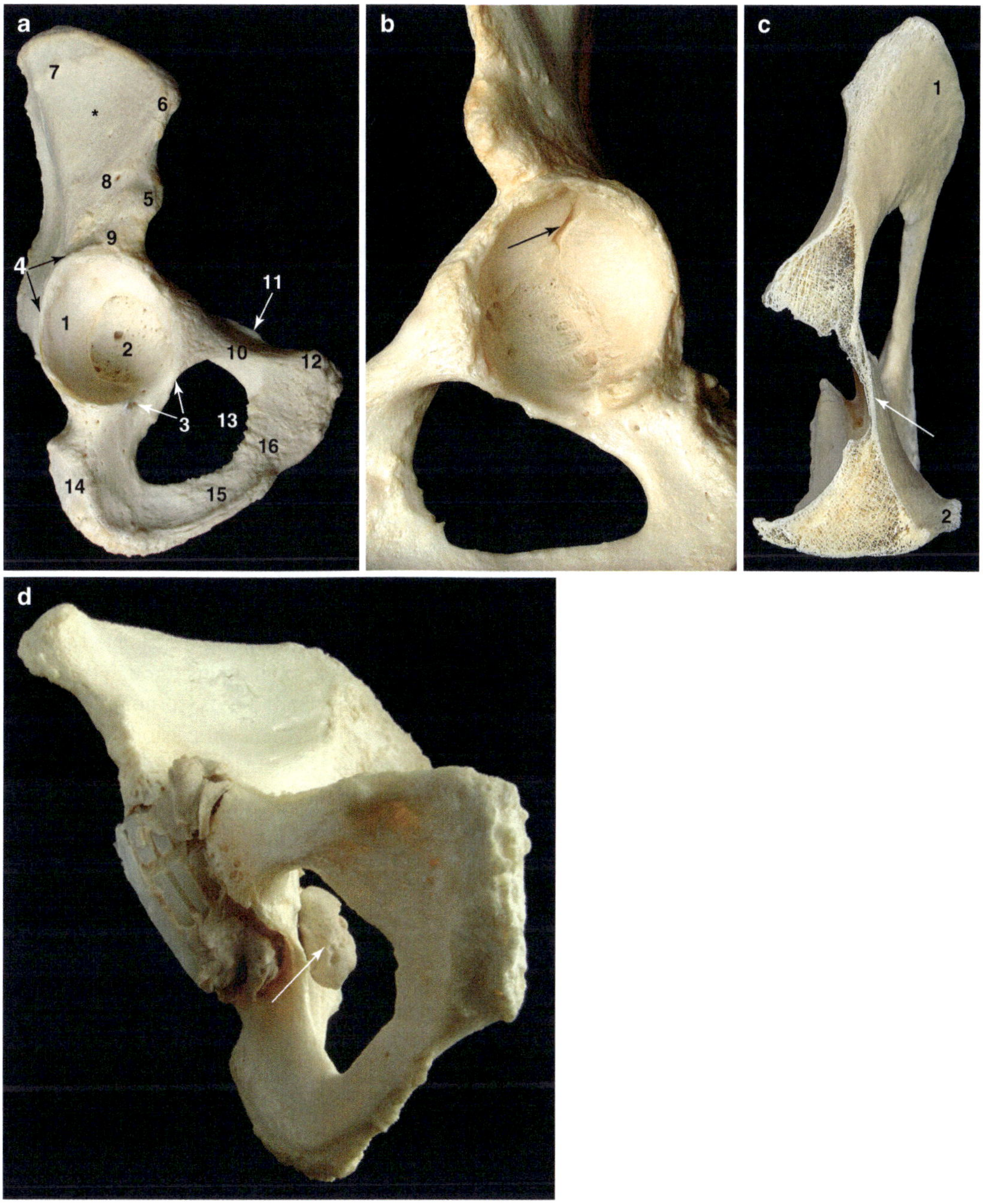

Fig. 1.6 (**a**) Innominate bone with insight of the acetabulum. **1**: Facies lunata, **2**: Fossa acetabuli, **3**: Incisura acetabuli, **4**: Limbus acetabuli, **5**: Spina iliaca anterior inferior, **6**: Spina iliaca anterior superior, **7**: Linea glutaea anterior, **8**: Linea glutaea inferior, **9**: Sulcus supraacetabularis, **10**: Ramus superior ossis pubis, **11**: Pecten ossis pubis, **12**: Tuberculum pubicum, **13**: Foramen obturatum, **14**: Tuber ischiadicum, **15**: Ramus ossis ischii, **16**: Ramus inferior ossis pubis. The star indicates the origin of the M. glutaeus medius between the Linea glutaea superior and the Linea glutaea inferior. (**b**) Insight of the left acetabulum. The arrow indicates a typical cleft in the superior region of the lunate area. This is a congenital anatomical variation. (**c**) Horizontal section of the acetabulum. The arrow indicates the very thin floor of the acetabular fossa. (**d**) Innominate bone with implanted acetabular cup. The arrow indicates a typical transacetabular cement cone

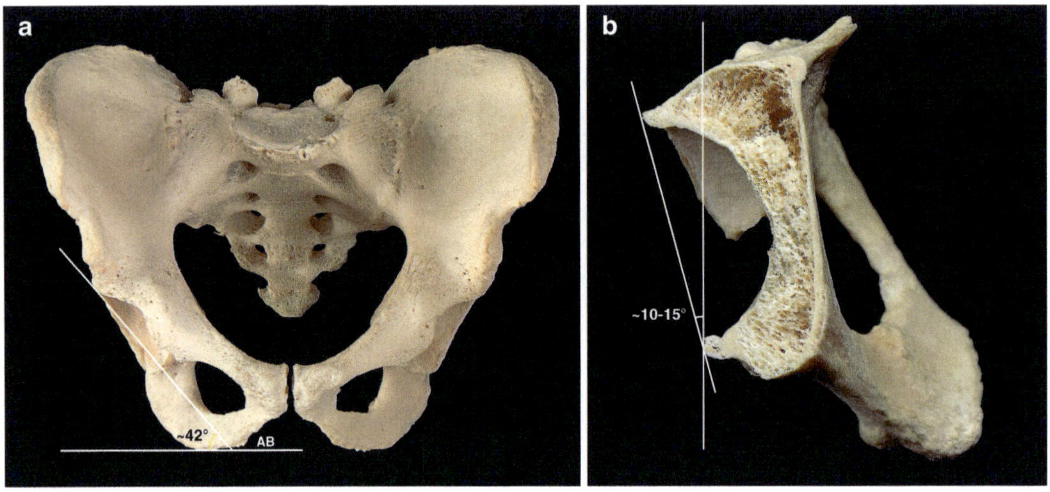

Fig. 1.7 (**a**) Normal horizontal inclination of the acetabulum. (**b**) Normal sagittal anteversion of the acetabulum

ally (Fig. 1.7a). The rim is interrupted at the anterior inferior margin, so that the acetabular notch is formed. This notch is bridged by the transverse acetabular ligament. The normal acetabular fossa has a characteristic orientation, which is defined by the horizontal inclination and the sagittal anteversion. The horizontal inclination is 42°, whereas the sagittal anteversion should be 10–15° (Fig. 1.7a, b). Together with the regular antetorsion of the femur (~12°) this geometry enables hip flexion up to 90° without femoroacetabular impingement. These anatomic features must be considered during total hip replacement.

The inner surface of the acetabulum shows the lunate area (Fig. 1.6a), which is covered with hyaline cartilage. This cartilage has its maximal thickness in the lateral region near the acetabular rim and especially at the anterior acetabular roof, which is due to the high pressure loading in this region [23]. The lunate area has a narrow anterior cornu and a broader posterior one [24]. In some cases the lunate area shows a typical cleft at its superior part (Fig. 1.6b), which can be recognized in X-rays. A separation of the anterior or posterior cornu by a cleft is also found. The center of the acetabulum, a rough area without hyaline cartilage, is the deepest point of the acetabulum. In this area several nutrient canals are present. Often the floor of the fossa acetabuli is very thin (Fig. 1.6c), showing also dehiscences, especially in old patients. These defects as well as large osseous canals for the vessels can be important when implanting a cemented cup. In some cases the cement drains through the dehiscences into the small pelvis, forming an irregular and bizarre cement protrusion, a so-called transacetabular cement cone [25] (Fig. 1.6d). This protrusion as well as the heat, generated by the polymerizing cement, can affect the obturator nerve running at the medial border of the acetabulum.

As an anatomical variation an isolated ossicle can occur at the superior margin of the acetabulum in 5% [26]. This ossicle is known as "Os ad acetabulum." The origin of this element can be due to different circumstances. It can be a congenital variation (persisting superior epiphysis), an arthrotic, isolated osteophyte or a stress fracture of the limbus acetabuli. The designation of this element as os acetabuli should be avoided, because this term should only be used for the intercalated osseous islands appearing within the triradiate cartilage.

1.4 Intraarticular Structures

Three intraarticular structures must be mentioned: the round ligament, the fat pad in the acetabular fossa, and the acetabular labrum.

1.4.1 The Round Ligament

This ligament originates with three parts. The anterior one is coming from the anterior cornu of the lunate area, the posterior one is originating from the posterior cornu, and the middle originates from the transverse acetabular ligament. It is inserting at the flat fovea capitis femoris and is sheathed by a thin tube of synovial tissue, the so-called inner synovial funnel [27]. The mechanical properties seem to be of no importance. Because of its length (3.5 cm) it is not able to stabilize the hip joint. But if the joint is moving, the cartilaginous surface of the femoral head is moving under this ligament, so that the synovial fluid is greased and mixed up. Therefore the ligament seems to be important for the lubrication of the hip joint and for the exchange of synovial fluid components. Furthermore the ligament contains arterial vessels, arising from the obturator artery as well as from the medial circumflex femoral artery. These vessels are according to Trueta important for the nutrition of the epiphysis in young individuals with preserved epiphyseal plate.

1.4.2 The Acetabular Fat Pad

In the fossa acetabuli a strongly vascularized, extrasynovial fat pad, the pulvinar acetabulare ("Havers' gland" of former times) can be seen (Fig. 1.8a). This pad is lying in the deepest part of the acetabulum and is important for the production of synovial fluid, necessary for the nutrition of the exhaustive areas of hyaline cartilage cover-

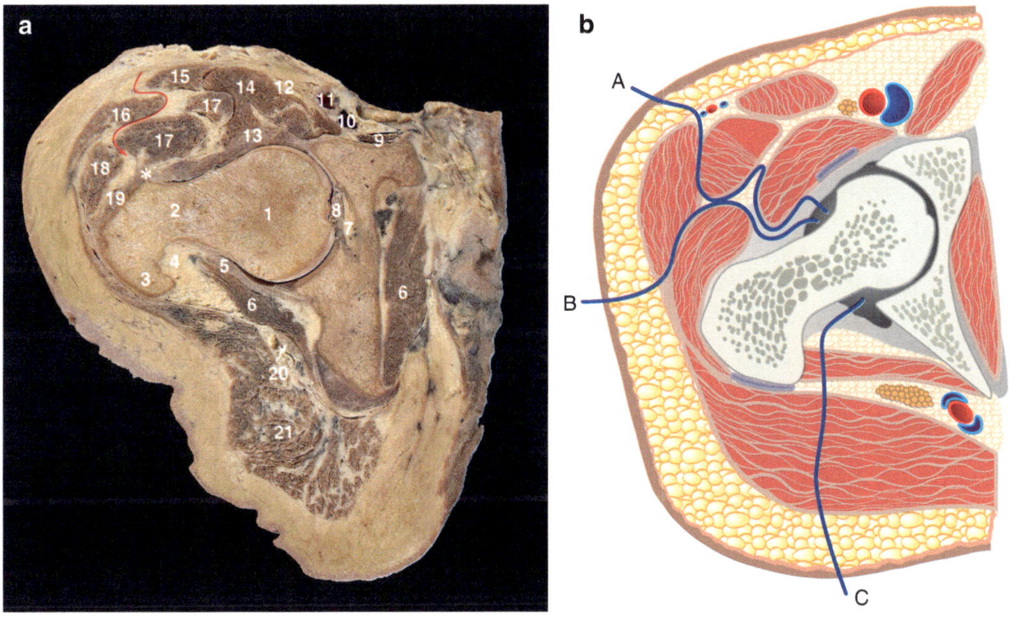

Fig. 1.8 (**a**) **1**: Caput femoris, **2**: Collum femoris, **3**: Trochanter major, **4**: Fossa trochanterica, **5**: posterior articular capsule, **6**: M. obturatorius internus, **7**: Pulvinar acetabulare in acetabular fossa, **8**: Lig. capitis femoris, **9**: M. pectineus, **10**: V. femoralis, **11**: A. femoralis, **12**: N. femoralis, **13**: anterior articular capsule, **14**: M. iliopsoas, **15**: M. sartorius, **16**: M. tensor fasciae latae, **17**: M. rectus femoris, **18**: M. glutaeus medius, **19**: M. vastus lateralis, **20**: N. ischiadicus, **21**: M. glutaeus maximus. The **star** indicates the insertion of the articular capsule at the intertrochanteric line. Notice that the ventral area of the femoral neck is completely intraarticular! **The red arrow** indicates the anterior approach, using Smith-Peterson's interval. (**b**) Schematic drawing of a horizontal section of the hip joint. The different possibilities of surgical approaches are indicated by arrows. **A**: Anterior approach using Smith-Peterson's interval. **B**: Lateral approach using Watson-Jones's interval. **C**: Posterior transgluteal approach with dissection of the short external rotators

ing the femoral head and the lunate area of the acetabulum. Furthermore this soft, yielding structure enables free movement of the round ligament, and prevents damage of this structure by compression, squeezing, and friction forces.

1.4.3 The Acetabular Labrum

A fibrocartilaginous lip, the acetabular labrum, is sitting with its broad base on the acetabular limbus and on the transverse acetabular ligament. The sharp margin of the acetabular labrum projects freely into the articular space (Fig. 1.9). The labrum is closely related to the surface of the femoral head, so that the inner articular space is hermetically closed. In this space a negative pressure is held up, so that the atmospheric pressure is able to hold the femoral head into the acetabulum. This was impressively demonstrated by the classical experiment of the Weber brothers. The acetabular rim together with the acetabular labrum is called acetabular limbus. Unfortunately the acetabular labrum is often termed as "limbus acetabuli," which is a typical misnomer. Due to the limbus acetabuli the whole acetabulum is deepened, so that the femoral head is fixed sufficiently in the cup. Furthermore the labrum contains numerous nerve fibers and receptors, so that it can be seen as important structure for proprioception [28]. At the outer side the perilimbic or perilabral recess is formed between the rim of the acetabular fossa and the articular capsule, which inserts at the basis of the labrum. The term "perilimbic recess" is not quite correct, because the recess is interrupted in the region of the transverse acetabular ligament. In arthrographies the perilimbic recess is the morphologic base of the "Rose-Thorne-Projection" [29]. Often the labrum is separated from the articular cartilage by a discrete cleft [30], which is known as "Labrumfurche" (Fig. 1.9) [31]. The surgical removal of the labrum is possible [31].

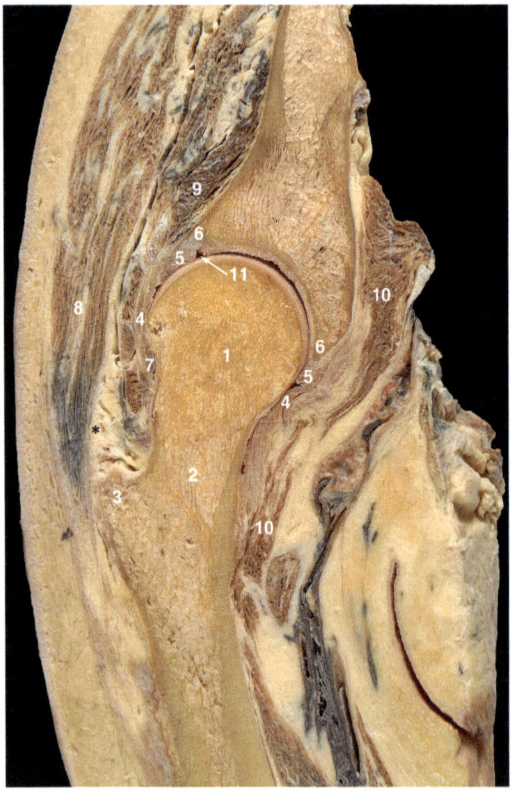

Fig. 1.9 Frontal section of the hip joint. **1**: Caput femoris, **2**: Collum femoris, **3**: Trochanter major, **4**: Capsula articularis, **5**: Labrum acetabulare, **6**: Limbus acetabuli, **7**: Zona orbicularis, **8**: M. glutaeus medius, **9**: M. glutaeus minimus, **10**: M. iliopsoas, **11**: "Labrumfurche". The **star** indicates the corpus adiposum between M. glutaeus medius and M. glutaeus minimus

1.4.4 The Transverse Ligament of the Acetabulum

The acetabular incisure is crossed by a strong ligament, which consists of a superficial and a deep part. Both parts are separated by a thin layer of connective tissue. The transverse ligament is functionally a tension-band-wiring-structure, which limits the widening of the acetabular margin during loading [32]. In cases of severe degenerative changes the ligament can ossify completely.

1.5 Ligaments

The strong ligaments of the hip joint are adding stability to the already strong osseous stabilization. The ligaments are arranged as a ligamentous screw, which is stretched and taut by retroversion. The screw limits all movements except the flexion. In the standing position the screw prevents the dorsal tilting of the pelvis. Furthermore the screw is relieved in slight abduction, external rotation, and flexion. All ligaments are components of the fibrous articular capsule. Anteriorly this very thick capsule (1–1.5 cm) inserts at the intertrochanteric line (Fig. 1.8a), dorsally in the region between medial and the lateral third of the femoral neck. Due to this condition, fractures of the femoral neck can be partly intracapsular and partly extracapsular fractures. Some innermost fibers of the fibrous capsule are reflecting medially and are forming retinacula on the femoral neck. These retinacula of Weitbrecht are running over the femoral neck towards the subcapital sulcus and are containing vessels supplying the femoral neck and head. Weitbrecht's retinacula are covered by synovial layer, so that typical folds or frenula capsulae are formed. These frenula are normally located at three positions: anterior, medial, and lateral. The mighty medial (posteroinferior) fold is also known as "Frenulum Amantini" or "Plica pectineofovealis" and occurs in 75% of specimens [2]. The retinacular vessels are exposed to intracapsular pathologies, for example, an intracapsular hematoma, so that they can be compressed and the vascularization of the femoral head can also be altered and disturbed seriously. The synovial layer of the articular capsule inserts at the lateral margin of the hyaline cartilage of the femoral neck and just before the lateral osseous insertions of the fibrous capsule, so that the outer synovial funnel is formed [27].

The ligamentous screw is formed by the following ligaments:

1.5.1 Iliofemoral Ligament (of Bertin or Bigelow)

This ligament is the strongest ligament of the human body and has a tensile strength of ~350 kp. It originates from the inferior anterior iliac spine and fans out in a lateral (transversal) and a medial (descending) limb, so that a reversed V-shaped structure results. The ligament inserts at the whole length of the intertrochanteric line. Additionally the lateral (or superior) part (iliotrochanteric ligament) has a strong osseous insertion at the femoral tubercle (also called innominate tubercle) (Fig. 1.3a) at the superior end of the intertrochanteric line.

1.5.2 Pubofemoral Ligament

The triangular pubofemoral ligament originates from the superior pubic ramus, especially from the iliopectineal eminence and fans out into the medial part of the articular capsule and the medial part of the iliofemoral ligament. Finally it ends at the inferior end of the intertrochanteric line. This ligament is the weakest ligament of the ligamentous screw and limits abduction, extension, and external rotation.

1.5.3 Ischiofemoral Ligament

This ligament strengthens the dorsal part of the articular capsule and originates from the dorsocaudal rim of the acetabulum. It inserts in the region of the trochanteric fossa and some fibers are running into the zona orbicularis.

1.5.4 Zona Orbicularis

The zona orbicularis is a thickened, ~0.5–1 cm broad circular structure weaved in to the articular capsule, which is formed by deeply placed circular fibers fanning out of the pubofemoral and the ischiofemoral ligaments. The zona orbicularis surrounds the narrowest area of the femoral neck and has no osseous insertion. The femoral head is sticked through this zona orbicularis like a button through the button hole, so that lateral dislocation of the femoral head is prevented. Functionally the zona orbicularis is a synergist to the labrum.

1.6 Muscles

The hip joint is surrounded by a lot of important muscles. These muscles are covering the joint completely, so that it cannot be palpated. The following muscle groups must be considered.

1.6.1 Dorsolateral Muscles

1.6.1.1 M. Glutaeus Maximus (Fig. 1.8a)

The gluteus maximus muscle is composed of thick muscular fibers which are running from craniomedial to laterocaudal. Furthermore the muscle is covered by a thin fascia which sends collagenous septa into the muscle belly, so that the thick muscle fibers are completely sheathed. This is important, because inflammations can spread in these sheathes, so that an early and intensive tension pain occurs. The muscle presents a wide-spread origin from the posterior area of the iliac bone behind the posterior gluteal line, from the lumbodorsal aponeurosis, from the lateral margin of the sacral and coccygeal bone and with deep fibers from the sacrotuberous ligament. The superior part inserts at the iliotibial tract, whereas the inferior one is fixed at the gluteal tuberosity. This distal insertion can also reach the lateral intermuscular septum and is therefore also connected to the linea aspera. The muscle consists of a sacroiliac and a coccygeal part, which are separated in early development and merge in the fetal period. The muscle is innervated by the inferior gluteal nerve. This nerve has a rather constant entrance point on the inner surface of the muscle positioned in a region which is relatively stationary during the different movements of the leg. This is an important fact, because the nerve will not be damaged by the normal hip motions.

1.6.1.2 M. Glutaeus Medius (Figs. 1.9 and 1.10a, b)

This muscle originates from the banana-shaped external area of the os ilium between the iliac crest and the anterior and posterior gluteal line and furthermore from the external labium of the iliac crest. Additionally there is a strong fiber origin from its fascia, covering the anterior part of the muscle. Often the anterior margin of the muscle is fused with the tensor fasciae latae muscle. The gluteus medius muscle inserts at the lateral surface

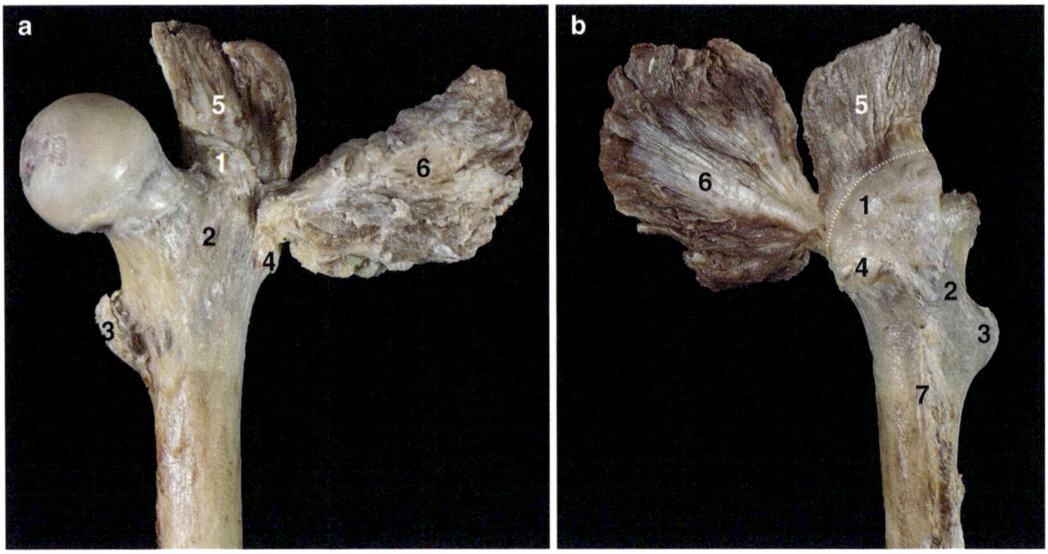

Fig. 1.10 (**a**) Anterior aspect of proximal femur with its relationship to the gluteus medius and minimus muscles. **1**: Trochanter major, **2**: Linea intertrochanterica, **3**: Trochanter minor with iliopsoas tendon, **4**: Tuberculum innominatum, **5**: M. glutaeus medius (underside), **6**: M. glutaeus minimus (underside). Notice, that the tip of the greater trochanter is not occupied by the medial gluteus muscle. The gluteus minimus inserts at a distinct area somewhat above the innominate tubercle. (**b**) Lateral aspect of proximal femur and its relationship to the gluteus medius and minimus muscle. **1**: Trochanter major, **2**: Crista intertrochanterica, **3**: Trochanter minor, **4**: Tuberculum innominatum, **5**: M. glutaeus medius (upper side), **6**: M. glutaeus minimus (upper side), **7**: Tuberositas glutaea. Notice the oblique insertion (punctated line) of the gluteus medius at the outer circumference of the greater trochanter

of the trochanter major. The insertion completely covers the lateral area and the insertion line descends obliquely, from posterocranial to anterocaudal. The medially bended tip of the trochanter is not covered by this insertion (Fig. 1.10a, b). The muscle is innervated by the superior gluteal nerve.

M. Tensor Fasciae Latae

From the viewpoint of developmental history this muscle is a separation of the gluteus medial muscle. The tensor originates from the external surface of the anterior superior iliac spine and inserts at the iliotibial tract of Maissiat as well as at the fascia lata. Often a dorsal, in some cases strongly developed, tendinous slip can be seen, which is inserting at the iliofemoral ligament or at the anterior inferior iliac spine. This tendinous slip is a relic of an additional former head of the tensor muscle [33, 34]. The muscle is innervated by the superior gluteal nerve. The innervating thin nerve is coming out of the gluteus minimus muscle and enters the tensor from the dorsal side. The whole muscle is sheathed in a thick fascia.

1.6.1.3 M. Glutaeus Minimus (Fig. 1.10a, b)

This fan-shaped muscle originates from the external area of the os ilium, between the anterior and inferior gluteal line. Additionally there are further origins from its fascia. The tendon inserts at the ventral margin of the trochanter major. In some cases the muscle is divided into two parts. The anterior part is also called gluteus quartus muscle, if it is completely separated. The posterior part is characterized by an impressive aponeurosis. Connections with surrounding muscles (piriformis, gemelli, vastus lateralis muscles) may be present. The muscle is innervated by the superior gluteal nerve.

1.6.2 Deep External Rotators (Pelvitrochanteric Muscles, Medial Group)

1.6.2.1 M. Piriformis (Figs. 1.11 and 1.15)

The piriformis muscle originates normally with three parts from the anterior area of the sacral bone, from the articular capsule of the sacroiliac joint and in some cases from the osseous surroundings of the greater sciatic foramen. The muscle exits through this foramen and the tendon inserts at the superior tip of the trochanter major. Between the tip of the trochanter and the piriformis tendon the bursa m. piriformis is intercalated. The muscle is innervated by direct branches from the sacral plexus or by muscular rami from the sciatic nerve. In about 25% the muscle is perforated by the peroneal part of the sciatic nerve, so that an intrapiriform foramen for the nerve fibers is established. The piriformis muscle has a high tendency for shrinkage and shortening.

1.6.2.2 M. Obturatorius Internus (Fig. 1.8a)

This muscle originates from the inner surface of the obturator membrane and its osseous surroundings. The muscle develops a typical gliding tendon, which runs out of the minor sciatic incisure and uses the osseous margin of the os ischii between the sciatic spine and the tuber ischiadicum as hypomochlion. The osseous margin in this area is covered by hyaline cartilage and separated from the tendon by the bursa ischiadica m. obturatorii interni. The tendon of the internal obturator muscle is deflected at the hypomochlion in an acute angle, runs than horizontally over the dorsal articular capsule of the hip joint and inserts at the anteromedial margin of the trochanter major, anterior to the fossa trochanterica. Between the articular capsule and the tendon is also a bursa, the bursa subtendinea m. obturatorii interni, intercalated, which can communicate with the bursa ischiadica m. obturatorii interni. The muscle is innervated by sacral plexus branches.

1.6.2.3 Mm. Gemellus Superior and Inferior (Fig. 1.11a, b)

The superior gemellus muscle originates from the ischial spine, whereas the inferior one originates from the superomedial corner of the tuber ischiadicum. Both muscles fuse with the tendon of the internal obturator muscle and are inserting together with this tendon in the trochanteric fossa. These little muscles show a lot of variations and can be substituted by fibrous bands. According to developmental history they belong to the internal obturator muscle and can be seen

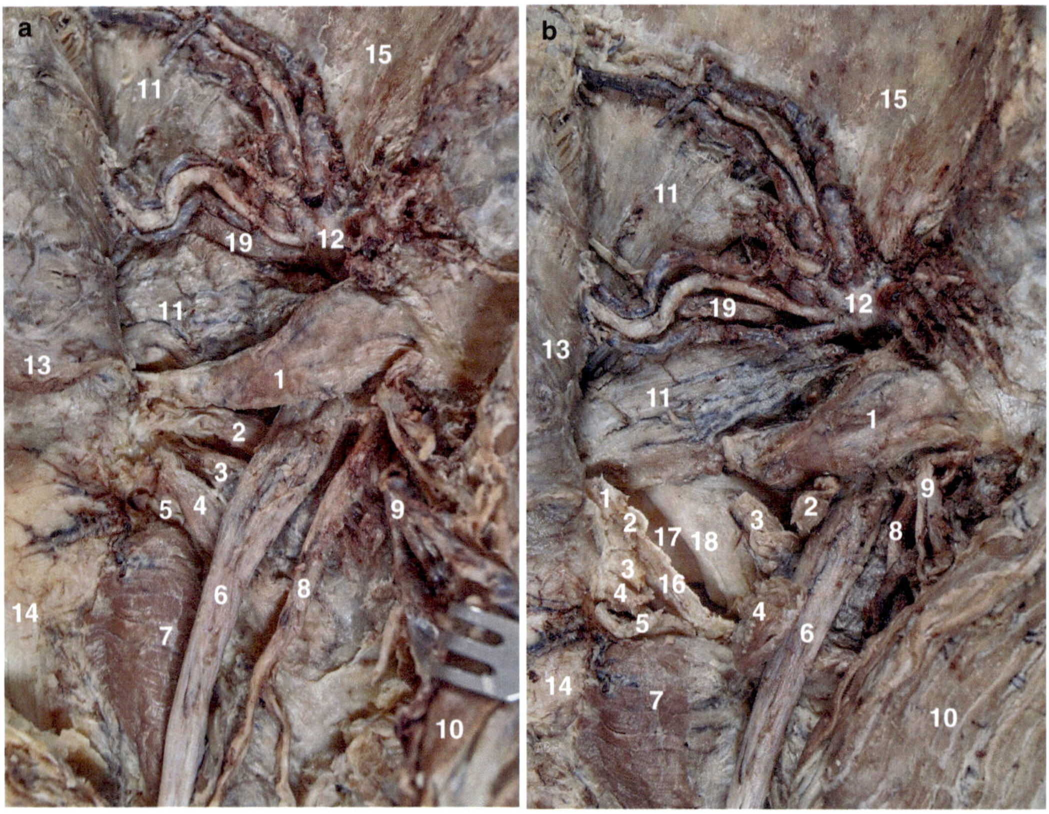

Fig. 1.11 (**a**, **b**) Left gluteal region (deep). In (**b**) the short rotators are dissected and tilted laterally. **1**: M. piriformis, **2**: M. gemellus superior, **3**: tendon of M. obturatorius internus, **4**: M. gemellus inferior, **5**: R. profundus of A. circumflexa femoris medialis, **6**: N. ischiadicus, **7**: M. quadratus femoris, **8**: N. cutaneus femoris posterior, **9**: Vasa glutaea inferiora and N. glutaeus inferior, **10**: M. glutaeus maximus, **11**: M. glutaeus minimus, **12**: Vasa glutaea superiora, **13**: M. glutaeus medius (removed), **14**: Trochanter major, **15**: area of origin or the M. glutaeus medius, **16**: Capsula articularis (opened), **17**: Caput femoris, **18**: Labrum acetabulare, **19**: N. glutaeus superior

as additional external heads of this muscle [35]. Both gemelli are innervated by direct branches originating from the sacral plexus.

1.6.2.4 M. Quadratus Femoris (Figs. 1.11 and 1.15)

This thick muscle runs from the lateral margin of the tuber ischiadicum to the trochanteric crest, where it causes the quadrate tubercle. Caudally the muscle belly is separated from the adductor magnus muscle by the transverse ramus of the medial circumflex artery. The dissection of the muscle can cause severe bleedings from these branches, so that separation of the muscle should be avoided, if possible. The muscle lies on the trochanter minor and often an inconstant bursa is found between these two structures. The muscle is innervated by the inferior gluteal nerve and by rami musculares branching directly from the tibial part of the sciatic nerve.

1.6.3 Adductors

1.6.3.1 M. Gracilis

This muscle is a two-joint muscle and originates from the anterior area of the inferior ramus of the pubic bone and inserts at the medial region of the tibia as a component of the pes anserinus superficialis. The muscle is innervated by the obturator nerve.

1.6.3.2 M. Pectineus (Fig. 1.13)

This nearly quadrangular muscle originates from the pecten ossis pubis and the pubic tubercle and inserts at the pectineal line of the proximal femur. The pectineal muscle forms the floor of the femoral triangle of Scarpa and in some cases the muscle shows a superficial and a deep portion and is therefore bilaminarily architectured. The muscle is double innervated from the femoral as well as from the obturator nerve. If an accessory obturator nerve is present, it can also contribute to the muscle innervation.

1.6.3.3 M. Adductor Longus

This triangular muscle originates from the corpus ossis pubis and inserts at the middle third of the medial labium of the linea aspera. It is in the plane of the pectineal muscle and contributes also to the floor of the femoral triangle of Scarpa. Beneath this muscle and on the anterior surface of the adductor brevis muscle the anterior ramus of the obturator nerve can easily be found. The muscle is innervated by the obturator nerve.

1.6.3.4 M. Adductor Brevis

This muscle is originating from the inferior ramus of the pubic bone and inserts at the proximal third of the medial labium of the linea aspera. Behind this muscle the posterior ramus of the obturator nerve is positioned. The muscle is also supplied by the obturator nerve.

1.6.3.5 M. Adductor Magnus

This strong muscle originates from a semicircular line from the inferior ramus of the pubic bone, from the inferolateral part of the tuber ischiadicum and from the ramus ossis ischii. The muscle inserts at the labium mediale of the linea aspera and additionally with a strong round tendon at the adductor tubercle of the medial condyle. In some cases the superior part of the muscle is separated and forms an isolated muscle belly. This variation is termed as M. adductor minimus. The great adductor muscle is double innervated by the tibial nerve and the posterior ramus of the obturator nerve.

1.6.3.6 M. Obturatorius Externus

This triangular and thick muscle originates from the external surface of the obturator membrane and the medial part of the osseous margin of the obturator foramen. The muscle runs towards the posterior part of the collum femoris and inserts at the posterior area of the fossa trochanterica. The insertion can be a deepening (Fig. 1.2b). Furthermore the tendon can produce a typical fibroostosis (Fig. 1.2c). The tendon of this muscle is directly lying at the posterior articular capsule. In some cases a bursa can be intercalated, which is communicating with the hip joint. The whole muscle shows a spiral conformation and becomes innervated by the posterior branch of the obturator nerve. The posterior branch of this nerve often pierces the muscle belly, whereas the anterior branch appears at its superior margin.

All these adductor muscles are forming a typical stratigraphic architecture. In the superficial layer the pectineal and adductor longus muscles are positioned. Beneath this in the middle layer the short adductor muscle can be exposed. In the deepest layer the adductor magnus muscle and in some cases the adductor minimus are positioned. This typical topography with the intercalated branches of the obturator nerve (before and beneath the adductor brevis) is important when performing medial approaches, e.g. according to Ludloff or Ferguson.

1.6.4 Ischiocrural Muscles ("Hamstrings")

1.6.4.1 M. Biceps Femoris

This muscle presents two heads: the long head originates from the inferomedial part of the tuber ischiadicum, whereas the short head originates from the lateral labium of the linea aspera of the middle part of the femur. The long head often merges with the semitendinosus tendon in the region of the ischial tuberosity, so that a common tendon is formed. Both heads are inserting together at the caput fibulae but are differently innervated. The long head is supplied by the tibial part of the sciatic nerve, whereas the short head is innervated by the peroneal part of the sciatic nerve or the common peroneal nerve.

1.6.4.2 M. Semitendinosus

It originates together with the long head of the biceps femoris muscle (common head) from the medial area of the tuber ischiadicum and also from an adjacent small area of the sacrotuberous ligament. This connection is important, because the muscle influences the sacroiliac joint by this connection [36]. In the mid-thigh the muscle belly forms a round tendon, which inserts at the medial metaphyseal tibial surface, somewhat behind the sartorius and distally to the gracilis tendon. The muscle is innervated by muscular branches originating from the tibial part of the sciatic nerve.

1.6.4.3 M. Semimembranosus

It originates with a small, membranous tendon from the superolateral area of the tuber ischiadicum. Then the muscle forms a massive muscle belly, which fans out into five tendinous slips (pes anserinus profundus). These slips are inserting at several structures of the knee region. The muscle is innervated by muscular branches coming from the tibial part of the sciatic nerve.

1.6.5 Anterior Femoral Muscles

1.6.5.1 M. Sartorius

It originates from the anterior superior iliac spine, runs over the anterior area of the thigh towards the medial tibial condyle, where it is inserting as a component of the superficial pes anserinus. The sartorius muscle is an important landmark, because it is the medial border of the Smith-Petersen-Interval. The muscle is innervated by the femoral nerve. It is important, that the muscular branches are entering the muscle belly only at the medial margin, so that it should only be dislocated to the medial site, in order not to disturb its innervation.

1.6.5.2 M. Rectus Femoris (Fig. 1.12)

This muscle originates with two heads. One head (the caput rectum) comes from the anterior inferior iliac spine, whereas the other (the caput reflexum) originates from the supraacetabular sulcus (Fig. 1.12). The muscle lies superficially at the ventral area of the thigh, runs downwards and inserts with a short tendon at the base of the patella and furthermore with the patellar ligament at the tibial tuberosity.

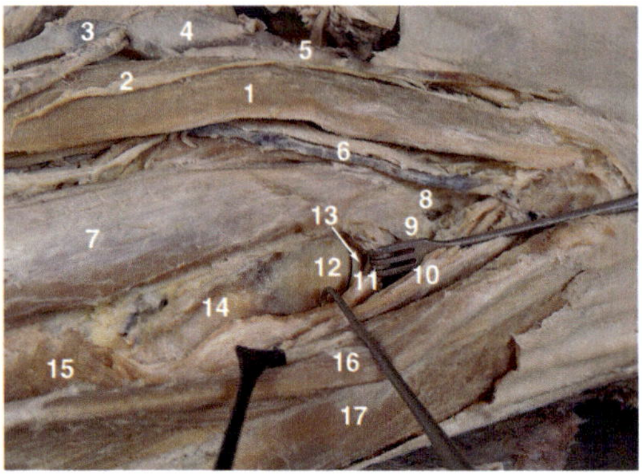

Fig. 1.12 Anatomy of the anterior approach using the Smith-Peterson-interval: **1**: M. sartorius, **2**: N. cutaneus femoris lateralis, **3**: V. saphena magna, **4**: V. femoralis, **5**: A. femoralis, **6**: A. and V. circumflexa lateralis: R. ascendens (running above the rectus femoris muscle as an anatomical variation), **7**: M. rectus femoris, **8**: M. rectus femoris: Caput rectum, **9**: M. rectus femoris: Caput reflexum, **10**: Mm. glutaeus medius und minimus fused together, **11**: Capsula articularis, **12**: Caput femoris, **13**: Labrum articulare, **14**: Collum femoris, **15**: M. vastus lateralis, **16**: M. tensor fasciae latae, **17**: M. glutaeus medius

1.6.5.3 Medial, Intermedial, and Lateral Vastus Muscle

These muscles have no direct topographic relationship to the hip joint, but they are visible by performing anterior or lateral approaches, so that they are mentioned here. Together with the rectus femoris muscle these muscles form the quadriceps femoris muscle. All these muscles are innervated by the femoral nerve. In the triangular space, bordered by the m. tensor fasciae latae, the vastus lateralis and the rectus femoris, the branching of the lateral circumflex artery can be found. Here the important descending ramus can also be exposed (vastus-lateralis-flap) (Fig. 1.13).

1.6.5.4 M. Iliopsoas (Fig. 1.13)

The iliopsoas muscle is composed by the fan-like iliac muscle, originating out of the iliac fossa, and by the psoas major muscle, originating with a superficial and a deep portion from the spine. The superficial portion of the illiopsoas muscle originates from the lateral area of the 12. thoracic vertebra and from the lateral areas of the lumbar

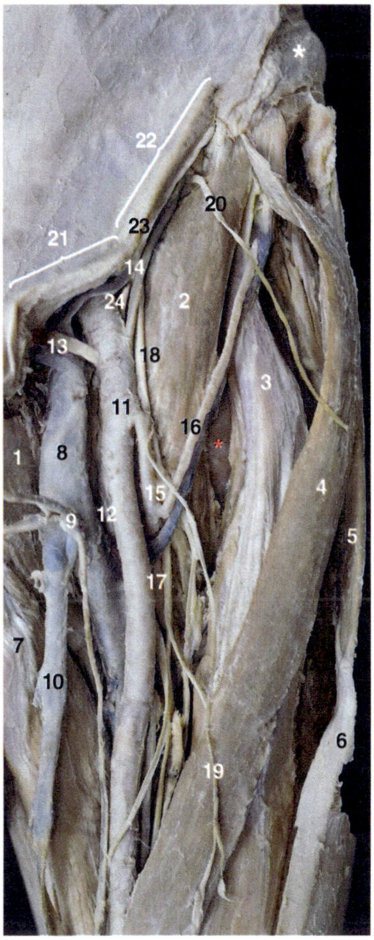

Fig. 1.13 **Red star**: Caput femoris: exposed by removing a part of the articular capsule, **white star**: Spina iliaca anterior superior, **1**: M. pectineus, **2**: M. iliopsoas, **3**: M. rectus femoris, **4**: M. sartorius, **5**: M. tensor fasciae latae, **6**: Tractus iliotibialis, **7**: M. adductor longus, **8**: V. femoralis, **9**: veins of the "venous star" tilted medially, **10**: V. saphena magna, **11**: A. femoralis, **12**: A. femoralis profunda, **13**: A./V. epigastrica inferior, **14**: A./V. circumflexa ilium profunda, **15**: A. circumflexa femoris lateralis, **16**: R. ascendens der A. circumflexa femoris lateralis, **17**: R. descendens der circumflexa femoris lateralis, **18**: N. femoralis, **19**: R. cutaneus femoris anterior, **20**: N. cutaneus femoris lateralis, **21**: Lacuna vasorum, **22**: Lacuna musculorum, **23**: Lig. inguinale, **24**: Arcus iliopectineus

vertebral bodies and from the intercalated intervertebral discs. The deep portion originates from the costal processes of the lumbar vertebrae. Between the superficial and the deep part the lumbar plexus is intercalated. After all three parts have fused the muscle exits through the lacuna musculorum and its strong, flat tendon inserts at the minor trochanter. The tendon uses the femoral head and the thick ventral part of the articular capsule as hypomochlion. According to this topography a bursa, the iliopectineal bursa, is intercalated between the two structures. In about 25% the bursa iliopectinea communicates with the hip joint. The muscle is innervated by direct muscular branches from the lumbar plexus and from the femoral nerve. A slight flexion of the hip joint relaxes the iliopsoas muscle, so that a medial dislocation can be easily performed during an anterior approach.

1.6.5.5 General Considerations

The hip joint is eccentrically sheathed by the above muscles. On the ventral side only a thin muscle coverage is found, whereas the dorsal part is covered by a mighty mass of muscles. The whole muscular coverage presents two muscular gaps, which can be used for surgical approaches. Such approaches do not damage muscular structures. On the ventral side such a gap is bordered by the tensor fasciae latae and the sartorius muscle. This gap is designated as Smith-Petersen-Interval (Fig. 1.8b). On the lateral side such a gap is positioned between the tensor fasciae latae and the gluteus medius muscle. This gap is known as Watson-Jones-Interval (Fig. 1.8b). Cranially the Watson-Jones-Interval is often not clearly bordered, but caudally the margins of bordering muscles are diverging, so that the interval can be identified more clearly.

1.7 Bursae

In the region of the hip joint several bursae can be found. In some cases these bursae are exhaustive spaces and are of clinical interest. Beside the more or less constantly occurring bursae several inconstant entities can be observed. The following entities are well defined and should be considered:

Bursa trochanterica m. glutaei maximi intercalated between the tendon of the glutaeus maximus muscle and the major trochanter.

Bursa trochanterica m. glutaei medii superficialis intercalated between trochanter major and the tendon of the glutaeus medius muscle.

Bursa trochanterica m. glutaei medii profunda intercalated between the piriform tendon and the tendon of the glutaeus medius muscle.

Bursa trochanterica m. glutaei minimi intercalated between the tendon of the glutaeus minimus muscle and the minor trochanter.

Bursa iliopectinea this bursa is intercalated between the iliopsoas tendon and the anterior articular capsule of the hip joint. The tendon uses the femoral head as a hypomochlion in this region and the bursa communicates with the hip joint in about 25%.

Bursa subtendinea iliaca this bursa lies between the iliopsoas tendon and the minor trochanter. In some cases there is a communication to the iliopectineal bursa.

Bursae intermusculares mm. glutaeorum these bursae are often multiple (2–3) and they are intercalated between the glutaeus maximus tendon and the linea aspera.

Bursa trochanterica subcutanea between skin and trochanter major (innominate tubercle) above the superficial fascia.

Bursa trochanterica subfascialis lies between superficial fascia and trochanter major (innominate tubercle).

Bursa ischiadica m. glutaei maximi lies between glutaeus maximus muscle and tuber ischiadicum.

Bursa m. piriformis this bursa lies between the piriform tendon and the bone.

Bursa ischiadica m. obturatorii interni this bursa is intercalated between the tendon of the obturatorius internus muscle and the osseous crest of the os ischii, acting as hypomochlion for the tendon.

Bursa m. obturatorii externi this bursa is positioned between the tendon of the external obturatorius muscle and the collum femoris. The bursa can communicate with the articular cavity of the hip joint.

Bursa m. bicipitis femoris superior this bursa can be found between the origins of the long head of the biceps femoris muscle and the semimembranosus muscle.

1.8 Vessels

On the ventral side of the sacroiliac joint the common iliac artery divides into the internal and the external iliac artery. Both arteries are important for the vascularization of the hip joint and the surrounding soft tissues. After passing the inguinal ligament the external iliac artery becomes the femoral artery and supplies the lower extremity. The internal iliac artery branches into parietal and visceral arteries. The following parietal arteries are of importance for the hip joint.

1.8.1 Parietal Branches of the Internal Iliac Artery (Figs. 1.11 and 1.14)

1.8.1.1 A. Iliolumbalis

This artery divides behind the psoas muscle into lumbar and iliac branches. The main iliac branch communicates with the deep circumflex iliac artery. A nutrient branch of the iliac division enters the iliac bone and contributes from the inner side to the vascular supply of the anterior part of the facies lunata and the superior acetabular edge.

1.8.1.2 A. Glutaea Superior (Fig. 1.11)

The superior gluteal artery runs through the suprapiriform foramen and divides into a superficial and a deep ramus. The superficial ramus lies between the gluteal maximus and the gluteal medius muscle, whereas the deep ramus is positioned between the gluteus medius and the glu-

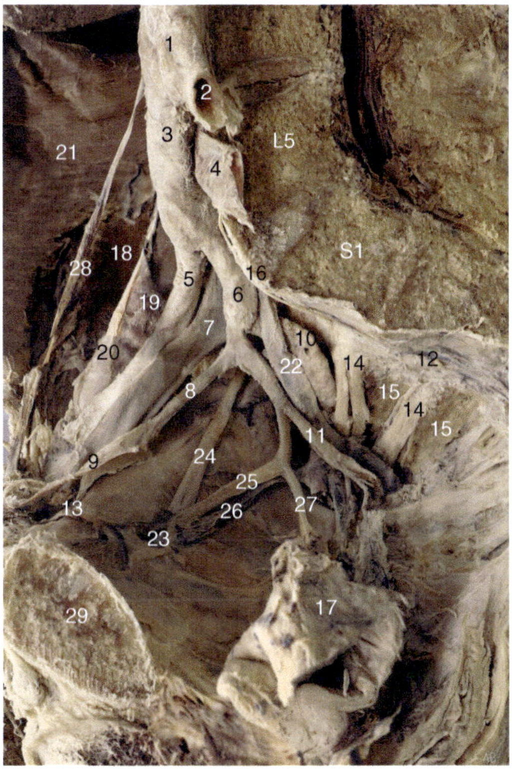

Fig. 1.14 **1**: lateral wall of the pelvis, exhibiting the nervous and vascular structures. Aorta abdominalis, **2**: A. iliaca communis sin., **3**: A. iliaca communis dex., **4**: V. iliaca communis sin., **5**: A. iliaca externa, **6**: A. iliaca interna, **7**: V. iliaca externa, **8**: A. umbilicalis: Pars patens, **9**: A. umbilicalis: Pars occlusa, **10**: A. glutaea sup., **11**: A. glutaea inf., **12**: A. sacralis mediana, **13**: R. pubicus, **14**: Plexus sacralis, **15**: M. piriformis, **16**: Promontorium, **17**: Vesica urinaria, **18**: M. iliacus, **19**: M. psoas major, **20**: M. psoas minor, **21**: M. transversus abdominis, **22**: V. iliaca interna, **23**: Canalis obturatorius, **24**: N. obturatorius, **25**: A. obturatoria, **26**: V. obturatoria, **27**: A. vesicalis inferior, **28**: A. testicularis, **29**: Symphyse

teal minimus muscle. Both rami of the superior gluteal artery are supplying the gluteal muscles.

1.8.1.3 A. Glutaea Inferior (Fig. 1.11)

The inferior gluteal artery runs through the infrapiriforme foramen and supplies mainly the gluteus maximus muscle. A small rudimentary artery branches off and accompanies the sciatic nerve as the sciatic artery. This vessel was the former main vessel of the lower extremity and therefore in some cases it persists as a large vessel.

1.8.1.4 A. Obturatoria (Fig. 1.14)

The obturator artery is accompanied by the obturator vein below and by the obturator nerve above. The artery lies at the lateral wall of the pelvis and runs antero-inferiorly towards the obturator canal at the superior margin of the obturator foramen. Passing the obturator canal the vessel divides into the anterior and posterior branch. An acetabular branch from the posterior branch runs through the acetabular incisure beneath the transverse acetabular ligament, supplies the pulvinar acetabulare, and enters the round ligament of the femoral head. This artery is termed A. ligamenti capitis femoris or the "medial epiphyseal vessel according to Trueta." This vessel is important for the vascularization of the femoral head [37, 38]. In about 14.9% the acetabular ramus can also be a branch of the medial circumflex artery [39]. In about 25% the obturator artery branches completely from the inferior epigastric artery. In these cases it runs about the posterior area of the pubic bone towards the obturator canal. This topographic situation is termed as "corona mortis." The obturator artery can also originate from the superior gluteal or inferior gluteal artery.

1.8.2 Femoral Artery (Fig. 1.13)

The femoral artery is the continuation of the external iliac artery distal to the inguinal ligament. This important vessel is positioned in the femoral triangle of Scarpa and can be identified just beneath the middle of the inguinal ligament. The artery is bordered laterally by the iliopsoas muscle and the femoral nerve; medially it crosses the pectineus and adductor longus muscles. Within the femoral triangle the deep femoral artery originates from the femoral artery (~3.5 cm below the inguinal ligament). After this origin the femoral artery is often termed as "superficial femoral artery." Regularly the deep femoral artery branches off the medial circumflex and the lateral circumflex artery and the perforating branches I-III.

The medial circumflex femoral artery, usually smaller than the lateral circumflex femoral artery, should be the first branch of the deep femoral artery and runs behind the femoral vessels and than under the pectineus muscle to the dorsal side of the femoral neck.

The medial circumflex artery divides into five branches:

R. superficialis supplies the skin of the femoral triangle and the superficial layer of the adductor muscles.

R. profundus runs beneath the trochanter minor between the quadratus muscle and the iliopsoas muscle to the dorsal side of the thigh.

R. acetabularis enters the acetabular fossa under the transverse acetabular ligament and supplies pulvinar acetabulare. Furthermore this artery enters the round ligament of the femoral head and supplies the femoral head epiphysis together with the ramus coming from the obturator artery.

R. ascendens runs towards the trochanteric fossa and supplies the obturatorius externus, the adductor brevis, adductor longus, and adductor magnus muscles.

R. descendens or transversus anastomoses with the transverse branch of the lateral circumflex artery, and is therefore a part of the "cruciate anastomosis."

The lateral circumflex femoral artery runs behind the sartorius and rectus femoris muscles laterally and divides into three branches:

R. ascendens runs upward, following the intertrochanteric line, supplies the trochanter major and anastomoses with branches from the medial circumflex artery, the superior gluteal artery, and the deep iliac circumflex artery. By the anastomosis with the medial circumflex femoral artery a vascular ring, surrounding and supplying the femoral neck, is formed.

R. descendens runs behind the rectus femoris muscle distally and supplies the vastus lateralis muscle.

R. transversus the usually small transverse branch passes to the intermedius vastus muscle, pierces the lateral vastus lateral muscle and establishes an anastomosis with the inferior gluteal, the medial circumflex and first perforating artery. This anastomosis is also called the "cruciate anastomosis."

According to the complicated vascularization of the femoral head, vascular diseases of the head can easily occur. Therefore the distinct vascular patterns of arteries and veins must be carefully considered during surgery.

The vascular anatomy of the femoral head and neck is described differently by different authors and with different nomenclatures. A detailed description can be found in the investigations of Trueta & Harrison [37], Trueta [38], and Hipp [40].

1.9 Nerves

The hip and the hip joint are supplied by branches of the lumbar as well as of the sacral plexus. The lumbar plexus is intercalated between the superficial and deep part of the psoas major muscle. The sacral plexus lies at the posterior pelvic wall in front of the piriformis muscle and beneath the branches of the internal iliac artery.

1.9.1 Branches of the Lumbar Plexus

1.9.1.1 N. Femoralis (Fig. 1.13)

This nerve appears at the lateral border of the psoas major muscle, then lies in the rim between the iliac and psoas major muscle and exits the pelvis through the lacuna musculorum. In this space the nerve is between the medial border of the iliopsoas muscle and the iliopectineal arch, which belongs to the fascia of the iliopsoas muscle. In front of the thigh the femoral nerve divides into an anterior and a posterior division. The anterior division branches off the cutaneous nerves and the muscular branch for the sartorius muscle. The posterior division raises the saphenous nerve, some muscular branches and thin vascular branches for the femoral artery. Lesions of the femoral nerve during hip surgery can be caused by malpositioned instruments, e.g. Hohmann-retractors [41].

1.9.1.2 N. Obturatorius (Fig. 1.14)

Only the obturator nerve is running medial to the psoas major muscle in the space between this muscle and the vertebral column (triangle of Marcille). The obturator nerve than descends at the lateral pelvic wall normally lying on the obturator internus muscle and above the obturator vessels. Here the nerve can be harmed by cement cones penetrating the acetabular floor (Fig. 1.6d). Just before the nerve runs into the obturator canal, it divides into an anterior and a posterior branch. The anterior branch lies on the anterior surface of the adductor brevis muscle, whereas the posterior branch can be found behind this muscle.

In about 29% an accessory obturator nerve can be seen [42]. This nerve runs also in Marcille's triangle, crosses the superior pubic ramus and lies behind the pectineus muscle, where it anastomoses with the regular obturator nerve. After crossing the superior pubic ramus, the obturator accessorius nerve divides into some branches. One of these branches supplies the articular capsule of the hip joint while the others are muscular branches.

1.9.1.3 N. Cutaneus Femoris Lateralis (Fig. 1.13)

The lateral cutaneus femoral nerve also appears at the lateral border of the psoas major muscle and than crosses the iliacus muscle and runs to the medial border of the anterior superior iliac spine. In this region the nerve exits the abdominal cavity in the most lateral corner of the lacuna musculorum.

The lateral cutaneus femoral nerve than descends, covered by the fascia lata for about 7 cm. After piercing the thick fascia the nerve runs subcutaneously, to supply the anterolateral area of the thigh.

According to Ghent [43] four typical situations can be seen:

- Type 1: the nerve pierces the inguinal ligament.
- Type 2: the nerve runs under the inguinal ligament and is medial to the anterior superior iliac spine.
- Type 3: the nerve pierces the sartorius muscle (rare).
- Type 4: the nerve runs over the anterior superior iliac spine to the lateral area (very rare observation).

The lateral femoral cutaneous nerve can be compressed under the inguinal ligament as well as by piercing the fascia lata (Meralgia paresthetica). In serious cases a neurolysis can be performed. The nerve is in great danger during a direct anterior approach to the hip joint.

1.9.2 Branches of the Sacral Plexus

1.9.2.1 N. Ischiadicus (Figs. 1.11 and 1.15)

This big nerve exits the pelvis through the infrapiriform foramen and then runs between the greater trochanter and the ischial tuberosity caudally. The nerve crosses the internal obturator

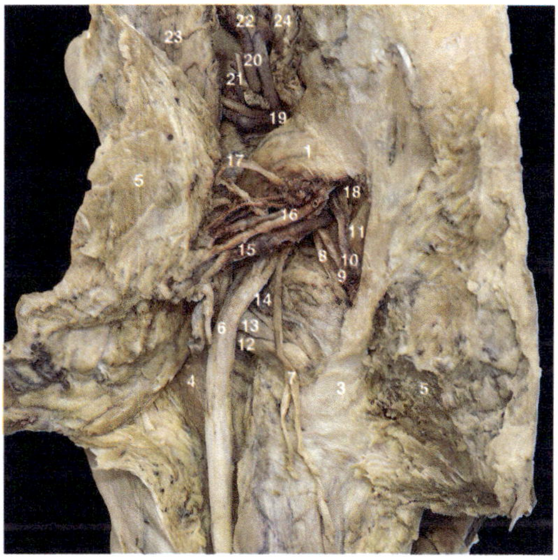

Fig. 1.15 Left gluteal region, exposed by removing the gluteus maximus laterally. **1**: M. piriformis, **2**: Lig. sacrotuberale, **3**: Tuber ischiadicum, **4**: M. quadratus femoris, **5**: M. glutaeus maximus, **6**: N. ischiadicus, **7**: N. cutaneus femoris posterior, **8**: N. pudendus, **9**: A. pudenda interna, **10**: V. pudenda interna, **11**: Spina ischiadica, **12**: M. gemellus inferior, **13**: M. obturatorius internus (tendon), **14**: M. gemellus superior, **15**: V. glutaea inferior, **16**: A. glutaea inferior, **17**: N. glutaeus inferius, **18**: Foramen infrapiriforme, **19**: Foramen suprapiriforme, **20**: V. glutaea superior, **21**: A. glutaea superior, **22**: N. glutaeus superior, **23**: M. glutaeus medius, **24**: M. glutaeus minimus

tendon, the gemellus superior, the gemellus inferior, and the quadratus femoris muscle. Furthermore the nerve is covered by the gluteus maximus muscle in this region and appears at its inferior margin. In the posterior region of the thigh the nerve divides into the peroneus communis and the tibial nerve. This division can also take place cranially in the pelvic region. In these cases (~15%) the peroneal part can perforate the piriformis muscle, so that an intrapiriform foramen is established. In very rare cases the peroneal part or even the whole sciatic nerve exits through the suprapiriform foramen, so that the nerve crosses the piriform muscle. In rare cases the intrapiriform foramen can cause a piriformis syndrome. In flexion the sciatic nerve is bent and stretched tightly over the posterior articular capsule. This intimate relationship exposes the nerve to trauma, especially dorsal luxations with or without acetabular rim fractures [2].

1.9.2.2 N. Cutaneus Femoris Posterior (Figs. 1.11 and 1.15)

The nerve exits the pelvic cavity through the infrapiriforme foramen, is in close relationship to the inferior gluteal vessels and lies under the gluteus maximus muscle. It descends at the dorsal side of the thigh, lying on the long head of the biceps muscle, just medial to the sciatic nerve. It is important that the posterior cutaneous femoral nerve is running beneath the fascia lata. The nerve branches off the inferior clunium nerves, which are bending around the inferior margin of the gluteus maximus muscle in order to supply the skin in the inferolateral gluteal region. The posterior femoral cutaneous nerve also can penetrate the piriform muscle as a variation.

1.9.2.3 N. Pudendus (Fig. 1.15)

This nerve is composed by the ventral branches of the second, third, and fourth sacral spinal nerve. It exits the pelvic cavity through the infrapiriform foramen, lying on the sacrospinal ligament or the ischial spine just medial to the internal pudendal vessels. Then the nerve passes the minor sciatic foramen. Together with the internal pudendal vessels the nerve now runs into the pudendal canal of Alcock, on the lateral wall of the ischiorectal fossa. In this region the nerve is in danger, if cement cones are penetrating the acetabular fossa (Fig. 1.6d).

1.9.2.4 N. Glutaeus Superior (Figs. 1.11, 1.15, and 1.16)

This nerve is formed by the fourth and fifth lumbar spinal nerve and by the first sacral spinal nerve. The superior gluteal nerve exits the pelvis through the suprapiriform foramen and runs between the gluteus medius and minimus muscles, supplying these muscles. One branch of the superior gluteal nerve runs through the gluteus minimus muscle and exits at its anterior border. This branch enters the m. tensor fasciae latae medially in order to supply this muscle [33].

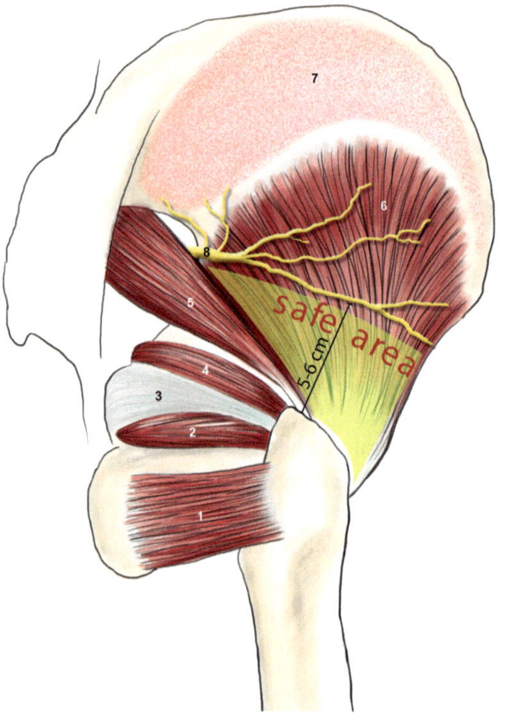

Fig. 1.16 Schematic drawing to explain the Skizze "safe area". Notice, that the inferior branch of the superior gluteus nerve runs ~5–6 cm above the greater trochanter. **1**: M. quadratus femoris, **2**: M. gemellus inferior, **3**: M. obturatorius internus (Sehne), **4**: M. gemellus superior, **5**: M. piriformis, **6**: M. glutaeus minimus, **7**: field of origin of the M. glutaeus medius, **8**: N. glutaeus superior

1.9.2.5 N. Glutaeus Inferior (Fig. 1.15)

This nerve, formed by the fifth lumbar and the first and second sacral spinal nerve, exits the pelvis through the infrapiriforme foramen. The nerve divides into several branches, supplying the gluteus maximus muscle. The entrance point is rather constant in the medial third and ~5 cm far from the midline [33]. Within the muscle, anastomoses are formed by the main branches, so that deleting one branch can be partly compensated. In some cases the nerve can pierce the piriform muscle.

According to Hilton's law the hip joint will be innervated by all nerves which supply muscles, moving the joint. Therefore articular branches are spreading off from the following nerves:

- N. femoralis
- N. ischiadicus
- N. obturatorius and obturatorius accessorius
- N. glutaeus superior
- N. glutaeus inferior

The distributions of these nerves define four innervation quadrants: anterior, anteromedial, posterolateral, and posteromedial. Beside these regular nerves additional nerves can participate in the innervation of the capsule in a great variety of combinations. This explains that an exclusive blocking of the obturator nerve does not always result in a complete anesthesia of the hip joint [44, 45].

1.10 Topographical Aspects for Surgical Approaches

The topographical aspects are important for the different approaches (anterior, lateral, and dorsolateral) to the hip joint (Fig. 1.8b).

1.10.1 Dorsolateral Region

In the dorsolateral region the gluteus maximus muscle with its broad fibers and its thin fascia can easily be identified. The quadrangular structure of the gluteus maximus is also known in surgery as the "gluteal lid of Henry." At its inferior margin the sciatic nerve and the medially positioned posterior cutaneous femoral nerve can be seen. Just behind the greater trochanter the gluteus maximus inserts at the iliotibial tract. After removing the gluteus maximus the deeper layer can be seen (Fig. 1.11a, b). Cranially lies the gluteus medius muscle. After removing this muscle the gluteus minimus can be exposed. In the deep layer we can identify the piriformis muscle centrally. At its superior margin the superior gluteal vessels as well as the superior gluteal nerve can be seen. At its inferior margin the structures of the infrapiriforme foramen are exiting the pelvic cavity. From lateral to medial the following structures can be identified: sciatic nerve, posterior cutaneous femoral nerve, inferior gluteal vessels and nerve, and the pudendal nerve and vessels. These gluteal vessels must be handled with care. If they are lacerated, a retraction towards the pelvic cavity takes place and the vessels cannot be reached from the external approach. Therefore a severe bleeding occurs in the pelvic cavity. Furthermore the external rotators can be seen. From cranial to caudal: superior gemellus, internal obturator tendon, inferior gemellus, and quadratus femoris muscle. Just beneath the short external rotators the articular capsule of the hip joint is reached. If possible, the quadratus muscle should not be dissected, because the deep branch of the medial circumflex artery can bleed severely. Furthermore a thick arterial branch can be seen often at the superior margin of the quadratus muscle, which can also bleed severely.

5–6 cm above the tip of the greater trochanter the so-called safe area can be defined (Fig. 1.16). Normally the superior gluteal nerve is running above this zone, so that it will not be in danger in this region [46].

1.10.2 Anterior Region (Figs. 1.12 and 1.13)

Beneath the inguinal ligament the iliopectineal arch separates the lateral lacuna musculorum from the medial lacuna vasorum. The iliopsoas muscle as well as the femoral nerve exit through the lacuna musculorum. The nerve lies at the medial margin of the muscle. In the lateral corner of the lacuna musculorum the lateral cutaneous femoral nerve exits also and descends beneath the fascia lata. Medially to the iliopectineal arch the femoral artery is positioned and then the femoral vein is coming out of the lacuna vasorum. Squeezing the femoral vein during hip arthroplasty may result in a thrombosis [47].

Between the tensor fasciae latae and sartorius muscle Smith-Petersen's interval can be opened. In this region branches of the lateral circumflex artery can cause severe bleedings. Beneath the sartorius muscle the rectus muscle is positioned. This muscle originates with two heads from the anterior inferior iliac spine as well as from the supraacetabular sulcus. If a dissection of these heads is necessary the separation should also be performed in a distance of ~1.5 cm from the osseous origin. This technique makes the later refixation easier. The lateral margin of the iliopsoas tendon is often attached to the iliofemoral ligament. The sharp dissection of this connection makes the exposition of the hip joint easier [2].

References

1. Harty M. The anatomy of the hip joint. In: Tronzo RG, editor. Surgery of the hip joint. Philadelphia: Lea & Febiger; 1973.
2. Harty M. Some aspects of the surgical anatomy of the hip joint. JBJS. 1966;48-A:197–202.
3. Harty M. The Calcar femorale and the femoral neck. JBJS. 1957;39-A:625–30.
4. Kummer B. Biomechanik. Deutscher Ärzteverlag Köln. 2005.
5. Pauwels F. Atlas zur Biomechanik der gesunden und kranken Hüfte. Berlin, Heidelberg: Springer; 1973.
6. Kielbasinski Podlaszewska O, Bekvala J, Williams RL, Adds PJ. The innominate tubercle of the femur: application to anterior surgical approaches to the hip. Clin Anat. 2017;30:578–84.
7. Finnegan M. Non-metric variation of the infracranial skeleton. J Anat. 1978;125:23–37.
8. Schmorl G. Die pathologische Anatomie der Schenkelhalsfraktur. Münch Med Wochenschr. 1924;71:1381–5.
9. Laros GS. Intertrochanteric fractures. In: McCollister Evarts C, editor. Surgery of the musculoskeletal system, vol. 2. New York: Churchill Livingstone; 1983.
10. Ward FO. Outlines of human osteology. London: Henry Renshaw; 1838.
11. Bertolini R, Leutert G. Atlas der Anatomie des Menschen. Bd. 1: Arm und Bein. Leipzig: Thieme; 1978.
12. Carlsson AS, Nilsson BE. The relationship of bone mass and loosening of the femoral component in total hip replacement. Acta Orthop Scand. 1980;51: 285–8.
13. Merkel F. Der Schenkelsporn. Centralblatt F Med Wiss. 1873;27:417–8.
14. Ackermann SE. Der Merkelsche Schenkelsporn. Experimentelle und klinische Untersuchungen. Medical Dissertation, RWTH University Aachen, Germany. 1994.
15. Fick R. Handbuch der Anatomie und Mechanik der Gelenke unter Berücksichtigung der bewegenden Muskeln. 1. Teil: Anatomie der Gelenke. In: Handbuch der Anatomie des Menschen, Hrsg: v. Bardeleben K, Gustav Fischer Jena; 1904.
16. Walmsley T. Observations on certain structural details of the neck of the femur. J Anat. 1915;49:305–13.
17. Odgers PNB. Two details about the neck of the femur: (1) the Eminentia (2) the empreinte. J Anat. 1931;65:352–62.
18. Angel JL. The reaction area of the femoral head. Clin Orthop. 1964;32:130–42.
19. Ganz R, Beck M, Leunig M, Nötzli HP, Siebenrock KA. Femoroazetabuläres impingement. In: Orthopädie und Orthopädische Chirurgie (Hrsg. Wirth CJ und Zichner L). Band: Becken, Hüfte (Hrsg. Tschauner C). New York: Thieme Stuttgart; 2004.
20. Pitt MJ, Graham AR, Shipman JH, Birkby W. Herniation pit of the femoral neck. Am J Roentgenol. 1982;138:1115–21.
21. Imhäuser G. Die Pfannenbodendicke bei der Protrusio acetabuli und der Hüftverrenkung. Z Orthop. 1947;76:251–3.
22. Scheuer L, Black S. Developmental juvenile osteology. San Diego: Academic; 2000.
23. Oberländer W. Die Beanspruchung des menschlichen Hüfgelenkes. Die Verteilung der Knorpeldicke im Acetabulum und ihre funktionelle Bedeutung. Anat Embryol. 1977;150:141–53.
24. Oberländer W, Kurrat H-J, Breul R. Untersuchungen zur Ausdehnung der knöchernen Facies lunata. Z Orthop. 1978;116:675–82.
25. Heller KD, Prescher A, Holbeck M, Forst R. Bone cement penetration of the acetabulum in total hip replacement. An experimental study. Int Orthop. 1996a;20:315–20.
26. Schmidt H, Braun S. Zur Ätiologie des Pfannenrandknochens am Hüftgelenk (Os ad acetabulum). Med Welt. 1961;36:1843–7.
27. Anderhuber F. Entwicklungsgeschichte und Anatomie. In: Orthopädie und Orthopädische Chirurgie (Hrsg. Wirth CJ und Zichner L). Band: Becken, Hüfte (Hrsg. Tschauner C). New York: Thieme Stuttgart; 2004.
28. Kim YH, Azuma H. The nerve endings of the acetabular labrum. Clin Orthop. 1995;320:176–81.
29. Grech P. Hip arthrography. London: Chapman & Hall; 1977.

30. Putz R, Schrank C. Anatomy of the labrocapsular complex. Orthopade. 1998;27:675–80.
31. Conn KS, Villar RN. Die Labrumläsion aus der Sicht eines arthroskopischen Hüftchirurgen. Orthopade. 1998;27:699–703.
32. Löhe F, Eckstein F, Sauer T, Putz R. Structure, strain and function of the transverse acetabular ligament. Acta Anat. 1996;157:315–23.
33. Frohse F, Fränkel M. Die Muskeln des menschlichen Beines. In: Handbuch der Anatomie des Menschen (Hrsg. K. von Bardeleben) Gustav Fischer; 1913.
34. Thiel W. Photographischer Atlas der praktischen Anatomie. Bd. 1: Bauch, untere Extremität. New York: Springer; 1996.
35. Shinohara H. Gemelli and obturator internus muscles: different heads of one muscle? Anat Rec. 1995;243:145–50.
36. Hayek H. Über den Ursprung der ischiokruralen Muskulatur vom Os sacrum. Ergh z Anat Anz. 1960;106/107:139–41.
37. Trueta J, Harrison MHM. The normal vascular anatomy of the femoral head in adult man. J Bone Surg. 1953;35B:442–61.
38. Trueta J. The normal vascular anatomy of the human femoral head during growth. J Bone Surg. 1957;39B:358–94.
39. Weathersby PD. The origin of the artery of the ligamentum teres femoris. JBJS. 1959;41A:261–3.
40. Hipp E. Die Gefässe des Hüftkopfes. Anatomie, Angiographie und Klinik. Beilagenheft zu Bd. 96 der Zeitschrift für Orthopädie. Stuttgart: Enke; 1962.
41. Heller KD, Prescher A, Birnbaum K, Forst R. Femoral nerve lesion in total hip replacement: an experimental study. Arch Orthop Trauma Surg. 1998;117:153–5.
42. Eisler P. Der Plexus lumbosacralis des Menschen. Abhandlung der naturforschenden Gesellschaft zu Halle. 1892;17:280–364.
43. Ghent WR. Further studies on meralgia paresthetica. Can Med Assoc J. 1961;85:871–5.
44. Birnbaum K, Prescher A, Hessler S, Heller K-D. The sensory innervation of the hip-joint. An anatomical study. Surg Radiol Anat. 1997;19:371–5.
45. Heßler S. Innervation des Hüftgelenkes. Medical Dissertation, RWTH University Aachen, Germany. 2001.
46. Perez MM, Llusa M, Ortiz JC, Lorente M, Lopez I, Lazaro A, Perez A, Götzens V. Superior gluteal nerve: safe area in hip surgery. Surg Radiol Anat. 2004;26:225–9.
47. Heller KD, Forst J, Prescher A. Proximale Beinvenenthrombose nach totalendoprothetischem Ersatz des Hüftgelenkes via transglutäalem Zugang—experimentelle Leichenstudie zum Einfluß der Beinlagerung. Orthopädische Praxis. 1996b;32:61–4.

The Minimally Invasive Direct Anterior Approach to the Hip

2

Wolf R. Drescher

2.1 Introduction

The direct anterior approach (DAA) was first described by Hueter in 1870 [1]. The DAA is the only true intermuscular and internervous approach to the hip [2]. In recent years, this approach has enjoyed increasing attention as it seems to reduce soft-tissue damage, to reduce pain [3], and to improve early recovery, and suggests a lower dislocation risk [4]. There have been several modifications to its original description, two of which seem to be favored internationally. Matta has described a direct anterior single-incision approach technique requiring a specially modified fracture table especially for facilitating the preparation of the femur and insertion of the femoral stem [5]. Lovell has described a similar technique using a standard operating table [6].

The author has started using the DAA technique around 10 years ago, and has implanted 2000 THAs via the DAA using a standard operating table. He has implemented the DAA as the standard approach for primary THA in his department combined with a modified fast-track treatment pathway [7, 8].

W. R. Drescher (✉)
Department of Orthopedics, RWTH Aachen University Hospital, Aachen, Germany

Orthopedic Surgery of the Lower Limb and Arthroplasty, Rummelsberg Hospital, Schwarzenbruck, Germany
e-mail: wolf.drescher@sana.de

2.2 Surgical Technique

The patient is placed on a radiolucent standard operating room table in the supine position. The hip rotation center should be placed at the hinge of the operating table to allow for 20° hyperextension. This can be practically ensured by palpating the trochanteric tip. No perineal post is used. Normal single-use surgical draping of the operative hip is used to allow full range of motion during the procedure. C-arm fluoroscopy is done intraoperatively when the original cup and the femoral probe implants are in place, and before wound closure.

The author always draws the important landmarks of surface anatomy in order to insure that the skin incision is precisely in the best place, and is the shortest possible. The skin incision originates 2–3 cm laterally and 2 cm distally from the anterior superior iliac spine, and extends slightly obliquely 5–6 cm distally directing towards the lateral femoral epicondyle. By choosing to start the skin incision 2–3 cm laterally, the lateral cutaneous femoris nerve is avoided (Fig. 2.1).

After subcutaneous hemostasis, the outer layer of the fascia of the tensor fasciae latae muscle is exposed, and longitudinally incised in the middle of the muscle with the scissors. The anterior portion of this muscle is then bluntly loosened out of the anterior circumference of its fascial sheath (Fig. 2.2).

W. R. Drescher et al. (eds.), *Advances in Specialist Hip Surgery*,
https://doi.org/10.1007/978-3-030-61830-8_2

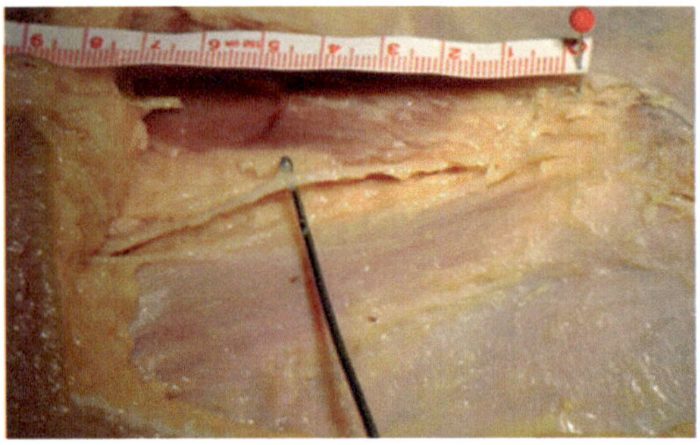

Fig. 2.1 Left cadaver hip from lateral view: The lateral cutaneous femoris nerve runs subcutaneously from the medial side of the anterior superior iliac spine (red needle) towards distal laterally directly over the gap between the sartorius medially and the tensor fasciae latae muscle laterally

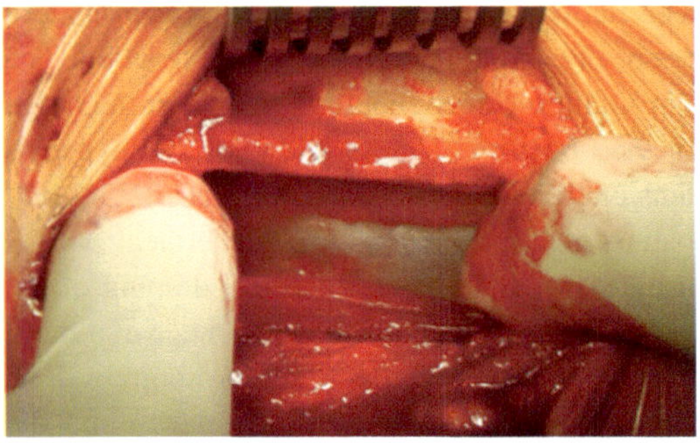

Fig. 2.2 The fascia is incised over the midpoint of the tensor fasciae latae muscle belly, and the anterior portion of this muscle bluntly loosened out of its fascial sheath. Medially, the rectus femoris muscle can be seen

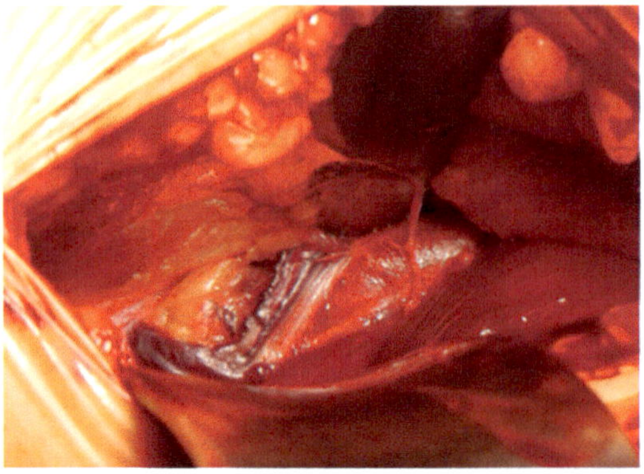

Fig. 2.3 The ascending branch of the lateral femoral circumflex artery with the adjacent veins lies in depth the distal part of the wound and must be ligated or cauterized

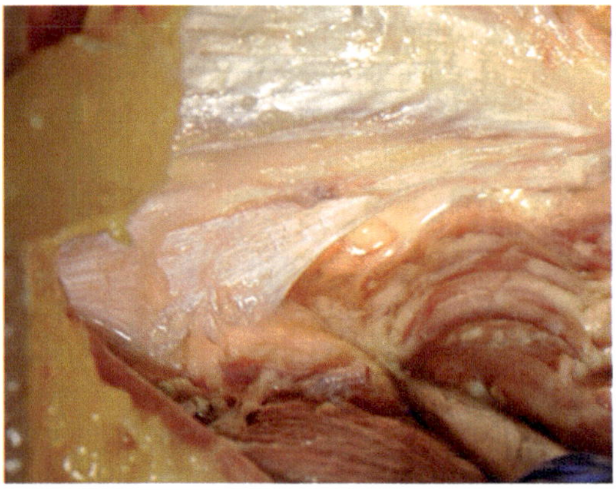

Fig. 2.4 The fascial arch of the reflect part of the rectus femoris muscle is well palpable in the depth of Hueter interval, and serves as a good anatomic orientation

A blunt liver retractor is inserted in order to retract the muscle belly of the tensor fascia latae muscle laterally. Additionally, a long Langenbeck retractor holds the rectus femoris muscle medially in order to gain insight into Hueter interval (Fig. 2.3). In its depth, the branches of the lateral femoral circumflex vessels cross. These must be ligated or coagulated in order to secure a dry surgical field.

The fascial arch of the reflect part of the rectus femoris muscle lies directly beneath the branches of the lateral femoral circumflex vessels (Fig. 2.4). The bow-shaped cranial border of this fascial arch extends laterally and can be well palpated and used as an anatomic orientation.

The fascial arch of the reflect part of the rectus femoris muscle is afterwards incised towards distally. This facilitates the access to the anterior hip joint capsule beneath the origin of the reflect part of the rectus femoris muscle (Fig. 2.5). A blunt Hohmann retractor is inserted through this "channel" in order to be placed on the medial capsule. Sometimes, the reflect part of the rectus femoris muscle has to be elevated from the anterior capsule by a Cobb's rasp.

A second blunt Hohmann retractor is obliquely inserted into the intertrochanteric fossa. At this point, the standard procedure is that either a capsule excision is done or it is opened in a "T"-shaped classic fashion [6] with an anterior acetabular retractor placed underneath the rectus femoris muscle and on the anterior acetabulum.

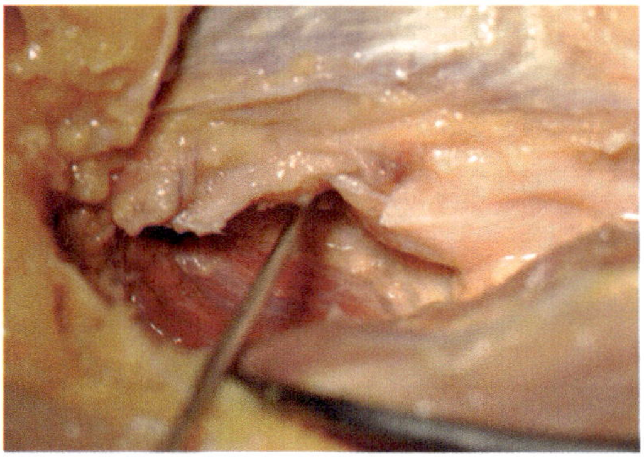

Fig. 2.5 After incision of the fascial arch of the reflect part of the rectus femoris muscle, a "channel" can be visualized between the rectus muscle and the underlying hip joint capsule with a Cobb's rasp

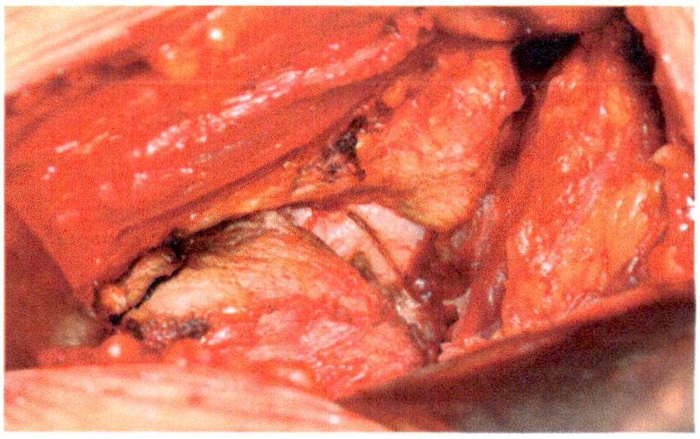

Fig. 2.6 Right hip seen anterolaterally: The capsule incision is started craniolaterally (left in the figure), and runs C-shaped on the lateral femoral head and upper neck into the anterolateral trochanteric fossa. Furthermore, a first capsule release is done on the inside of the major trochanter. The second capsule incision runs parallely above the cranial border of the vast lateral muscle (almost perpendicular to the first capsule incision in the right third of the figure). In the center of the figure, the remaining cartilage of the femoral head shines through. Medially is the rectus femoris muscle

In a modification, this author performs a C-shaped electric knife incision of the hip joint capsule starting from the laterocranial acetabular socket down to the trochanteric fossa (Fig. 2.6). At its insertion on the inner side of the major trochanter, the capsule is released back to the posterior portion of the femoral neck. Perpendicular to the femoral neck axis, a second capsule incision is performed parallel with the cranial border of the vast lateral muscle. This technique of capsulotomy leaves the anterior capsule and reflect part of the rectus femoris muscle intact, and facilitates the closure of the capsule after implantation.

The two blunt Hohmann retractors are moved into the intracapsular space. A (double) neck osteotomy is then performed with the oscillating saw (and the resulting bony neck slice extracted). The tensor fascia latae muscle should be protected with a blunt retractor during the neck osteotomy. An MIS Hohmann retractor with bowed shape is inserted into the craniomedial hip joint space in order to mobilize the lose femoral head. This is then extracted by means of a corkscrew.

Consequently, the MIS Hohmann retractor is placed beneath the rectus femoris muscle directly onto the anterior acetabular rim in a direction perpendicular to the inguinal ligament. The inferior part of the hip joint capsule is released down to the lesser trochanter. Positioning the leg in a "lazy figure-of-four" position facilitates this step.

A Müller retractor is then placed behind the dorsal acetabular rim in order to hold the femoral neck down and get a good overview of the acetabulum (Fig. 2.7). The blunt liver retractor is still in place to protect and hold the tensor fasciae latae muscle to the side. The preparation of the acetabulum and insertion of the cup are then done conventionally. The author uses a conventional straight, not-special MIS reamers and a straight cup inserter, for this step.

For preparation of the proximal femur, the author places the Müller retractor on the medial

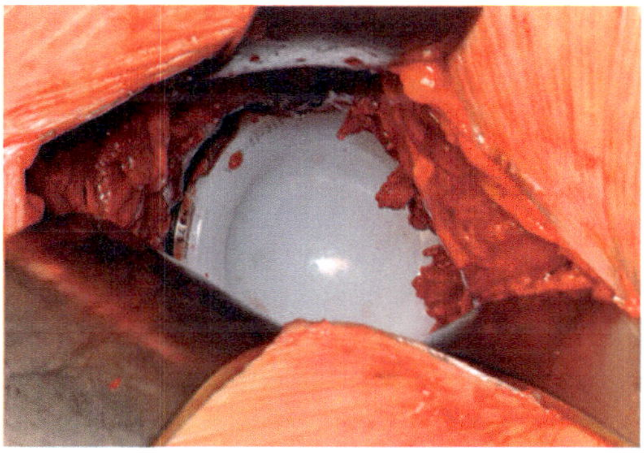

Fig. 2.7 Right hip seen anterolaterally: With the skin incision in the right place, and the three retractors carefully positioned as pictured, acetabular reaming and cup positioning can be easily performed with conventional straight instruments

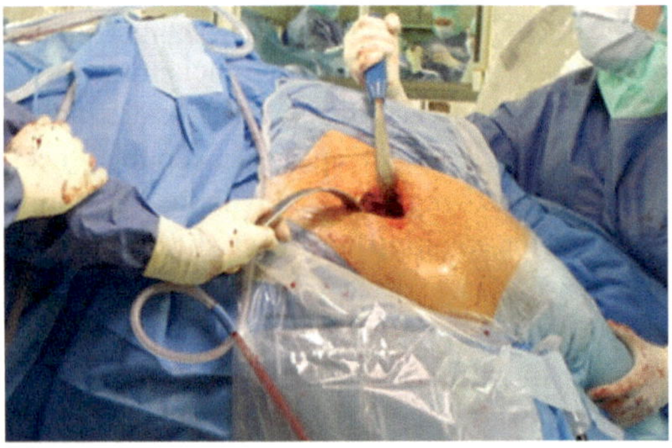

Fig. 2.8 For femoral preparation, the hip is externally rotated and adducted with the knee kept in straight position. The hip is hyperextended by lowering the foot part of the operating room table 15–20°

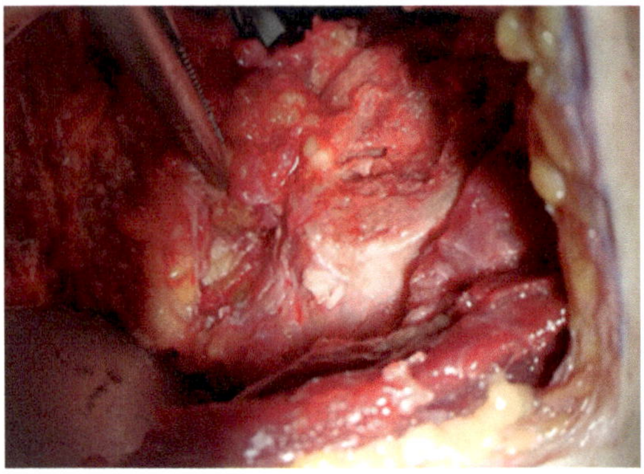

Fig. 2.9 Right cadaveric hip seen craniolaterally: The hip joint capsule has been stepwise released starting in the trochanteric fossa from anterior, and advancing further posterior. The proximal femur will then move towards the surgeon from behind the acetabulum. The capsule is then held to the side by the two-tipped MIS retractor, but not excised

side of the femoral neck. The hip is then externally rotated 90° and adducted by placing the leg below the contralateral leg (Fig. 2.8). During this maneuver, it is important to keep the knee straight. The foot part of the operating room table is then lowered 15–20° in order to achieve hyperextension of the hip.

A double-tipped MIS retractor is then positioned on the outer facet of the greater trochanter, between the hip joint capsule and minimal gluteal muscle. The aim of this retractor is to elevate the externally rotated proximal femur. Only little force should be used on the retractors especially in elderly, osteopenic patients. After drying the site, the capsule is released subperiosteally in the trochanteric fossa from anterior to posterior until the yellow fat pad by electric knife (Fig. 2.9). By slightly pulling on the proximal femur with a Kocher hook inserted into the femoral neck trabecular bone, the proximal femur is stepwise elevated from behind the dorsal acetabular wall during the capsular release. Care has to be taken not to perform the capsule release too far posterior in order not to detach the piriform, internal obturator, and gemelli muscles. After successful performance of this step, the osteotomized femoral neck "is looking at the operator" who is now working from cranially.

The consequent femoral preparation can be started with a straight box chisel. Further, it requires double-offset MIS handles in order to pass by the lateral os ilium and not to harm the tensor fasciae latae muscle with the broaches (Fig. 2.10).

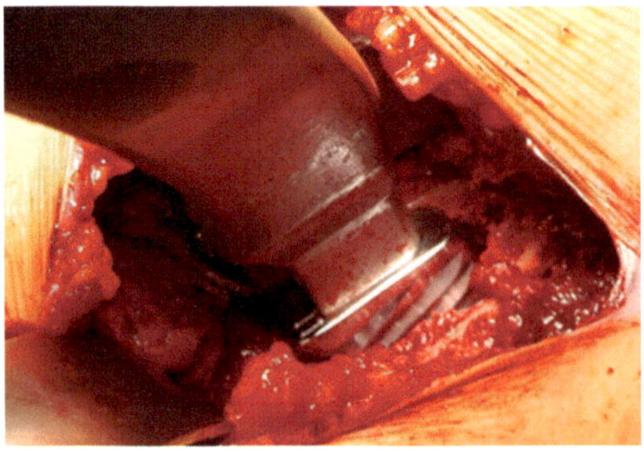

Fig. 2.10 Right hip: The double-offset handle facilitates the broaching of the proximal femur

After broaching is complete, the trial femoral neck and head components can be mounted. The foot of the operating table should then be slightly raised. The trial implant can be reduced by the first assistant pulling on the leg and the operator pushing on the head component with the special inserter. We then test for rotational stability in hyperextension of the hip. Afterwards, the foot part of the operating table is raised to neutral position, and the full stability, impingement, and leg length testing are performed as well as fluoroscopy with the C-arm in two plains. After sat-

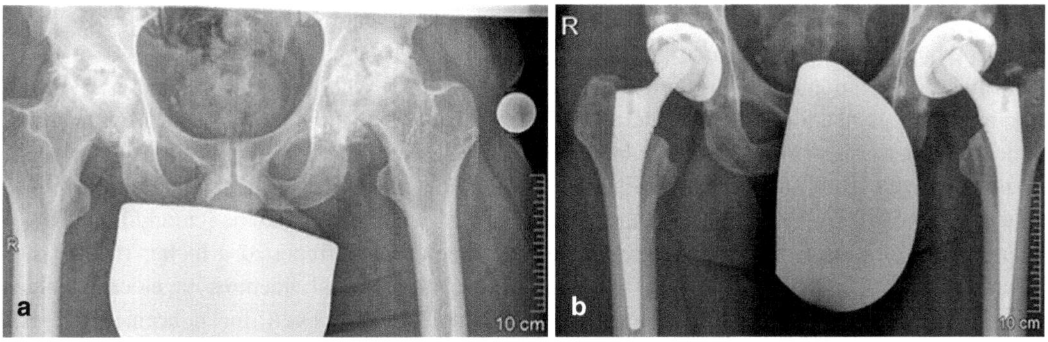

Fig. 2.11 (**a**, **b**) 50-Year-old male patient with severe pain and reduced quality of life because of bilateral arthritis of the hips. The author performed a single-setting bilateral cementless THA via the direct anterior approach. After 5 days, the patient was discharged for 3 weeks of rehabilitation. 6 weeks postoperatively, the patient returned to work

isfactory testing, the hip is dislocated by pulling laterally with a small Kocher hook around the trial neck component. The trial femoral implant is removed, and the original inserted in the same position as described above. Again, stability, impingement, and leg length are checked. The final implant position is documented by C-arm fluoroscopy. The hip joint capsule is closed with single resorbable stitches. Wound closure includes suture of the outer fascia of the tensor fasciae latae muscle. After normal subcutaneous suture, the skin is closed. Mobilization with full weight bearing is started in the afternoon of the same day. A pelvic overview and axial X-ray control are done 2 days postoperatively (Fig. 2.11).

The experience of this author with the DAA is that all types of primary femoral stems can be implanted with a double-offset broach handle. This includes short, straight, anatomic stems in cemented or uncemented fashion. In case of cementing, a bowed inserter facilitates the placement of the cement stopper. For the further cementing steps, conventional instruments can be used.

2.3 Discussion

During the last years, minimally invasive total hip arthroplasty via the direct anterior approach (DAA) has gained increasing popularity throughout the orthopedic community. It could be shown that it contributes to less surgery-related muscle damage [9]. Creatine kinase, an established serum marker for skeletal muscle damage, was significantly lower immediately after THA surgery via the DAA compared to the posterior approach to the hip. Clinically, a superior early hip function was observed for the DAA compared to the direct lateral approach to the hip for THA [10]. Hip function was assessed by the timed up and go test and the Harris hip score in this study. Also, less pain as registered by visual analogue scale on the day of surgery and the following days was reported [3].

This author has started using the direct anterior approach to the hip 10 years ago, and up to date performed 2000 of these procedures. Since 6 years, he has been implementing this approach as the standard surgical approach for primary THA together with a fast-track recovery pathway in his own department comparable to that of Free et al. [8]. The DAA and the fast-track recovery pathway [7] act in a symbiotic fashion: The minimally invasive DAA has less impact on the patient than the conventional approaches. This facilitates mobilization on the day of surgery and accelerates recovery during the following days. The primary THA patients of this author operated via DAA have only little blood loss and do not need cell saver or blood transfusions.

During almost daily performance, the author has introduced the above-described modification of preserving the anterior hip joint capsule and reflect part of the rectus femoris muscle (Fig. 2.6). With this modification, either posterior or anterior instability is not found among the author's patients. Posterior instability has been described in a randomized series of 50 THAs via the DAA compared to 50 THAs performed via the direct lateral approach [10]. A risk factor for posterior instability seems to be an excessive capsular release with detachment of the piriformis, internal obturator, and gemelli muscles which should be avoided by not releasing too far posteriorly. Anterior instability consequent to the DAA has been described by Meneghini et al. [11].

A prolonged learning curve for adopting the direct anterior approach has been experienced by some authors [12]. Spaans et al. reported on a consecutive series of their first 46 THAs performed via DAA. Before starting this operation technique, the surgeons had an internal education and training on cadavers that was supervised by an experienced orthopedic surgeon who had used the DAA for 5 years. In this initial series, they reported a higher rate of complications compared to their usual posterolateral approach. Complications needing revision were cup migration/dislocation, a femoral stem collapse, and a quadriceps muscle weakness. Spaans et al. did not observe an improvement after 46 cases.

A higher complication rate has also been reported by other authors in a community hospital series of 247 THAs implanted via the DAA by 5 surgeons [13]. They reported 23 early major complications comprising 14 proximal femoral/greater trochanter fractures, 2 femoral shaft fractures, 2 deep infections, 2 nerve palsies, and 3 immediate reoperations for leg length discrepancy.

In contrast, Free et al. reported neither a different learning curve nor higher complication rates when transitioning from lateral or posterior approaches [8]. With careful and detailed preparation, it could be shown that the transition from another approach to the DAA can be safely performed [14].

The group of Yamamoto has reported a reduced motor-evoked potential amplitude of the femoral nerve immediately after placement of the anterior acetabular retractor in 77% of DAA cases [15]. Although this reduction appeared reversible, and the manual muscle test revealed no pathology postoperatively, the retractor on the anterior acetabular wall should be positioned with special attention to the femoral nerve.

Berend et al. reported a higher risk of periprosthetic femoral fractures in elderly women when using the DAA for noncemented THA implantation [16]. This author therefore strictly adheres to cementing the elderly female patient group also via the DAA.

On the other hand, in-hospital morbidity and postoperative revisions were found to be less in the DAA group compared to the posterior approach in a study from the Hospital of Special Surgery [4]. Ponzio et al. reported a shorter length of stay and procedure time, lower blood transfusion rate, and increased discharge to home rate in DAA patients compared to the posterior approach. The incidence of revision for dislocation was 1.5% for the posterior approach vs. 0.4% for the DAA.

In a report from the Norwegian Arthroplasty Register, the revision rates associated with the MIS anterior approach were not increased and implant survival was not different compared with those of the conventional posterior and direct lateral approaches [17].

Obese patients with a body mass index (BMI) above 35 receiving THA via the DAA were shown to have higher complication and early reoperation rates compared with nonobese patients with a BMI less or equal to 25 [18]. These were mostly due to wound infection and dehiscence. However, these rates were found to be comparable to the rates of the standard surgical approaches.

For this author, the DAA is also the approach of choice for a carefully selected healthy and younger group of patients who desire single-setting bilateral THA (Fig. 2.11). The literature does not report higher complication rates for single-setting bilateral compared to unilateral THA in patient groups with equivalent comorbidities [19].

The DAA may also be a credible and safe option for trauma patients with femoral neck fracture, with excellent functional outcomes, less surgery-related complications, and lower short-term and long-term mortality, than those reported in the literature [20].

In conclusion, our experience and the literature suggest that the direct anterior approach for THA is a technically demanding procedure. When starting to use the DAA, careful rehearsal of the anatomy of the hip should be done, ideally at an anatomic institute, in order to shorten the learning curve. Surgeons starting to learn this approach should prepare themselves by first visiting a high-quality cadaver course, and visiting a surgeon experienced in the technique. Additionally, the first surgeries should be assisted by an experienced surgeon in the DAA until the learning surgeon feels safe.

Under these conditions, the DAA is a safe approach with several advantages in the early phase: less soft-tissue damage, less pain, less blood loss, better early hip function, reduced length of stay, a shorter incision length, and a less visible scar are the advantages which make the DAA the standard approach for primary THA of this author.

Acknowledgement The author would like to thank professor Andreas Prescher, MD, PhD, Dept. of Anatomy, RWTH Aachen University Hospital, Germany, for great help in making the cadaver figures in this chapter.

References

1. Rachbauer F, Kain MS, Leunig M. The history of the anterior approach to the hip. Orthop Clin North Am. 2009;40(3):311–20. https://doi.org/10.1016/j.ocl.2009.02.007.
2. Kennon RE, Keggi JM, Wetmore RS, Zatorski LE, Huo MH, Keggi KJ. Total hip arthroplasty through a minimally invasive anterior surgical approach. J Bone Joint Surg Am. 2003;85-A(Suppl 4):39–48.
3. Mjaaland KE, Kivle K, Svenningsen S, Pripp AH, Nordsletten L. Comparison of markers for muscle damage, inflammation, and pain using minimally invasive direct anterior versus direct lateral approach in total hip arthroplasty: a prospective, randomized, controlled trial. J Orthop Res. 2015;33(9):1305–10. https://doi.org/10.1002/jor.22911.
4. Ponzio DY, Poultsides LA, Salvatore A, Lee YY, Memtsoudis SG, Alexiades MM. In-hospital morbidity and postoperative revisions after direct anterior vs. posterior total hip arthroplasty. J Arthroplast. 2018;33(5):1421–1425.e1421. https://doi.org/10.1016/j.arth.2017.11.053.
5. Matta JM, Shahrdar C, Ferguson T. Single-incision anterior approach for total hip arthroplasty on an orthopaedic table. Clin Orthop Relat Res. 2005;441:115–24.
6. Lovell TP. Single-incision direct anterior approach for total hip arthroplasty using a standard operating table. J Arthroplast. 2008;23(7 Suppl):64–8. https://doi.org/10.1016/j.arth.2008.06.027.
7. Husted H, Otte KS, Kristensen BB, Orsnes T, Wong C, Kehlet H. Low risk of thromboembolic complications after fast-track hip and knee arthroplasty. Acta Orthop. 2010;81(5):599–605. https://doi.org/10.3109/17453674.2010.525196.
8. Free MD, Owen DH, Agius PA, Pascoe EM, Harvie P. Direct anterior approach total hip arthroplasty: an adjunct to an enhanced recovery pathway: outcomes and learning curve effects in surgeons transitioning from other surgical approaches. J Arthroplast. 2018;33(11):3490–5. https://doi.org/10.1016/j.arth.2018.06.033.
9. Bergin PF, Doppelt JD, Kephart CJ, Benke MT, Graeter JH, Holmes AS, Haleem-Smith H, Tuan RS, Unger AS. Comparison of minimally invasive direct anterior versus posterior total hip arthroplasty based on inflammation and muscle damage markers. J Bone Joint Surg Am. 2011;93(15):1392–8. https://doi.org/10.2106/JBJS.J.00557.
10. Brismar BH, Hallert O, Tedhamre A, Lindgren JU. Early gain in pain reduction and hip function, but more complications following the direct anterior minimally invasive approach for total hip arthroplasty: a randomized trial of 100 patients with 5 years of follow up. Acta Orthop. 2018;89(5):484–9. https://doi.org/10.1080/17453674.2018.1504505.
11. Meneghini RM, Elston AS, Chen AF, Kheir MM, Fehring TK, Springer BD. Direct anterior approach: risk factor for early femoral failure of cementless total hip arthroplasty: a multicenter study. J Bone Joint Surg Am. 2017;99(2):99–105. https://doi.org/10.2106/JBJS.16.00060.
12. Spaans AJ, van den Hout JA, Bolder SB. High complication rate in the early experience of minimally invasive total hip arthroplasty by the direct anterior approach. Acta Orthop. 2012;83(4):342–6. https://doi.org/10.3109/17453674.2012.711701.
13. Woolson ST, Pouliot MA, Huddleston JI. Primary total hip arthroplasty using an anterior approach and a fracture table: short-term results from a community hospital. J Arthroplast. 2009;24(7):999–1005. https://doi.org/10.1016/j.arth.2009.04.001.
14. Yuasa T, Maezawa K, Sato H, Maruyama Y, Kaneko K. Safely transitioning to the direct anterior from posterior approach for total hip arthroplasty. J Orthop. 2018;15(2):420–3. https://doi.org/10.1016/j.jor.2018.03.013.

15. Ishimatsu T, Kinoshita K, Nishio J, Tanaka J, Ishii S, Yamamoto T. Motor-evoked potential analysis of femoral nerve status during the direct anterior approach for total hip arthroplasty. J Bone Joint Surg Am. 2018;100(7):572–7. https://doi.org/10.2106/JBJS.17.00679.
16. Berend KR, Mirza AJ, Morris MJ, Lombardi AV Jr. Risk of periprosthetic fractures with direct anterior primary total hip arthroplasty. J Arthroplast. 2016;31(10):2295–8. https://doi.org/10.1016/j.arth.2016.03.007.
17. Mjaaland KE, Svenningsen S, Fenstad AM, Havelin LI, Furnes O, Nordsletten L. Implant survival after minimally invasive anterior or anterolateral vs. conventional posterior or direct lateral approach: an analysis of 21,860 total hip arthroplasties from the Norwegian Arthroplasty Register (2008 to 2013). J Bone Joint Surg Am. 2017;99(10):840–7. https://doi.org/10.2106/JBJS.16.00494.
18. Antoniadis A, Dimitriou D, Flury A, Wiedmer G, Hasler J, Helmy N. Is direct anterior approach a credible option for severely obese patients undergoing total hip arthroplasty? A matched-control, retrospective, clinical study. J Arthroplast. 2018;33(8):2535–40. https://doi.org/10.1016/j.arth.2018.03.071.
19. Lanting BA, Odum SM, Cope RP, Patterson AH, Masonis JL. Incidence of perioperative events in single setting bilateral direct anterior approach total hip arthroplasty. J Arthroplast. 2015;30(3):465–7. https://doi.org/10.1016/j.arth.2014.09.021.
20. Dimitriou D, Helmy N, Hasler J, Flury A, Finsterwald M, Antoniadis A. The role of total hip arthroplasty through the direct anterior approach in femoral neck fracture and factors affecting the outcome. J Arthroplast. 2019;34(1):82–7. https://doi.org/10.1016/j.arth.2018.08.037.

Part II

Maturity Disorders of the Hip

3 Hip Dysplasia: Osteotomies Around the Hip in Childhood

Walter Michael Strobl

3.1 Definition

Osteotomies around the hip are surgical procedures performed to correct disorders of biomechanical alignment of the hip joint in order to achieve normal distribution of load, equilibrium of muscle forces, as well as normal growth of cartilage and bone structures by cutting and redirecting either the proximal femur only, the pelvis only, or both bones.

3.2 Classification

Osteotomies around the hip may be classified according to the following:

1. Anatomic location: High femoral neck, intertrochanteric, transtrochanteric, subtrochanteric femoral osteotomies, incomplete shelf osteotomies, acetabuloplasties, periacetabular osteotomies, complete single-, double-, and triple-pelvic osteotomies
2. Time and indication of surgery: Preventive, reconstructive, or salvage procedures

3.3 Indication

Osteotomies around the hip may be indicated in the following:

1. Developmental or congenital dislocations or severe dysplasia of hip: Pemberton's innominate osteotomy, Salter's innominate osteotomy, Steel's triple innominate osteotomy, shelf osteotomies, and acetabuloplasties, combined with femoral varization/derotation osteotomy, as salvage procedure: Chiari's osteotomy
2. Neuromuscular and other secondary dislocations, painful or unstable hips: Pemberton's or Dega's or modified osteotomies and acetabuloplasties, combined with femoral varization/derotation/shortening osteotomies, as salvage procedure: Schanz angulation osteotomy
3. Congenital or developmental deformities like coxa vara, coxa retrotorta: femoral valgization and derotation osteotomies
4. Deformities following slipped capital femoral epiphysis: Dunn's intracapsular cuneiform osteotomy, extracapsular base-of-neck osteotomy, compensatory basilar osteotomy of femoral neck, ball-and-socket trochanteric osteotomy
5. LCP disease: Salter's innominate osteotomy, and/or femoral varization/derotation osteotomy, as salvage procedure: Chiari's osteotomy
6. Osteonecrosis of femoral head: Sugioka's transtrochanteric osteotomy, and/or femoral varization/derotation.

W. M. Strobl (✉)
MOTIO Institute for Pediatric Orthopaedics and Neuro-Orthopaedics, Vienna, Austria
e-mail: walter.strobl@motio.org

W. R. Drescher et al. (eds.), *Advances in Specialist Hip Surgery*,
https://doi.org/10.1007/978-3-030-61830-8_3

7. Early stages of osteoarthritis: Pauwels type I varus osteotomy, Pauwels type II valgus osteotomy
8. Non-united fractures of femoral neck: McMurray's osteotomy, Dickson's high geometric osteotomy, Schanz angulation osteotomy, unstable intertrochanteric fractures: Dimon-Hughston osteotomy, Sarmiento osteotomy.

3.4 Normal Development of Hip in Childhood

While maturing in childhood, hip joints change their shape step by step. Physiologically, head and acetabulum are not congruent in newborn children in order to allow squeezing of the child's pelvic region during the process of birth. The acetabulum is smaller than the femoral head. Within the first months of life, hips mature quickly. The acetabulum grows faster than the femoral head and while its shape changes it covers more and more of the femoral head. This causes the joint to become increasingly stable during the first years of life.

Prerequisites for this development are a normal genetic disposition, normal development of soft tissue like ligaments and joint capsule, normal movement due to normal motor development, normal weight-bearing in early toddler age, lack of muscle weakness, lack of laxity of ligaments, and no adverse involuntary movement like spasticity or dystonia (Fig. 3.1).

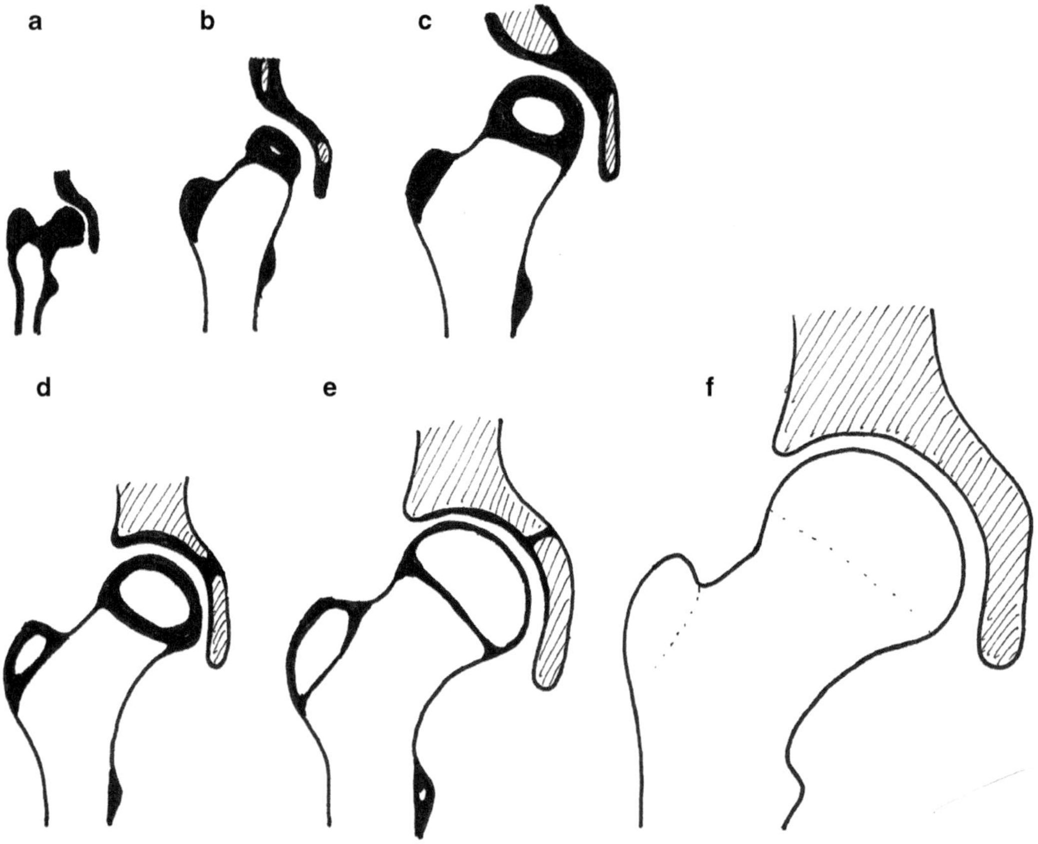

Fig. 3.1 Normal development of hip congruity and diminishing plasticity of cartilage in the age of (**a**) newborn, (**b**) 3 months, (**c**) 1 year, (**d**) 4 years, (**e**) 8 years, (**f**) 18 years. ©WM Strobl

3.5 Most Common Disorder: Hip Dysplasia and Unstable Hip

Developmental dysplasia of the hip (DDH) has been one of the most demanding pediatric orthopedic diseases for generations. Today, combined clinical and ultrasound screening and very early conservative interventions in the first months of life by splints have dropped the incidence of severe late dysplasias and dislocations significantly. In countries with qualified prevention programs, only few children are in need of surgical interventions by osteotomies around the hip (Fig. 3.2).

In several diseases of either the muscles or the central as well as the peripheral nerve system, the abovementioned prerequisites of normal hip development are lacking. So today screening and early detection of pathophysiologic processes of the maturing hip in systemic neurogenic, muscular, and other diseases have become the most challenging tasks of the pediatric orthopedic specialist (Fig. 3.3).

Risk factors for the development of unstable hip joints are:

1. Hereditary dysplasia of hip joints like DDH
2. Teratologic deformities of pelvis and lower extremities like PFFD
3. Hyperlaxity of capsule or ligaments like in Down syndrome or Ehlers-Danlos syndrome
4. Muscle inactivity like in arthrogrypotic syndromes
5. Muscle force imbalance due to motor disorders like muscle diseases
6. Muscle force imbalance due to sensorimotor disorders like CP, spina bifida, and SMA (Fig. 3.4)
7. Muscle force imbalance due to sensory/proprioceptive deficit like neuropathies
8. Avascular disorders of femoral head and acetabulum like in LCP disease

3.6 Most Common Indication: Cerebral Palsy

Not only in countries with screening for DDH, unstable hips in cerebral palsy (CP) are the most common indication for osteotomies around the hip. CP is used as term for a group of frequent developmental disorders with an incidence of approximately 3 per 1000 newborns. CP is defined as sensorimotor disorder caused by an early pre-, peri-, or postnatal damage of the maturing brain. Depending on the location and extent of the brain lesion, different patterns of sensorimotor deficits will be observed. In the more common severe types of CP hip instability and dislocation, especially nonambulatory children with GMFCS IV and V (Gross Motor

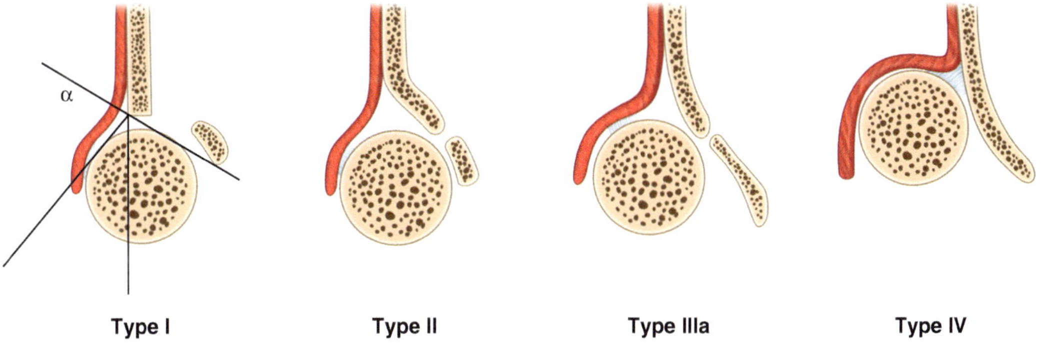

Fig. 3.2 Neonatal ultrasound screening indicating type I normal, type II immature/dysplastic, type III decentered, type IV dislocated hip. ©WM Strobl

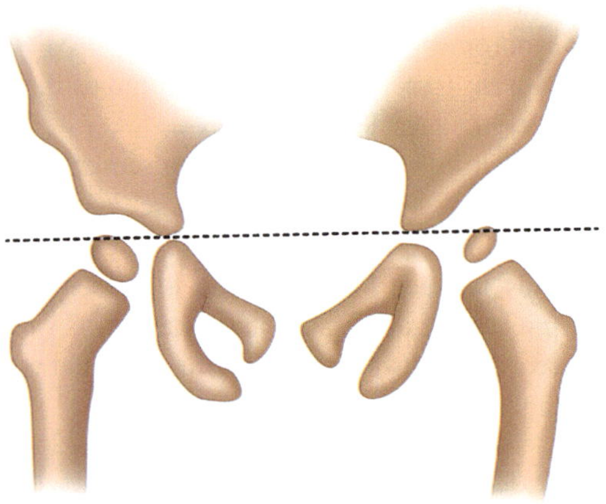

Fig. 3.3 Dysplastic acetabulum and decentered femoral head in unstable hip. ©WM Strobl

Function Classification System), hip instability may be diagnosed in up to 100% [1–3].

Damage to the central nervous system causes lack of motor control and weakness of certain muscle groups leading to imbalanced forces over joints. Thus, normal maturing of the hip joint is inhibited. The force of the overactive spastic hip adductors and flexors combined with weakness of stabilizing abductors and extensors promotes lateralization of the femoral head and decentration of the hip joint. So changes of the musculoskeletal system may be regarded as a secondary damage.

Biomechanics explain forces and the resulting type of musculoskeletal damage. The vector of

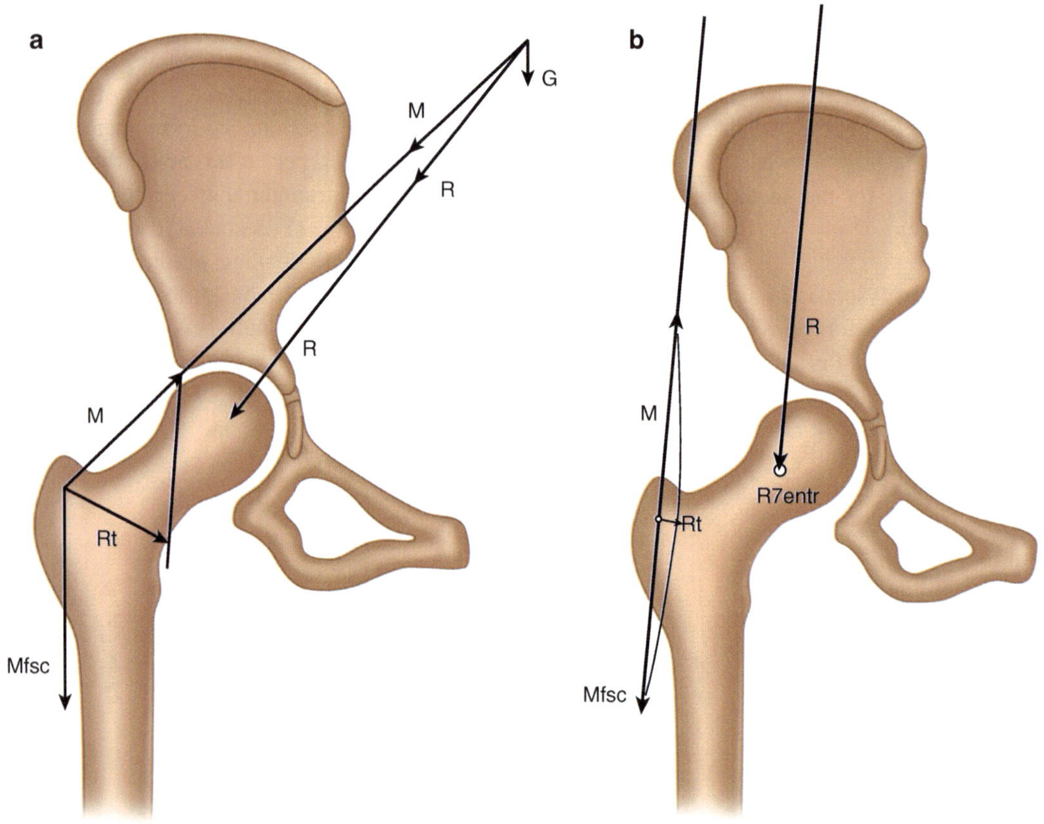

Fig. 3.4 Normal forces centering (**a**) and pathological forces dislocating (**b**) the hip joint. ©WM Strobl

the resulting force is directed in a lateral, superior, and posterior direction and, in most cases, defects of the acetabular rim are in this position. In addition, the shape of the proximal femur follows the altered function. Physiological high neck-shaft angles and high femoral anteversion in newborn children decrease during the first years of life due to increasing muscle power and weight bearing. Altered biomechanical forces reduce this development and cause increased neck-shaft angles and femoral anteversion, forming hip types of coxa valga and coxa antetorta. Additionally the second head of the femoral rectus muscle, the caput reflexum, and the lateral capsule of the hip joint, which are toughly stretched, cause a deformity of the femoral head. Because of the even increasing power of the overactive muscles and increasing weakness of paretic muscles this pathomechanism and the progress of hip dislocation are regarded to be irreversible. Quality of life will become significantly reduced [4–6]. By that point, conservative treatment may influence the migration of femoral head and progressive dislocation but it is not able to stop it [7].

In this stage, conservative treatment like exercises or splints is unlikely to improve the development. If only high muscular tension or spasticity has been diagnosed without muscular shortening, local injections of botulinum toxin may help to improve the balance of muscular forces.

If structural musculoskeletal changes have already occurred, botulinum toxin and splints are not effective and surgical procedures are indicated [8]. Combined lengthening of the adductor and iliopsoas muscles followed by splints and exercises may be effective in improving the situation. However, it has turned out that not in any case this method is sufficient and the dislocation may be progressive.

Pain is no early indicator for altered biomechanical function of the hip joint. In early stages, pain may only be triggered by passive movement, whereas in progredient stages of dislocation, hip pain is reported by patients or caretakers commonly [9].

Concerning the treatment of children with CP, the role of surgery and its timing are still controversially discussed. Some authors have reported excellent long-term results with prevention programs including close surveillance, positioning, splints, and physiotherapy [10]. Others perform open or percutaneous muscle lengthening with good long-term results in patients with a radiologic migration percentage (MP) of less than 40% [11].

In the last decade, in cases of progredient stages of dislocations, commonly single-event multilevel surgery (SEMLS) was simultaneously performed with hip reconstruction surgery [12–14].

Not only in children with CP but also in Down syndrome, Ehlers-Danlos syndrome, lumbar level of myelomeningocele, arthrogrypotic syndromes, hereditary neuropathies, and other diseases with progressive, painful, or disabling hip dislocation, osteotomies around the hip and especially hip reconstruction surgery are widely regarded as golden standard for effectively achieving a stable and pain-free hip joint.

3.7 Osteotomies Around the Hip Improving Acetabular Coverage

The goal of preventive and reconstructive femoral or pelvic osteotomies is to restore normal functional anatomy, thus improving joint pressures and loading patterns. The goal of salvage osteotomies is to relieve pain and improve function sufficiently by remodeling to delay the need for total hip arthroplasty in adulthood.

Historical development of procedures:

1. König 1891: first surgery for improving coverage by distalizing lateral iliac cortical bone lap
2. Late 1890: first proximal femoral osteotomy
3. Albee 1915: short osteotomy to lever down cranial acetabular roof
4. Modified procedures: Jones 1920, Schede 1920, Lance 1925
5. Spitzy 1924: fixation of tibial graft at cranial acetabular margin
6. Wiberg 1944: long osteotomy to the triradiate cartilage
7. Chiari 1953: complete osteotomy and medialization of acetabulum and femur
8. Blavier 1962: first periacetabular pelvic osteotomy
9. Dega 1964: lateral acetabuloplasty by osteotomy to incisura ischiadica
10. Pemberton 1965: pericapsular curved pelvic osteotomy from ventral to incisura ischiadica
11. LeCoeur 1965: first triple osteotomy
12. Salter 1966: complete osteotomy with improving lateral and anterior coverage
13. Steel 1973: modified triple osteotomy
14. Sutherland 1977: double osteotomy
15. Wagner 1978: modified periacetabular spherical osteotomy
16. Tönnis 1981: modified triple osteotomy
17. Ganz 1988: modified periacetabular pelvic osteotomy PAO
18. Staheli 1992: modified shelf acetabuloplasty
19. Robb and Brunner 2006: Dega-like acetabuloplasty—also after triradiate cartilage closure

3.8 Complete Pelvic Osteotomies

Pelvic osteotomies may be defined as procedures that are **completely cutting the pelvic bone**. These procedures can be used for an easy three-dimensional redirection of the acetabular plane. Disadvantages are complete cutting of the pelvic bone with longer time of bone healing, rehabilitation, and a higher risk of loss of correction and development of pseudarthrosis. Due to postoperative temporary instability of the pelvis, these osteotomies may be performed only unilaterally. The radius of an enlarged acetabulum will not be reduced by this group of osteotomies. However, authors reported evidence that the shape of the femoral head and the acetabulum is adjusted by remodeling, and joint function improved following reconstructions including Salter's procedure [4, 13]. Commonly, pelvic osteotomies are performed in combination with proximal femoral varus osteotomies in children with severe hip dysplasia as well as all stages of hip dislocation (see hip reconstruction below).

In all innominate osteotomies, overcorrection should be avoided while treating acetabular dysplasia because it can create iatrogenic femoroacetabular impingement and have an adverse effect on the outcome Castaneda reported [15].

3.8.1 Chiari's Osteotomy: A Salvage Procedure for the Age Older Than 14 Years

In 1953, Chiari described a complete single-cut osteotomy following lateralization of the cranial portion of the iliac bone in order to improve lateral coverage of the femoral head [16].

Surgical technique: The osteotomy is performed at the superior margin of the acetabulum. Then the pelvis inferior to the osteotomy and the proximal femur is displaced medially. The line of osteotomy extends from closely superior to the lip of acetabulum into the sciatic notch. It can be curved to facilitate femoral head coverage. Parts of the hip joint capsule are interposed between the shelf and the femoral head (Fig. 3.5).

Indications are salvage procedures in selected children older than 14 years with severe dysplastic hips with incongruous joints, or when reduction of the head is not possible, and also in cases with osteoarthritis, where other osteotomies are not favored. Patient's selection by age, activities, goals, range of motion, leg length discrepancy, status of the homolateral knee, and radiographic

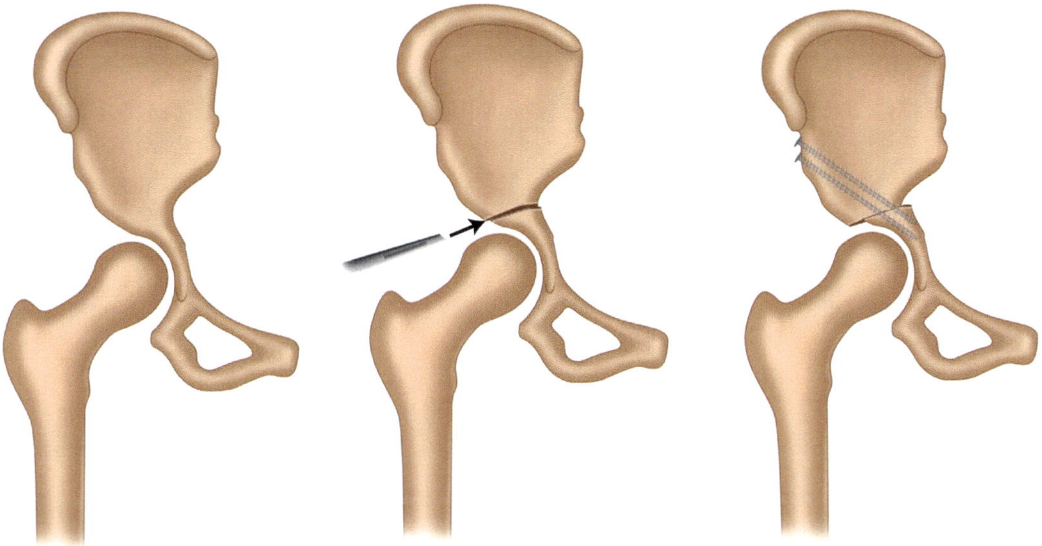

Fig. 3.5 Pre- and post-Chiari's osteotomy. ©WM Strobl

assessment is crucial for optimal outcome. Advantages are achieving hip stability in severe cases and decreasing lumbar lordosis with pain relief. Disadvantages of this procedure are no anterior coverage of the femoral head and a high risk of persistent abductor weakness.

3.8.2 Salter's Innominate Osteotomy: A Simple Procedure for Anterior-Lateral Coverage

In 1966, Salter described a complete osteotomy of the iliac bone superior of the acetabulum followed by ventrolateral tilting of the acetabular bone to improve head coverage anteriorly and laterally [17]. Indications of this procedure are several dysplastic disorders with a congruous shape of the hip joint, if less than 10–15° correction of radiological acetabular index is required.

Prerequisites are free range of motion especially of hip abduction, internal rotation, and flexion; no contracture of hip adductors and hip flexor muscles; radiologically normal level of the femoral head positioned opposite of the acetabulum; and patient's age between 18 months and 7 years.

Surgical technique: Skin incision parallel and 1 cm inferior to the iliac crest and superior anterior spina, preservation of cutaneous femoral lateral nerve, subperiosteal preparation of iliac crest to incisura ischiadica, cutting the iliac bone 2 cm superior to inferior anterior spina in line to the incisura ischiadica using a flexible Gigli saw. Then Salter's maneuver means abduction and flexion of the hip joint and anterior and lateral shifting of the roof of the acetabulum, and also filling the gap of osteotomy with a wedged bone graft extracting from femoral osteotomy or iliac crest, fixing with 3–5 Kirschner wires (Fig. 3.6).

Postoperatively hip spica cast is done or—compliance permitting—similar removable soft orthosis for 6 weeks, limited passive exercises are done starting 2 weeks after surgery, and 6 weeks postoperatively X-ray checkup is performed followed by full or temporary partial weight bearing on crutches depending on bone healing and body weight. Outcome measurement should be assessed by AP-view X-ray evaluating acetabular angle and center-edge angle.

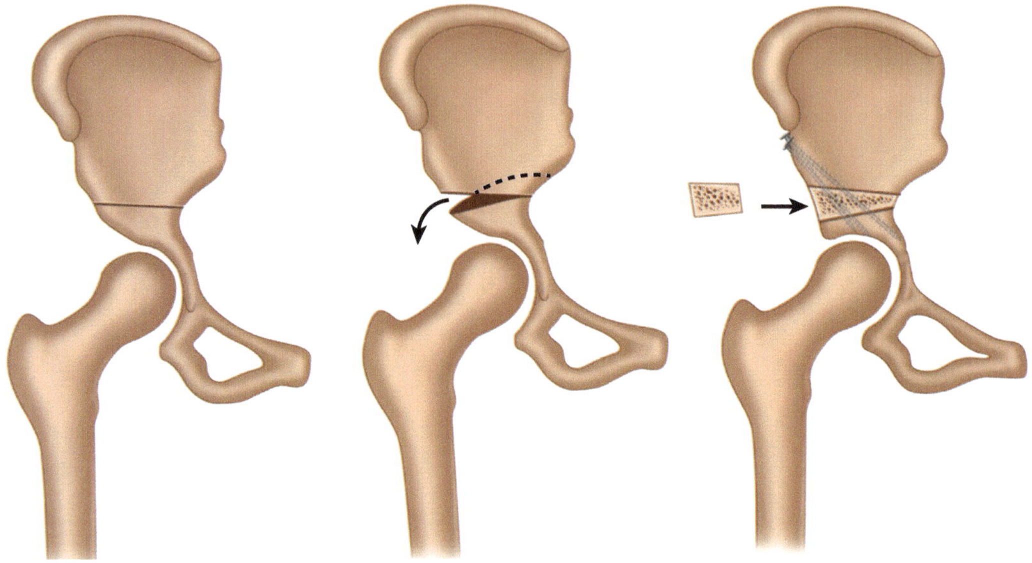

Fig. 3.6 Pre- and post-Salter's osteotomy. ©WM Strobl

3.8.3 Steel's and Others' Triple Osteotomy: A Simple and Efficient Covering Procedure

In 1965 LeCoeur was the first author publishing his experience with a triple-pelvic osteotomy to improve the coverage of the femoral head [18]. Eight years later, Steel described a pelvic triple osteotomy for older children with dislocation or subluxation of the hip in order to obtain a stable hip in anatomical position [19]. His procedure is indicated when other single-pelvic or femoral osteotomies are not able to achieve sufficient coverage. For the success of surgery, the articular surfaces of the joint must be congruous or become so when the acetabulum has been redirected, so that a functional, painless range of motion is achieved and a Trendelenburg gait is absent. In a significant enlarged acetabulum, Steel's osteotomy is not recommended, because the radius of the acetabulum will not be reduced by this procedure.

Surgical technique: Skin incisions at anterior, medial, and posterior aspects of the hip joint. It also includes subperiosteal preparation of the ischial bone, the superior pubic ramus, and the iliac bone superior to the acetabulum; cutting of three bones; and moving the free acetabular portion. The acetabulum is redirected, repositioned, and stabilized by bone graft and Kirschner wires or screws. In the bone graft, a wedge of bone will be extracted from most superior portion of iliac bone (Fig. 3.7).

Postoperatively hip spica cast is done for 6 weeks, or—compliance permitting—limited passive exercises starting 2 weeks after surgery. Six to eight weeks postoperatively, X-ray checkup is done followed by full or temporary partial weight bearing on crutches depending on bone healing and body weight. Outcome measurement should be assessed by AP-view X-ray evaluating acetabular angle and center-edge angle.

Steel's osteotomy is indicated in adolescents and skeletally mature adults with residual dysplasia and subluxation in whom remodeling of acetabulum is no longer anticipated. Advantages are an improved coverage of femoral head by articular cartilage and improved hip joint stability. Early mobilization without full immobilization is possible. Disadvantage of this procedure is the fact that it does not change the radial size of an enlarged acetabulum, and it may distort the pelvic

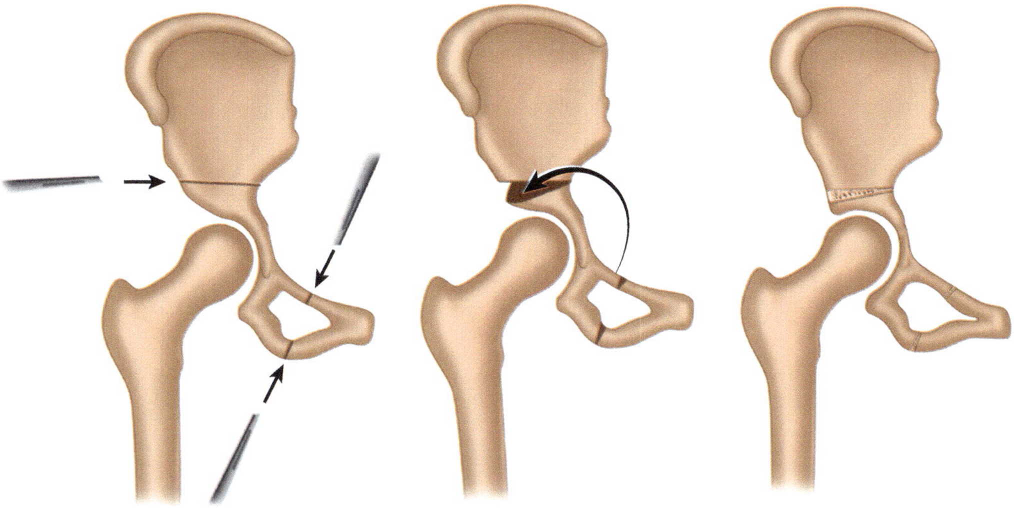

Fig. 3.7 Pre- and post-triple-pelvic osteotomy. ©WM Strobl

bone so that natural childbirth may be impossible in adulthood. The surgical technique is demanding and needs some learning curve.

Until now, several authors, for example Tönnis and Dungl, have described their modifications of triple-pelvic osteotomies. On the whole, principles of surgical anatomy did not change. Good long-term outcome studies have been published. In 2018, Farsetti et al. [20] concluded that Tönnis osteotomy represents a good treatment option: it is technically easy, enables direct visualization of the three osteotomies, and leads to few complications, and its learning curve is short. The absence of radiographic signs of osteoarthritis and hip congruency before surgery would be the basic requirements to achieve a successful result.

3.9 Shelf Procedures: Open or Endoscopic

3.9.1 Spitzy's Shelf Arthroplasty: A Simple and Effective Alternative over 8 Years

In 1924, Spitzy was the first author describing a shelf acetabuloplasty by inserting a tibial bone graft (Fig. 3.8). After introducing pelvic osteotomies and acetabuloplasties shelf procedures became to be used less commonly. However, Terjesen recently reported good short- and long-term effects of Spitzy's operation on hip pain and a 30-year survival (no THA) of 72% of the hips [21]. These results can be compared favorably with those of PAO and indicate that there is still a place for the shelf procedure in older children and young adults. Holm's study showed that Spitzy's shelf operation had satisfactory long-term outcome with hip survival in almost 90% at patient age of 40 years [22]. The results would indicate that Spitzy's shelf operation postpones total hip replacement. They considered Spitzy's shelf operation a good alternative in patients above 8 years. In younger children, the procedure would not be recommended due to increased frequency of graft resorption.

3.9.2 Staheli's Shelf Arthroplasty

In 1992, Staheli described a procedure to create a shelf increasing the volume of the acetabulum and the amount of coverage measured by CE angle [23]. It is indicated in cases of acetabular dysplasia when redirection is not sufficient. It is contraindicated in cases of dysplastic hips with spherical congruity that may be corrected by

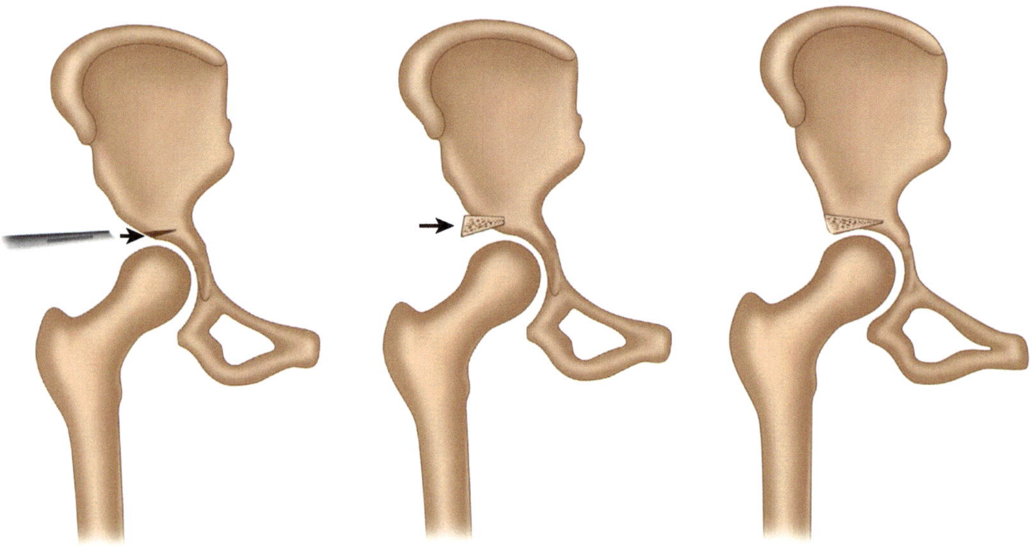

Fig. 3.8 Pre- and post-Spitzy's shelf procedure. ©WM Strobl

redirectional osteotomies. Patients should be 5 years or older.

Surgical technique: Skin incision 1 cm below the iliac crest and iliofemoral approach. The most critical part of the procedure is the exact placement of the acetabular slot right at the acetabular margin. There the shelf is fixed with layers of cancellous grafts bringing the reflected head of rectus femoris forward over the graft and suturing it in its original position.

Today, shelf arthroplasties are performed by arthroscopic approach in some centers. Uchida [24] reports promising clinical outcomes and return to sports-related activity for active patients with DDH following endoscopic shelf acetabuloplasty.

3.10 Acetabuloplasties and Periacetabular Osteotomies

Acetabuloplasties and periacetabular osteotomies may be defined as procedures that are **only partially cutting the pelvic bone by a single approach.** Cuts are performed periacetabularly in order to alter the shape of the incongruent acetabulum and/or redirect the plane of the acetabulum. These interventions improve the coverage of clearly defined parts of the acetabulum. They reduce pelvic stability less than complete osteotomies because the medial corticalis of the iliac bone is not affected. The pelvis remains more stable postoperatively, early mobilization is possible, rehabilitation process is shorter, and complication rate is lower, for example as stated by Karlen et al. [25]. Acetabuloplasties and periacetabular osteotomies may be performed bilaterally. Recently authors reported evidence that the shapes of the femoral head and the acetabulum are adjusted by remodeling and joint function improved following reconstructions including periacetabular acetabuloplasties. Braatz et al. [26] reported that high plasticity of the hip joint suggests that even if the femoral head is deformed and a persistent incongruency is expected after surgery, hip reconstruction can be recommended.

In the first years of life, good results could be observed after an incomplete acetabuloplasty in combination with open reduction. Carsi described it as a reliable adjunct to open reductions, and it would be followed by a rapid acetabular growth response that avoids secondary pelvic procedures. It would be a one-stop surgery with predictable outcome that can be performed in 0.5- to 2.5-year-old children [27]. Commonly, acetabuloplasties are performed in combination with proximal femoral varus osteotomies in children with severe hip dysplasia as well as all stages of hip dislocation (see hip reconstruction below).

3.10.1 Dega's Acetabuloplasty: For Effectively Diminishing Enlarged Acetabulums

In 1964, Dega described a procedure to reduce the radial shape of an enlarged acetabulum by improving the amount of coverage of the femoral head measured by CE angle. It is indicated in cases of acetabular dysplasia when redirection is not sufficient. It is contraindicated in cases of dysplastic hips with spherical congruity that may be corrected by redirectional osteotomies. Patients should be 5 years or older.

Surgical technique: Skin incision 1 cm below the iliac crest and iliofemoral approach. The most critical part of the procedure is the exact placement of the acetabular osteotomy above the acetabular margin. The roof of the acetabulum is distalized by the chisel, achieving a congruent shape of the joint. Then the gap is filled with one wedge-shaped bone graft or some layers of cancellous grafts. Intraoperatively passive range of movement of the hip joint is evaluated to secure dosed coverage of the head. The posterior column of the hemipelvis remains mechanically intact, allowing early mobilization. The shape of the pelvis stays unaltered, permitting a normal childbirth. Further advantages are the facts that correction can be obtained in all directions, including the medial and lateral planes, and blood supply to the acetabulum is preserved. Disadvantage is the demanding surgical technique with learning curve (Fig. 3.9).

In a recent study, Issin reports open reduction plus Dega's osteotomy to be a good option to regain acetabular coverage over the femoral head. It provides better radiographic results after a 5-year follow-up period in patients with a mean age of 25 months. Open reduction alone should not be performed unless the child had mildly dysplastic acetabulum according to Tönnis' definition [28].

In their 13–25-year long-term study El-Sayed et al. report favorable outcome in 76% of all patients treated with Dega's osteotomy [29].

Rampal reported a modified Dega's acetabuloplasty to be effective in correcting acetabular dysplasia in DDH. Functional and radiological results were good, with a low rate of acetabular retroversion (2/10), unlike with other techniques

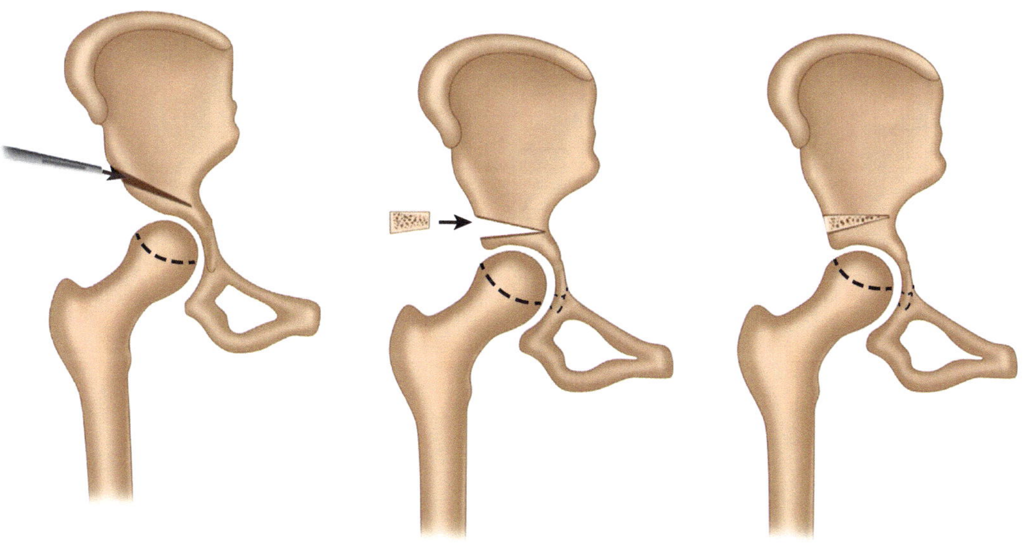

Fig. 3.9 Pre- and post-Dega's osteotomy. ©WM Strobl

[30]. In addition, Akgül found the Dega's osteotomy combined with anterior open reduction and femoral osteotomies to be a safe and effective acetabular osteotomy for surgical treatment of severe DDH such as Tönnis grade 3 and 4 dislocations [31]. Czubak reported Dega's osteotomy to be a safe and adequate procedure for the management of developmental dysplasia of the hip in walking patients with low complication rates. Restoring the acetabulum to normal or nearly normal would result in good medium-term results [32].

3.10.2 Pemberton's Pericapsular Osteotomy: For Better Congruity in Enlarged Acetabulums

Wiberg published a long osteotomy to the triradiate cartilage for the first time in 1944. In 1965, Pemberton described a pericapsular osteotomy of the iliac bone with significant reducing of the enlarged radial shape of the acetabulum. It is indicated in children with hip dislocation or dysplasia with enlarged acetabulum and small femoral head when more than 10–15° correction of acetabular index is required. Patient's age should be between 18 months and 10 years.

Surgical technique: Skin incision 1 cm below the iliac crest and iliofemoral approach. Important is the exact placement of the pericapsular osteotomy 1.5 cm cranial of the acetabulum. The osteotomy follows a curved line from slightly superior to the anteroinferior iliac spine anteriorly to the triradiate cartilage posteriorly. A curved chisel may be used. Radiological control is crucial, as the medial column of the iliac bone must not be cut. The triradiate cartilage is used as a hinge on which the acetabular roof is rotated anteriorly and laterally. Then a 1–2 cm-based bone wedge is placed and impacted in the bone gap; pin fixation is usually not required (Fig. 3.10).

Postoperatively hip spica cast is done or—compliance permitting—similar removable soft orthosis for 6 weeks, limited passive exercises are done starting 5–10 days after surgery, and 6 weeks postoperative X-ray checkup is performed followed by full or temporary partial weight bearing on crutches depending on bone healing and body weight. Outcome measurement should be assessed by AP-view X-ray evaluating acetabular angle and center-edge angle.

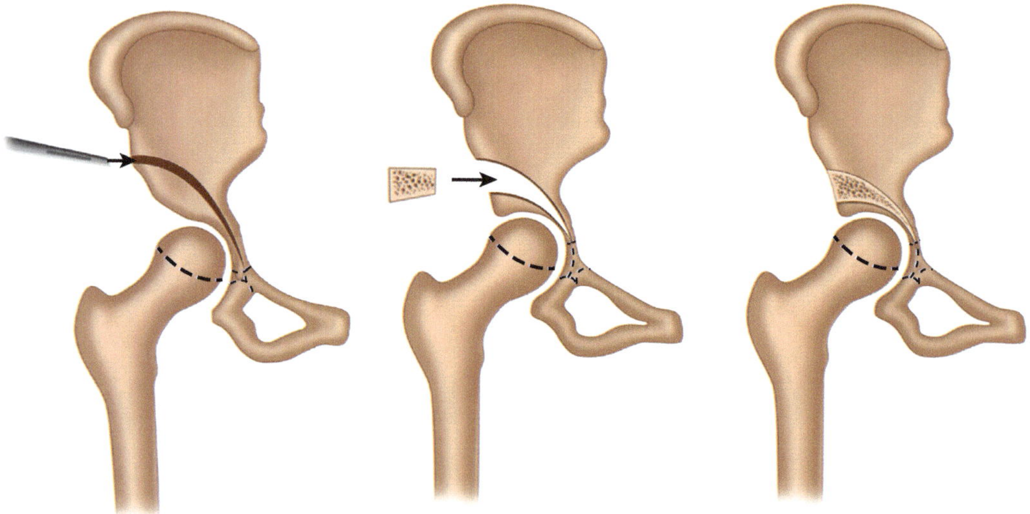

Fig. 3.10 Pre- and post-Pemberton's osteotomy. ©WM Strobl

Krieg and Hefti found good long-term results after Dega's and Pemberton's acetabuloplasty regarding prevention of a secondary coxarthrosis. They stated that correct indication is crucial since this surgical technique is more difficult compared to Salter's osteotomy but is also associated with a higher correction potential and a lower complication rate [33]. Baki concluded that the combination of single-stage medial open reduction and Pemberton's acetabuloplasty represents an effective method for developmental dysplasia of the hip in children older than 15 months of age [34]. Ertürk reported that children who underwent Pemberton's osteotomy achieved an improved radiological ADR compared with those who underwent Salter's osteotomy on an average follow-up of 5 years after innominate osteotomy [35].

3.10.3 Wagner's Spherical Pelvic Periacetabular Osteotomy

A modified technique of Blavier, who was the first author reporting a periacetabular osteotomy in 1962 [36], was described by Wagner in 1978 [37]. He differentiated three types of periacetabular pelvic osteotomies to improve the coverage of the femoral head in young adults. In spite of the assumed increased risk for osteonecrosis, Schramm found good long-term results following Wagner's spherical pelvic osteotomies [38].

3.10.4 Ganz Bernese Periacetabular Osteotomy PAO: For Effective Covering of the Spherical Hip

In 1988, Ganz described a periacetabular triple osteotomy performed by a single approach [39] (Fig. 3.11). This procedure is indicated in adolescents and adults with severe hip dysplasia that requires correction of congruency and containment of the femoral head with only incipient osteoarthritis. Its indication in cases of incongruent dysplastic hips is discussed controversially while it is contraindicated in cases with severely enlarged acetabulum when redirection is not sufficient to obtain stability of the joint. An advantage is the use of a single approach; only Smith Peterson approach is needed. The posterior column of the hemipelvis remains mechanically intact, allowing early mobilization. The shape of the pelvis stays unaltered, permitting a normal childbirth. Further advantages are the facts that correction can be obtained in all directions,

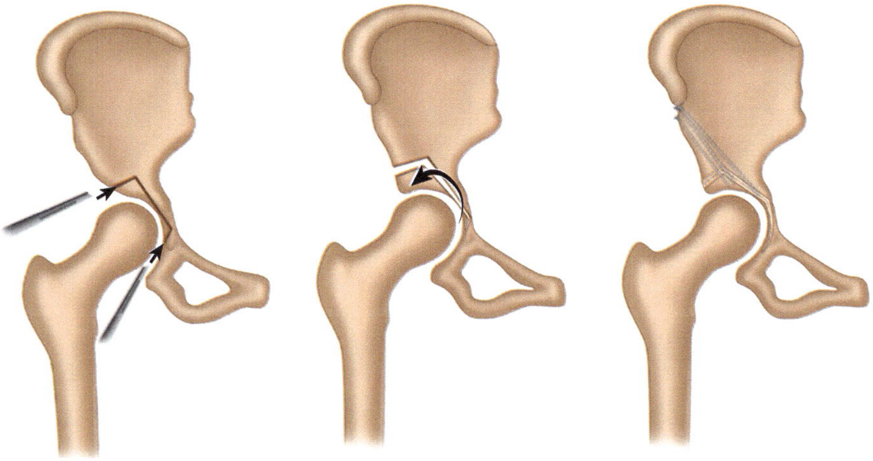

Fig. 3.11 Pre- and post-Ganz periacetabular osteotomy. ©WM Strobl

including the medial and lateral planes, and blood supply to the acetabulum is preserved. Lerch reports good long-term outcome and states the PAO to be the standard procedure for the surgical therapy of hip dysplasia in adolescents and adults with spherical acetabulum [40].

3.10.5 Modified Dega-Pemberton-Like Periacetabular Osteotomy: For More Congruity in Any Age

Over the last decades modified Dega's and Pemberton's techniques have also been used in patients with already closed triradiate cartilage. In 1994, Brunner and Baumann reported benefits of hip reconstruction including a Dega-like periacetabular osteotomy in patients with cerebral palsy [41]. In 2015, Rutz presented data on 168 hip reconstructions at a mean follow-up of 7 years that showed significant and clinically meaningful improvements in pain intensity and frequency as well as in clinical scores and hip coverage [42].

In 2006, Robb and Brunner were the first to describe a Dega-type osteotomy used in older children and adolescents where the triradiate cartilage is already closed (Fig. 3.12). They concluded that it is possible to perform a satisfactory pelvic osteotomy of this type in these patients after the triradiate cartilage has been closed [43]. There is evidence that the procedure improves the shape of an enlarged acetabulum and secures hip stability as part of a hip reconstruction surgery in adolescents and young adults with neuromuscular and other secondary hip dislocation. Long-term studies describe improvement of quality of life by pain relief and improved mobility following remodeling of cartilage of the femoral head and acetabulum [4, 26, 44].

Advantages are the three-dimensional reduction of an enlarged acetabulum and correction of its shape in order to achieve a stable congruent hip joint. Severe joint incongruity however requires some time for remodeling. The posterior column of the hemipelvis remains mechanically intact, allowing early mobilization. The shape of the pelvis stays unaltered, permitting a normal childbirth. Further advantages are the facts that correction can be obtained in all directions, including the medial and lateral planes, and blood supply to the acetabulum is preserved. Disadvantage is the demanding surgical technique with learning curve. Today this technique has become the golden standard for hip dysplasia and disloca-

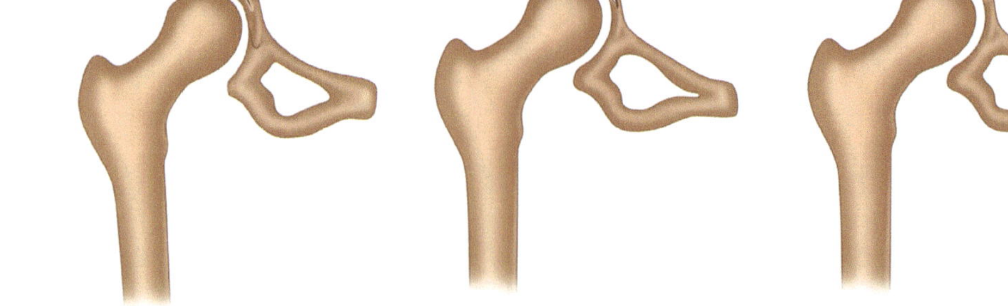

Fig. 3.12 Pre- and post-modified Dega-Pemberton-like periacetabular osteotomy. ©WM Strobl

tions in neuromuscular and systemic disorders with enlarged and aspherical acetabulum.

The similarly performed San Diego acetabuloplasty has the same results in patients with open and closed triradiate cartilage. Recently Murar reported that the San Diego pelvic osteotomy is equally effective in improving radiographic parameters in neuromuscular patients with both open and closed triradiate cartilage. Their study challenges the notion that closed triradiate cartilage is a contraindication to a San Diego pelvic osteotomy [45].

3.11 Proximal Femoral Osteotomies

Osteotomies of the proximal femur may be defined as surgical procedures aiming to improve biomechanical forces and weight transmission over the hip joint by angulation of the proximal femur related to the axis of the femoral shaft. The axis of the femoral shaft is shifted more in line with the direction of weight transmission.

Proximal femoral osteotomies are usually performed as combined three-dimensional effective procedures. However, they can be classified according to the major direction of their correction:

1. Varus osteotomy
2. Valgus osteotomy
3. Rotation osteotomy to achieve less or more femoral anteversion
4. Shortening or lengthening osteotomy

3.11.1 Varus Osteotomies of the Proximal Femur

Varus osteotomies achieve to restore joint congruity and decrease muscle forces around the hip by elevation and lateral movement of the greater trochanter while moving the abductor and psoas muscles medially. Varus osteotomy increases the weight-bearing area of femoral head while relaxing all three important muscle groups around the hip joint.

Indications for a single varus osteotomy are slightly or non-dysplastic hips with a spherical femoral head, valgus neck-shaft angle of more than 140°, center-edge angle of more than 15°, and fixed abduction deformity. Varus osteotomy with medial displacement of the femoral shaft relaxes the abductor, psoas, and adductor muscles; unloads the hip joint; and increases the weight-bearing surface.

Commonly varus osteotomies are performed in combination with acetabuloplasties or pelvic osteotomies in children with severe hip dysplasia as well as all stages of hip dislocation (see hip reconstruction below).

Proximal femoral varus osteotomies can be performed by four types of surgical techniques:

1. Close-wedge-type osteotomy provides excellent stable osseous apposition by transverse closing wedge. Its major disadvantage is shortening of the extremity.
2. Open-wedge-type osteotomy lengthens the extremity, but it is initially unstable. Bony apposition is limited and union may be delayed in adolescents and adults.
3. Half-wedge cut medially and transposed laterally obtains better stability and less shortening.
4. Ball-and-socket-type osteotomy achieves stability without leg length discrepancy, but extensive dissection is required and correction of complex deformities is technically demanding.

Surgical technique: Skin incision distal to greater trochanter parallel to the femur, preparation dorsal to lateral vastus of quadriceps muscle, subperiosteal preparation of proximal femur on intertrochanteric level of osteotomy. It also includes marking central femoral neck by Kirschner wire, placement of chisel or proximal screw for internal fixation plate, and cutting the femur by removing a medially based bone wedge according to the degree of varization. Alternatively, an open-wedge, half-wedge, or ball-and-socket type of osteotomy may be used. Apply the plate-and-screw fixation after three-dimensional correction. Medial displacement of 1 cm is recommended to keep the ipsilateral knee centered under the center of the femoral head and to maintain the mechanical axis of the leg. Shortening of abductor muscles may be indicated to avoid weakness during early postoperative rehabilitation.

The aim of the subtrochanteric derotation and varus osteotomy is to center the femoral head inside the joint cavity to form the normal shape of head and acetabulum by normal function. In patients with LCP the same principles are regarded to form the altered shape of the plastic epiphysis, keeping it well covered by the roof of the acetabulum and allowing the child to walk so that the redistributed intra-articular pressures will contribute to the molding of a more normal joint. Internal fixation allows early mobilization with crutches—compliance permitting—from 5 to 10 days after surgery. In toddlers, a spica cast is applied for 4–6 weeks followed by X-ray checking of bony union and by full weight-bearing exercise program.

Clinical outcome: Buxbom reports that hip migration stagnates within the first 5 weeks, indicating stability across the VDRO in most patients following varus derotation osteotomy combined with muscle-lengthening procedures [46].

Pauwels Y-shaped osteotomy is an osteotomy of the proximal femur to prevent painful osteoarthritis in adolescents and younger adults by converting static forces from shearing to impacting forces. In mild or moderate osteoarthritis, this salvage osteotomy can improve function and delay the need for total hip arthroplasty.

3.11.2 Valgus Osteotomies of the Proximal Femur

The normal femoral neck-shaft angle in infant is 120°–140°. In severe coxa vara deformity of the proximal femur (110° or less), reduction to a more physiologic angle is provided by a valgus osteotomy. A transverse osteotomy is done at the level of lesser trochanter with removing of a lateral wedge to correct neck-shaft angle to 135°–145°. Surgery is indicated in children older than 3 years of age to ease internal fixation technique.

Valgus subtrochanteric osteotomies are indicated in overcorrected coxa vara as well as in hip joint disorders like hinged abduction and coxa magna or combined with shelf augmentation and Chiari's pelvic osteotomy. They improve biomechanics of the hip joint by transferring the center of hip rotation medially from the superior aspect of the acetabulum to increase joint congruity and the weight-bearing area of the femoral head. Muscle relaxation is provided by release of psoas tendon and adductor muscles.

Prerequisites for excellent outcomes are knowledge of biomechanical cause, young age, good preoperative range of motion, and rigid internal fixation allowing early mobilization. There is still an increased risk for malunion and pseudarthrosis, depending on the age and systemic disease.

A special type of valgus osteotomy of the proximal femur is Dunn's femoral neck osteotomy in slipped capital femoral epiphysis.

Sugioka's transtrochanteric anterior rotational osteotomy is a special type of rotation osteotomy to improve weight bearing in non-deficient zones of cartilage in LCP disease and avascular necrosis.

Schanz and Lorenz osteotomies are subtrochanteric femoral osteotomies at the level of ischial tuber that achieve pelvic support by correcting flexion, adduction, and external rotation deformities. In these special valgization osteotomies, the proximal part of the femur is angled inward until it rests against the side wall of pelvis. Lurching of gait may be reduced, and the depression of the greater trochanter may improve the lever arm of the glutei. Disadvantages are no normal functional anatomy, shortening, and still an increased risk of osteoarthritic pain. Indications are rare cases of irreducible hip dislocations and severe deformities of the hip joint in adolescents and adults when hip reconstruction surgery is not indicated.

3.12 Combined Procedure: Surgical Hip Reconstruction

Hip reconstruction surgery may be defined as a bony procedure to reduce a subluxated or dislocated hip and help to permanently secure stability and function with free movement of the hip joint. It includes a femoral derotation-varization-shortening osteotomy, open or closed reduction of the femoral head, tense suture of the joint capsule, and improving of the bony coverage of the head by reconstruction of the acetabulum. For this step of acetabular improvement over the last decades, several procedures have been described.

Indications for hip reconstruction are hip instability and dislocation in DDH, late-onset DDH, ligament laxity, different neuromuscular movement disorders, and other systemic diseases.

Surgical technique (Fig. 3.13):

1. Clinical and radiological examination under anesthesia. Testing stability and dislocation mechanism of hip joint according to 3D MRI results. Evaluation of muscle lengths, contractures, and fixed deformities that may impede successful reconstruction of the hip.
2. Balancing of muscular forces over the hip joint by release of fixed contractures (for example adductor contracture or rectus femoris shortening) and preparation of muscle-shortening procedures (for example abductors, tensor fasciae latae, quadriceps) performed at the end of surgery.
3. Clinical and radiologic testing if closed reduction is now possible or open reduction will be necessary.
4. Open reduction of the hip dislocation and preparation of the (modified) Pemberton's osteotomy: Skin incision 1 cm below the iliac crest and iliofemoral approach. Subperiosteal preparation of the iliac crest to the ischial incisura. Preparation of the inferior anterior spina

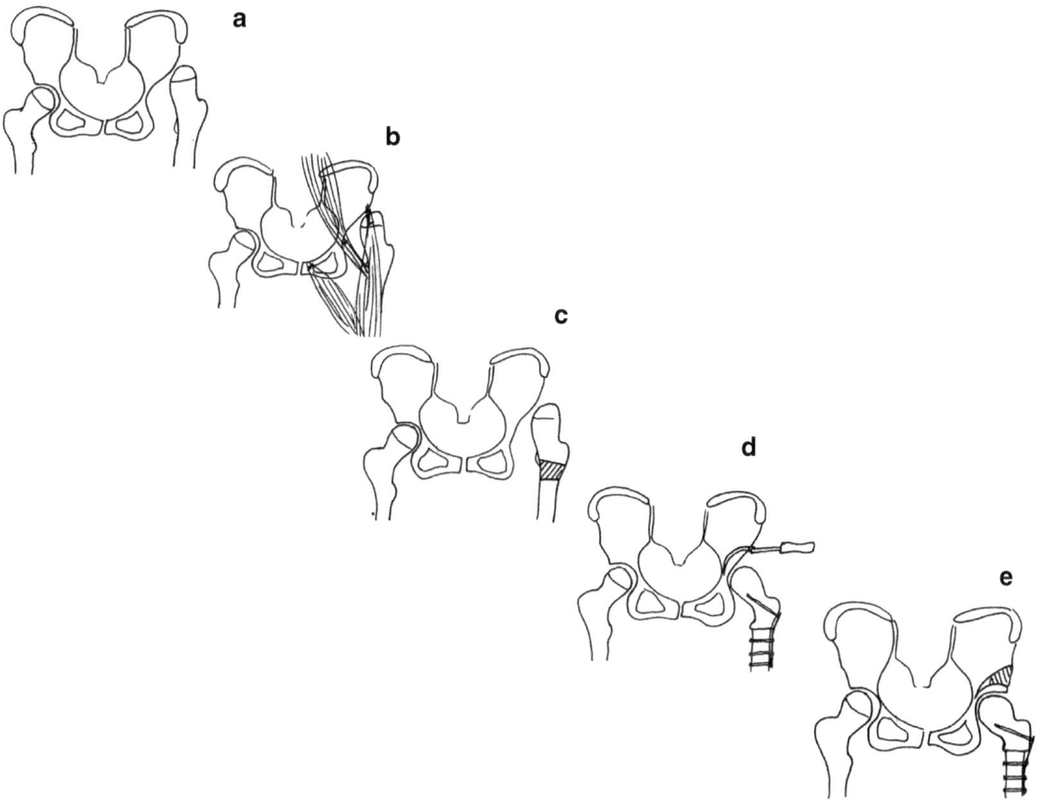

Fig. 3.13 Steps of hip reconstruction: (**a**) dislocated left hip, (**b**) muscle force-balancing surgery, (**c**) proximal varus derotation-shortening osteotomy, (**d**) open reduction and modified Dega-Pemberton-like periacetabular osteotomy, (**e**) impacting of bone graft and suture of capsule. ©WM Strobl

and release of the rectus tendon, securing it with a suture. Preparation and T-shaped opening of the joint capsule, dislocation of the head, removing of the capital femoral ligament, cleaning of the acetabulum, cutting of the transverse ligament, and testing of reduction of the femoral head. If open reduction is not possible at this point, it has to be observed during the following performance of proximal femoral correction osteotomy.

5. Skin incision distal to greater trochanter parallel to the femur, preparation dorsal to lateral vastus of quadriceps muscle, subperiosteal preparation of proximal femur on intertrochanteric level of osteotomy. Marking central femoral neck by Kirschner wire, and placement of chisel or proximal screw for internal fixation plate. Cutting the femur by removing a medially based bone wedge according to the degree of varization. Alternatively, an open-wedge, half-wedge, or ball-and-socket type of osteotomy may be used. Shortening of the femur is crucial—the higher the dislocation, the more the shortening is demanded. Apply the plate-and-screw fixation after three-dimensional correction. Medial displacement of 1 cm is recommended to keep the ipsilateral knee centered under the center of the femoral head and to maintain the mechanical axis of the leg. Shortening of abductor muscles may be indicated to avoid weakness during early postoperative rehabilitation.
6. Preparation of the sutures of the hip joint capsule as long as there is enough space before performing distalization of the acetabular roof.
7. (Modified) Dega-Pemberton's osteotomy: Important is the right placement of the pericapsular osteotomy 1.5 cm cranial of the acetabulum. The osteotomy follows a curved line from slightly superior to the anteroinferior iliac spine anteriorly to the triradiate cartilage posteriorly. A curved chisel may be used. Radiological control is crucial, as the medial column of the iliac bone must not be cut. The triradiate cartilage is used as a hinge on which the acetabular roof is rotated anteriorly and laterally. Then a 1–2 cm-based bone wedge is placed and impacted in the bone gap; pin fixation is usually not required.
8. Tense suture of the hip joint capsule, clinical and radiological evaluation of hip joint function and stability. In the case of free movement and lack of instability, shortening of overstretched and weak muscles and wound closure step by step.

Postoperatively: positioning in bilateral 20° hip abduction, hip extension, and secured neutral rotation by spica cast or—compliance permitting—similar removable soft orthosis (like an individual foam shell) for 6 weeks, limited passive exercises starting 2 days after surgery under epidural anesthesia, max. 60° hip flexion, free extension free abduction, no adduction, and only neutral rotation, first active exercises and sitting 2 weeks after surgery, 4–6 weeks postoperatively X-ray checkup followed by full or temporary partial weight bearing on crutches depending on bone healing and body weight. Outcome measurement should be assessed by AP-view X-ray evaluating acetabular angle and center-edge angle (Fig. 3.14).

Patient care and exercise programs need particular education (Fig. 3.15). Over the past decade, educational programs for patients and parents as well as for medical, therapeutic, and orthopedic-technical professions have been designed. Scripts about hip reconstruction explaining surgery and postoperative treatment step by step in easy language and including cartoons are recommended. Additionally, members of the therapeutic team should have the possibility to attend a multi-professional postgraduate program on neuro-orthopedics and disability management.

Recently, first outcome studies on early mobilization have been published. Gather et al. (2018) [47] reported successful hip reconstruction according to clinical and radiographic outcome parameters after early mobilization without cast therapy. Retrospectively, they evaluated 33 children with developmental hip dysplasia (DDH) and dislocation of the hip (Tönnis grades 1 to 4), who underwent hip reconstruction (Dega's acetabuloplasty, varization-derotation osteotomy,

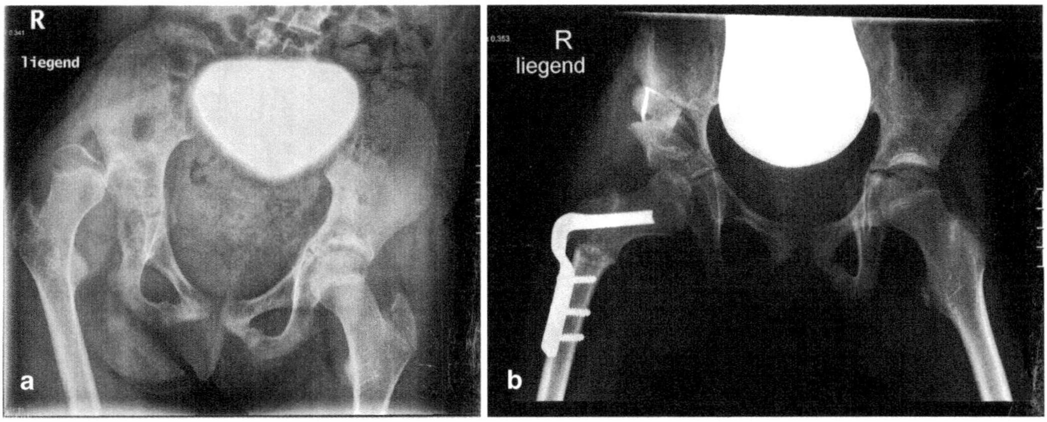

Fig. 3.14 Pre- (**a**) and post-hip reconstruction (**b**) in a girl, 13 years, with secondary hip dislocation. ©WM Strobl

and facultative open reduction), and summarized early mobilization to be recommended as an alternative treatment option after hip reconstruction in DDH. This strongly supports observations of the author who uses early mobilization following hip reconstruction in children with DDH and cerebral palsy older than 3 years of age.

For DDH, this procedure containing open reduction combined with femoral varus-derotation osteotomy and improvement of acetabular roof has become a golden standard of surgical treatment for children older than 18 months [13]. Carsi and Clarke reported that the addition of an incomplete periacetabular acetabuloplasty to all hips undergoing open reduction eliminated residual acetabular dysplasia, whereas it did not appear to have deleterious effects as evidenced by the similar AVN proportion [48]. Recently Cicekli and Dogan recommended this one-staged operative procedure for the treatment of patients with DDH of late onset [49].

Over the past three decades, this procedure has also become the treatment of choice for all stages of hip dislocations in neuromuscular and systemic diseases. In 1994, Brunner and Baumann reported benefits of hip reconstruction including a Dega-like periacetabular osteotomy in patients with cerebral palsy [41]. Rutz presented data on 168 hip reconstructions at a mean follow-up of 7 years that showed significant and clinically meaningful improvements in pain intensity and frequency as well as in clinical scores and hip coverage. Analysis of potential risk factors showed only the preoperative migration percentage to have a relevant influence on outcomes [42]. Mallet reported the one-stage hip reconstruction procedure including acetabuloplasty and femoral osteotomy without hip dislocation efficaciously corrected acetabulum dysplasia and successfully treated neurological hips in CP patients. Progressive recurrence of the valgus deformity of the proximal femur, attributable to adductor spasticity and gluteus medius weakness, would lead to a significant increase in the Reimers index. However, hip coverage remained >70% at maturity in 90% of the hips [50]. McNerney reported stable hips with good coverage in 95% of 104 hips 7 years after surgical treatment by hip reconstruction including open reduction, femoral osteotomy, and their San Diego acetabuloplasty [51]. In case of hip pain and femoral head deformity, Braatz's long-term study indicates that hip reconstruction surgery as a part of multilevel surgery improves pain and function in patients with CP and Tönnis IV hip dislocation, even if the hip joint is incongruent after operation. This incongruity improves over the long term [4]. If possible, a reconstruction procedure should be performed before the femoral head becomes deformed. High plasticity of the hip joint would suggest that even if the femoral head is deformed, hip reconstruction could be recommended.

Unstable hips in children with Down syndrome are also successfully treated by hip reconstruc-

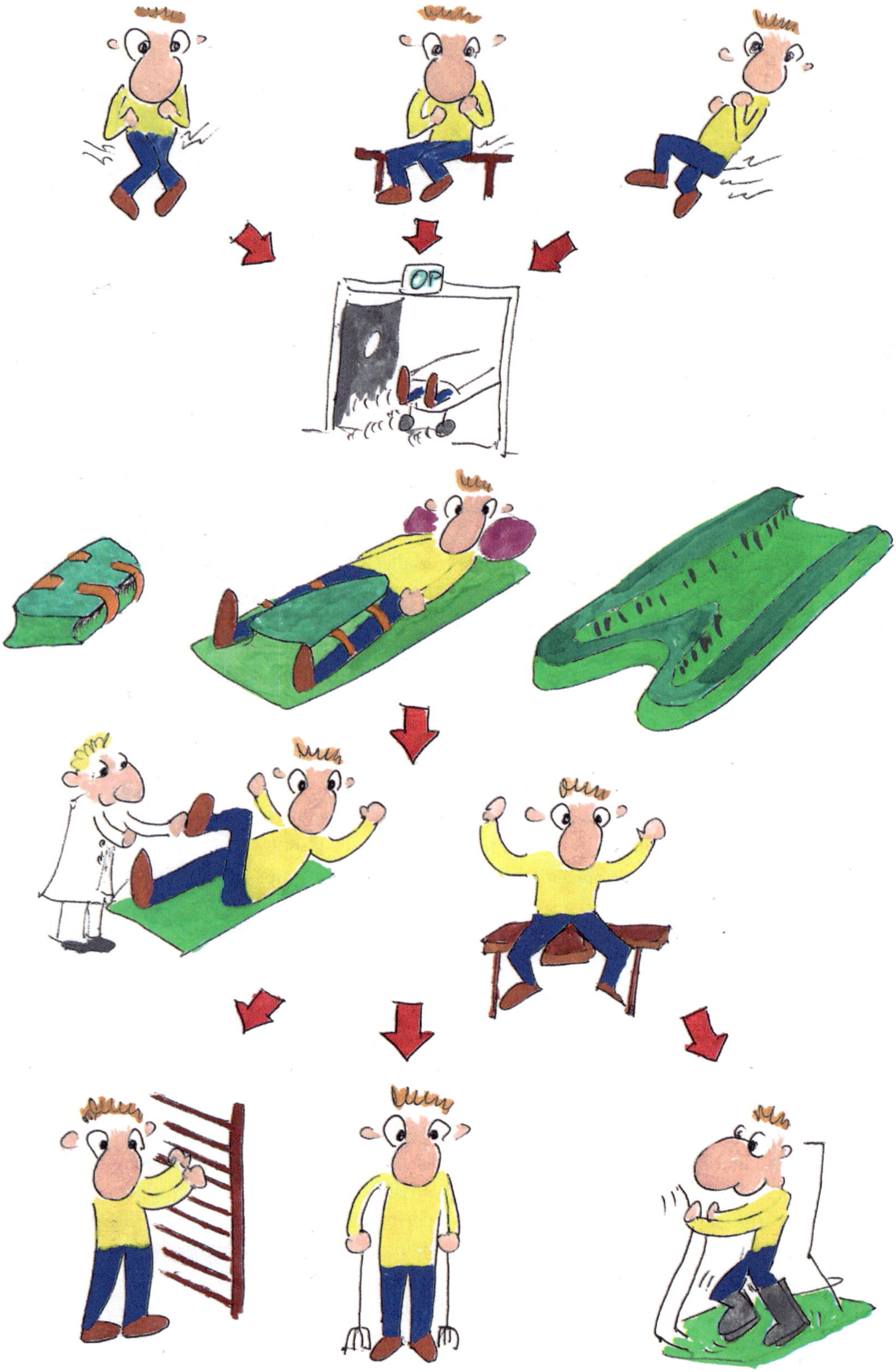

Fig. 3.15 Cartoons for instructing children and parents about surgery and postoperative early mobilization. ©WM Strobl

tion. Aly reported femoral varus derotation osteotomy combined with Dega's osteotomy to be efficient in the management of hip instability in Down syndrome, as it corrects hip biomechanics and increases posterior acetabular coverage [52].

Nevertheless, recent studies are discussing endoscopic assisted surgery in the treatment of irreducible hip dislocations. Eberhardt [53] and Xu [54] report arthroscopic treatment combined with acetabuloplasty and/or femoral osteotomy to have advantages of less trauma and better function preservation compared with the open reduction.

References

1. Graham HK. Classifying cerebral palsy. J Pediatr Orthop. 2005;25(1):127–8.
2. Palisano RJ, Hanna SE, Rosenbaum PL, et al. Validation of a model of gross motor function for children with cerebral palsy. Phys Ther. 2000;80:974–85.
3. Terjesen T. The natural history of hip development in cerebral palsy. Dev Med Child Neurol. 2012;54:951–7.
4. Braatz F, Eidemüller A, Klotz MC, Beckmann NA, Wolf SI, Dreher T. Hip reconstruction surgery is successful in restoring joint congruity in patients with cerebral palsy: long-term outcome. Int Orthop. 2014;38(11):2237–43. https://doi.org/10.1007/s00264-014-2379-x.
5. Moreau M, Drummond DS, Rogala E, Ashworth A, Porter T. Natural history of the dislocated hip in spastic cerebral palsy. Dev Med Child Neurol. 1979;21(6):749–53.
6. Soo B, Howard JJ, Boyd RN, Reid SM, Lanigan A, Wolfe R, Reddihough D, Graham KH. Hip displacement in cerebral palsy. J Bone Joint Surg Br. 2006;88-A:121–9.
7. Jung NH, Heinen F, Westhoff B, Doederlein L, Reissig A, Berweck S, Linder-Lucht M, Schandelmaier S, Mall V. German Abo study group. Hip lateralisation in children with bilateral spastic cerebral palsy treated with botulinum toxin type A: a 2-year follow-up. Neuropediatrics. 2011;42(1):18–23.
8. Graham HK, Boyd R, Carlin JB, Dobson F, Lowe K, Nattrass G, Thomason P, Wolfe R, Reddihough D. Does botulinum toxin a combined with bracing prevent hip displacement in children with cerebral palsy and "hips at risk"? A randomized, controlled trial. J Bone Joint Surg Am. 2008;90(1):23–33.
9. Boldingh EJ, Jacobs-van der Bruggen MA, Bos CF, Lankhorst GJ, Bouter LM. Determinants of hip pain in adult patients with severe cerebral palsy. J Pediatr Orthop B. 2005;14(2):120–5.
10. Hägglund G, Andersson S, Duppe H, Lauge-Pedersen H, Nordmark E, Westbom L. Prevention of dislocation of the hip in children with cerebral palsy. The first ten years of a population-based prevention programme. J Bone Joint Surg Br. 2005;87:95–101.
11. Miller F, Cardoso Dias R, Dabney KW, Lipton GE, Triana M. Soft-tissue release for spastic hip subluxation in cerebral palsy. J Pediatr Orthop. 1997;17(5):571–84.
12. Karol LA. Surgical management of the lower extremity in ambulatory children with cerebral palsy. J Am Acad Orthop Surg. 2004;12(3):196–203.
13. Sankar WN, et al. Long-term follow-up after one-stage reconstruction of dislocated hips in patients with cerebral palsy. J Pediatr Orthop. 2006;26(1):1–7.
14. Valencia FG. Management of hip deformities in cerebral palsy. Orthop Clin North Am. 2010;41(4):549–59.
15. Castañeda P, Vidal-Ruiz C, Méndez A, Salazar DP, Torres A. How often does femoroacetabular impingement occur after an innominate osteotomy for acetabular dysplasia? Clin Orthop Relat Res. 2016;474(5):1209–15. https://doi.org/10.1007/s11999-016-4721-7.
16. Chiari K. Pelvic osteotomy in hip arthroplasty. Wien Med Wochenschr. 1953;103(38):707–9.
17. Salter RB. Role of innominate osteotomy in the treatment of congenital dislocation and subluxation of the hip in the older child. J Bone Joint Surg Am. 1966;48(7):1413–39.
18. LeCoeur P. Ostéotomie isthmique de bascule. In: Chapchal G, editor. Internationale Symposium über Beckenosteotomie/Pfannendachplastik. Stuttgart: Thieme; 1965.
19. Steel HH. Triple osteotomy of the innominate bone. J Bone Joint Surg Am. 1973;55(2):343–50.
20. Farsetti P, Caterini R, De Maio F, Potenza V, Efremov K, Ippolito E. Tönnis triple pelvic osteotomy for the management of late residual acetabular dysplasia: mid-term to long-term follow-up study of 54 patients. J Pediatr Orthop B. 2018;28:202. https://doi.org/10.1097/BPB.0000000000000575.
21. Terjesen T. Residual hip dysplasia: is there a place for hip shelf operation? J Child Orthop. 2018;12(4):358–63. https://doi.org/10.1302/1863-2548.12.180042.
22. Holm AG, Reikerås O, Terjesen T. Long-term results of a modified Spitzy shelf operation for residual hip dysplasia and subluxation. A fifty-year follow-up study of fifty six children and young adults. Int Orthop. 2017;41(2):415–21. https://doi.org/10.1007/s00264-016-3286-0.
23. Staheli LT, Chew DE. Slotted augmentation in childhood and adolescence. J Pediatr Orthop. 1992;12:569–80.
24. Uchida S, Hatakeyama A, Kanezaki S, Utsunomiya H, Suzuki H, Mori T, Chang A, Matsuda DK, Sakai A. Endoscopic shelf acetabuloplasty can improve clinical outcomes and achieve return to sports-related activity in active patients with hip dysplasia. Knee Surg Sports Traumatol Arthrosc. 2018;26(10):3165–77. https://doi.org/10.1007/s00167-017-4787-0.

25. Karlen JW, et al. The Dega osteotomy: a versatile osteotomy in the treatment of developmental and neuromuscular hip pathology. J Pediatr Orthop. 2009;29(7):676–82.
26. Braatz F, Staude D, Klotz MC, Wolf SI, Dreher T, Lakemeier S. Hip-joint congruity after Dega osteotomy in patients with cerebral palsy: long-term results. Int Orthop. 2016;40(8):1663–8. https://doi.org/10.1007/s00264-015-3013-2.
27. Carsi B, Al-Hallao S, Wahed K, Page J, Clarke NM. Incomplete periacetabular acetabuloplasty. Acta Orthop. 2014;85(1):66–70. https://doi.org/10.3109/17453674.2014.886030.
28. Issin A, Öner A, Koçkara N, Çamurcu Y. Comparison of open reduction alone and open reduction plus Dega osteotomy in developmental dysplasia of the hip. J Pediatr Orthop B. 2016;25(1):1–6. https://doi.org/10.1097/BPB.0000000000000227.
29. El-Sayed MM, Hegazy M, Abdelatif NM, ElGebeily MA, ElSobky T, Nader S. Dega osteotomy for the management of developmental dysplasia of the hip in children aged 2-8 years: results of 58 consecutive osteotomies after 13-25 years of follow-up. J Child Orthop. 2015;9(3):191–8. https://doi.org/10.1007/s11832-015-0665-9.
30. Rampal V, Klein C, Arellano E, Boubakeur Y, Seringe R, Glorion C, Wicart P. Outcomes of modified Dega acetabuloplasty in acetabular dysplasia related to developmental dislocation of the hip. Orthop Traumatol Surg Res. 2014;100(2):203–7. https://doi.org/10.1016/j.otsr.2013.12.015.
31. Akgül T, Bora Göksan S, Bilgili F, Valiyev N, Hürmeydan OM. Radiological results of modified Dega osteotomy in Tönnis grade 3 and 4 developmental dysplasia of the hip. J Pediatr Orthop B. 2014;23(4):333–8. https://doi.org/10.1097/BPB.0000000000000059.
32. Czubak J, Kowalik K, Kawalec A, Kwiatkowska M. Dega pelvic osteotomy: indications, results and complications. J Child Orthop. 2018;12(4):342–8. https://doi.org/10.1302/1863-2548.12.180091.
33. Krieg AH, Hefti F. Acetabuloplasty—the Dega and Pemberton technique. Orthopade. 2016;45(8):653–8. https://doi.org/10.1007/s00132-016-3295-0.
34. Baki ME, Baki C, Aydin H, Ari B, Özcan M. Single-stage medial open reduction and Pemberton acetabuloplasty in developmental dysplasia of the hip. J Pediatr Orthop B. 2016;25(6):504–8. https://doi.org/10.1097/BPB.0000000000000360.
35. Ertürk C, Altay MA, Işikan UE. A radiological comparison of Salter and Pemberton osteotomies to improve acetabular deformations in developmental dysplasia of the hip. J Pediatr Orthop B. 2013;22(6):527–32. https://doi.org/10.1097/BPB.0b013e32836337cd.
36. Blavier L, Blavier J. Traitement de la subluxation de la hanche. Rev Chir Orthop. 1962;48:208–13.
37. Wagner H. Korrektur der Hüftgelenksdysplasie durch die sphärische Pfannenosteotomie. In: Chapchal G, editor. Internationales Symposium über Beckenosteotomie/Pfannendachplastik. Stuttgart: Thieme; 1965.
38. Schramm M, Hohmann D, Radespiel-Troger M, Pitto RP. The Wagner spherical osteotomy of the acetabulum. Surgical technique. J Bone Joint Surg Am. 2004;86-A(Suppl 1):73–80.
39. Ganz R, Klaue K, Vinh TS, Mast JW. A new periacetabular osteotomy for the treatment of hip dysplasias. Technique and preliminary results. Clin Orthop Relat Res. 1988;232:26–36.
40. Lerch TD, Steppacher SD, Liechti EF, Siebenrock KA, Tannast M. Bernese periacetabular osteotomy: indications, technique and results 30 years after the first description. Orthopade. 2016;45(8):687–94. https://doi.org/10.1007/s00132-016-3265-6.
41. Brunner R, Baumann JU. Clinical benefit of reconstruction of dislocated or subluxated hip joints in patients with spastic cerebral palsy. J Pediatr Orthop. 1994;14(3):290–4.
42. Rutz E, Vavken P, Camathias C, Haase C, Jünemann S, Brunner R. Long-term results and outcome predictors in one-stage hip reconstruction in children with cerebral palsy. J Bone Joint Surg Am. 2015;97(6):500–6. https://doi.org/10.2106/JBJS.N.00676.
43. Robb JE, Brunner R. A Dega-type osteotomy after closure of the triradiate cartilage in non-walking patients with severe cerebral palsy. J Bone Joint Surg Br. 2006;88(7):933–7.
44. Krebs A, Strobl WM, Grill F. Neurogenic hip dislocation in cerebral palsy: quality of life and results after hip reconstruction. J Child Orthop. 2008;2(2):125–31.
45. Murar J, Dias LS, Swaroop VT. San Diego pelvic osteotomy in patients with closed triradiate cartilage. J Child Orthop. 2018;12(5):461–71. https://doi.org/10.1302/1863-2548.12.180046.
46. Buxbom P, Sonne-Holm S, Ellitsgaard N, Wong C. Stability and migration across femoral varus derotation osteotomies in children with neuromuscular disorders. Acta Orthop. 2017;88(2):198–204. https://doi.org/10.1080/17453674.2016.1263110.
47. Gather KS, von Stillfried E, Hagmann S, Müller S, Dreher T. Outcome after early mobilization following hip reconstruction in children with developmental hip dysplasia and luxation. World J Pediatr. 2018;14(2):176–83. https://doi.org/10.1007/s12519-017-0105-7.
48. Carsi MB, Clarke NM. Acetabuloplasties at open reduction prevent acetabular dysplasia in intentionally delayed developmental dysplasia of the hip: a case-control study. Clin Orthop Relat Res. 2016;474(5):1180–8. https://doi.org/10.1007/s11999-015-4501-9.
49. Çiçekli Ö, Doğan M. Evaluation of surgical outcome in advanced age patients with developmental hip dysplasia. Int J Surg. 2018;52:44–9. https://doi.org/10.1016/j.ijsu.2018.02.020.
50. Mallet C, Ilharreborde B, Presedo A, Khairouni A, Mazda K, Penneçot GF. One-stage hip reconstruction in children with cerebral palsy: long-term results at

skeletal maturity. J Child Orthop. 2014;8(3):221–8. https://doi.org/10.1007/s11832-014-0589-9.
51. McNerney NP, Mubarak SJ, Wenger DR. One-stage correction of the dysplastic hip in cerebral palsy with the San Diego acetabuloplasty: results and complications in 104 hips. J Pediatr Orthop. 2000;20(1):93–103.
52. Aly AS, Al-Kersh MA. Femoral and Dega osteotomies in the treatment of habitual hip dislocation in Down syndrome patients—is it efficient or not? J Child Orthop. 2018;12(3):227–31. https://doi.org/10.1302/1863-2548.12.170130.
53. Eberhardt O, Wirth T, Fernandez FF. Arthroscopic reduction and acetabuloplasty for the treatment of dislocated hips in children of walking age: a preliminary report. Arch Orthop Trauma Surg. 2014;134(11):1587–94. https://doi.org/10.1007/s00402-014-2063-z.
54. Xu HF, Yan YB, Xu C, Li TQ, Zhao TF, Liu N, Huang LY, Zhang CL, Lei W. Effects of arthroscopic-assisted surgery on irreducible developmental dislocation of hip by mid-term follow-up: an observational study. Medicine (Baltimore). 2016;95(33):e4601. https://doi.org/10.1097/MD.0000000000004601.

4 Pelvic Osteotomies: The Periacetabular Osteotomy Technique for Patients with Developmental Dysplasia of the Hip

Joshua S. Bingham, Robert T. Trousdale, and Rafael J. Sierra

4.1 Introduction

Numerous osteotomies have been described in an attempt to improve hip joint mechanics in young patients with symptomatic dysplasia in the absence of secondary arthritis [1]. The Bernese periacetabular osteotomy (PAO) which was first described by Prof. Reinhold Ganz for the treatment of symptomatic hip dysplasia has become the pelvic osteotomy of choice at many institutions [2]. There are several well-described advantages associated with the PAO technique, particularly the ability to perform an optimal deformity correction in all planes through a single incision [2, 3]. Additionally, as the posterior column remains intact, the osteotomy is inherently stable, and in conjunction with the preservation of the abductor mechanism, accelerated rehabilitation with early weight bearing is possible after PAO [4].

As the anatomy of patients with dysplasia can vary significantly it is useful to be able to perform both large and small corrections in any plane. In dysplastic patients the major deformity is usually on the acetabular side. Generally the acetabulum is shallow and excessively anteverted with a lateralized hip center (Fig. 4.1; [5]). This deformity results in an anterior superior deficiency. However the acetabulum may also be deficient posteriorly secondary to acetab-

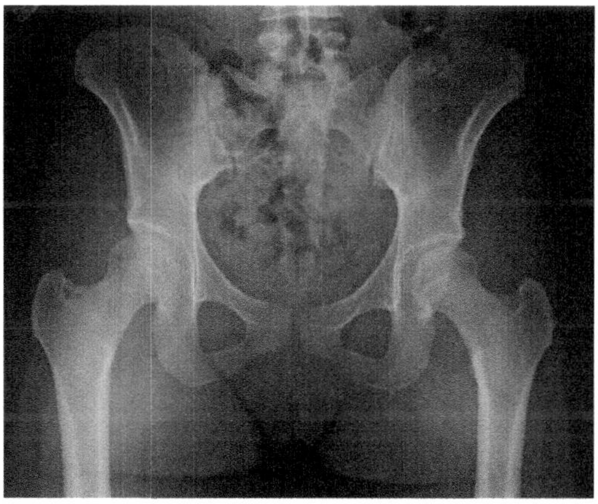

Fig. 4.1 AP pelvic radiograph demonstrating classic dysplasia of the right hip. The acetabulum is shallow, and the hip center is lateralized with both anterior and superior deficiency

J. S. Bingham
Department of Orthopedic Surgery, Mayo Clinic, Rochester, MN, USA

Department of Orthopedic Surgery, Mayo Clinic, Phoenix, AZ, USA
e-mail: bingham.joshua@mayo.edu

R. T. Trousdale · R. J. Sierra (✉)
Department of Orthopedic Surgery, Mayo Clinic, Rochester, MN, USA
e-mail: trousdale.robert@mayo.edu; sierra.rafael@mayo.edu

W. R. Drescher et al. (eds.), *Advances in Specialist Hip Surgery*,
https://doi.org/10.1007/978-3-030-61830-8_4

ular retroversion in up to 40% of patients [6]. On the femoral side, excessive anteversion and a high neck-shaft angle are common. Overall these anatomic abnormalities result in decreased contact area between the weight-bearing dome of the acetabulum and the femoral head.

Patients with dysplasia often have activity-related groin pain that is related to both instability of the femoral head and higher joint reactive forces secondary to the lateralized hip center. Trochanteric pain is also common and often associated with abductor fatigue while catching and mechanical symptoms may be indicative of chondral and/or labral pathology [7]. With an appropriate correction, the reoriented acetabular fragment allows a more normal load transmission through the cartilage surface area, and medialization of the hip center when needed lessens the joint reactive forces in the hip joint. By correcting the anatomic abnormalities and improving the biomechanics of the hip, a PAO in the right patient can reliably improve symptoms and result in excellent long-term survivorship (Table 4.1; [8–13]).

While there may be variations in patient anatomy and surgical technique, the overall goal of the procedure remains the same: Obtain adequate exposure of the innominate bone to safely enable four separate osteotomies to be performed, thereby allowing a complete detachment of the acetabulum from the intact pelvis while leaving the posterior column intact to reorient the acetabulum in all required planes. It is critical that these goals be achieved while minimizing the risk of intraoperative complications as PAOs are not without risk and complications can be high particularly when performed by surgeons without the appropriate training or while still in their learning curve [8, 14].

By having an intimate knowledge of the anatomy around the pelvis and recognizing the structures at risk, in general a PAO can be performed safely and in a reproducible fashion [15, 16].

4.1.1 Anatomic Structures at Risk

1. The lateral femoral cutaneous nerve (LFCN): Is at risk both during exposure and closure. Symptoms associated with the LFCN can occur in 75% or more of patients although symptoms resolve in most patients [15]. As such all patients should be made aware of this potential complication.
2. Obturator neurovascular structures: Are at risk during the dissection down to the ischium and during the superior pubic ramus osteotomy.

Table 4.1 Literature results of the Bernese periacetabular osteotomy for patients with hip dysplasia

Authors	Year	Number of hips	Mean patient age in years (range)	Mean follow-up in years (range)	Success rate (%)[a]	Results[b]
Trousdale et al.	1995	42	37 (11–56)	4 (2–8)	86	HHS improved by 24 points
Siebenrock et al.	1999	75	2 (13–56)	11 (10–14)	82	–
Clohisy et al.	2005	16	18 (13–32)	4 (2–8)	100	Merle d'Aubigné improved by 15 points
Cunningham et al.	2006	52	27	2 (2–8)	90	HHS improved by 6 points
Peters et al.	2006	83	31	3	96	WOMAC improved by 33 points
Garras et al.	2007	58	38 (13–48)	6 (1–13)	95	Merle d'Aubigné improved by 3 points
Steppacher et al.	2008	68	29 (13–56)	20 (19–23)	60	Merle d'Aubigné improved by 0.6 points

HHS Harris hip score, *WOMAC* Western Ontario and McMaster Universities Osteoarthritis Index
[a]Success is defined as procedures not requiring conversion to a total hip arthroplasty
[b]All results are mean values and indicate improvement from preoperative to postoperative

3. Medial femoral circumflex artery: Is at risk during exposure of the inferior ischial cut if dissection during the blind exposure of the ischium is carried distal from the cephalad edge of the obturator externus [17, 18].
4. Femoral neurovascular structures: Are at particular risk during the exposure of the superior pubic ramus and when excessive tension is applied to the psoas during exposure.
5. Sciatic nerve: Is at risk during the ischial and posterior iliac osteotomies if care is not taken to prevent the osteotomes from migrating too far laterally as these are blind cuts.

4.2 Alternative Treatments

The appropriate indication for a PAO is essential as there is a wide spectrum of anatomic abnormalities in dysplastic hips which vary based on the severity and type of deformity [1, 19]. Initially patients should be treated nonsurgically with physical therapy, anti-inflammatory medications, and activity modifications. The natural history of dysplasia should be discussed with the patient, and radiographs should be obtained every couple of years to monitor for the development of subsequent osteoarthritis. Surgical management should be reserved for patients with persistent symptoms in conjunction with marked structural abnormalities.

While a pelvic realignment osteotomy is the procedure of choice for most patients with symptomatic dysplasia, other surgical procedures should also be considered when appropriate. Poor candidates for a PAO include those patients with a lack of joint congruency on abduction films, significant cephalad migration of the femoral head, an open triradiate cartilage, and osteoarthritis with Tönnis grade two or higher [20]. While there is not a defined upper age limit, in general PAOs are rarely performed in patients greater than 45 years. Excellent long-term survivorship and maintenance of functional gains after PAO have been reported when performed in well-selected patients [9, 10].

4.3 Surgical Technique

Although the PAO technique has already been extensively described in the literature, the technique continues to evolve and the following is our preferred and current surgical technique.

4.3.1 Preoperative Planning

- In addition to a detailed history and clinical examination, standard AP pelvic and false-profile-view radiographs are obtained for all patients.
- Although not routine, a computerized tomography (CT) scan (1 mm slices and 3-dimensional reconstruction) of the pelvis with knee cuts can also be obtained and is particularly helpful in evaluating the femoral neck torsion if a femoral osteotomy is being considered in conjunction with the PAO. This would be considered in patients with severe dysplasia (possibly varus osteotomy), increased antetorsion (derotational retroverting osteotomy), or significant limitations in range of motion (derotational anteverting osteotomy).

4.3.2 Setup and Positioning

- The patient is placed on an image table.
- Regional spinal anesthesia is the preferred anesthetic option for most patients undergoing a PAO in conjunction with a local periarticular anesthetic.
- Intraoperative cell saver is routinely used rather than preoperative autologous blood donation.
- Tranexamic acid is administered intravenously (1 g prior at incision, and 1 g at closure).
- Intraoperative electromyography monitoring (EMG) of both the sciatic and femoral nerve is utilized to identify intraoperative pressure and tension on these structures (Fig. 4.2; [21]).
- Specialized osteotomes have been developed and are helpful at various stages of the procedure (Fig. 4.3).

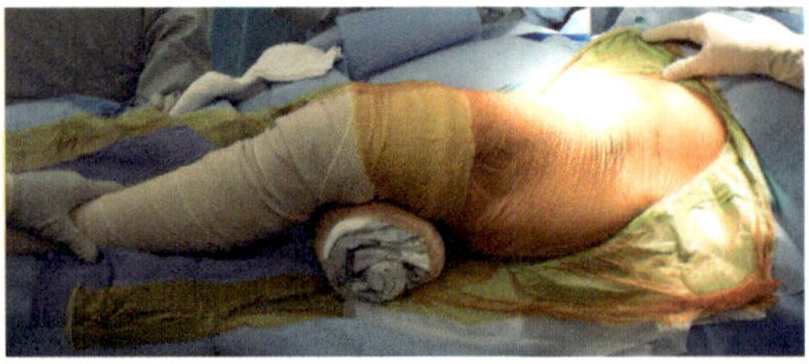

Fig. 4.2 Intraoperative photograph showing a patient draped for a periacetabular osteotomy to manage hip dysplasia with both fluoroscopic imaging and electromyographic monitoring equipment

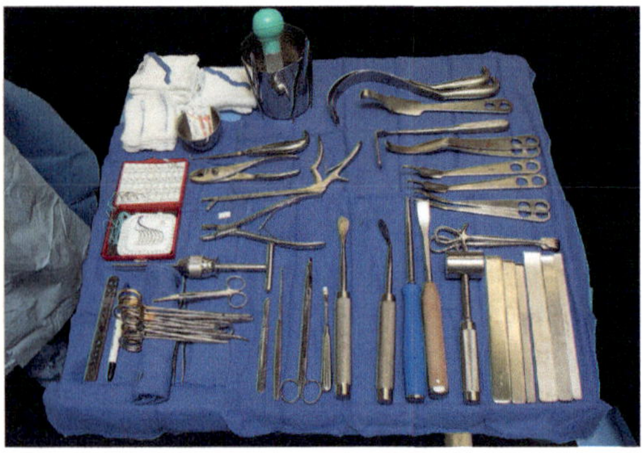

Fig. 4.3 Intraoperative photograph showing the back table setup for a periacetabular osteotomy with the various retractors and specialized osteotomes routinely used

4.3.3 Skin Incision and Exposure

- A modified Smith-Petersen approach, with a superficial Hueter approach, is utilized which spares the abductor muscles as the osteotomies are performed through the inner aspect of the pelvis [3].
- The incision begins just lateral to the border of the iliac crest and is carried distal and lateral to the anterior superior iliac spine (ASIS). The incision ends approximately 3 cm distal and anterior to the greater trochanter.
- The fascia is incised distally to the ASIS over the tensor fasciae latae (TFL), and the interval between sartorius and the TFL is developed with blunt dissection down to the anterior inferior iliac spine (AIIS).
- The entire origin of sartorius is subperiosteally reflected off the ASIS with electrocautery and tagged with a suture for later repair.
- The hip is flexed and adducted after which an angled Cobb elevator is utilized to expose the inner table of the pelvis from the sciatic notch to the quadrilateral surface.
- With the hip flexed and the inner table of the pelvis exposed, the iliopsoas tendon can be retracted medially to expose the pubis medial to the iliopectineal eminence. In order to protect the femoral neurovascular structures, the iliopsoas tendon should not be tenotomized. Once the iliopectineal eminence is clearly visible a sharp Hohmann can be placed medial in the pubis to aid in retraction.
- At this point the direct head of the rectus femoris can be reflected distally off the AIIS and an arthrotomy can be performed to address any central compartment pathology. However a rectus-sparing approach is currently our preference.
- Blunt dissection with curved scissors is carried out medial to the direct head of the rectus femoris and distally to develop a plan between the iliocapsularis and hip capsule. The scissors should be able to palpate the ischium at this point.

4.3.4 Procedure

- Utilization of intraoperative fluoroscopy at several critical points has made performing the pelvic osteotomies relatively routine and predictable.
- The osteotomies include a partial osteotomy of the ischium, a complete pubic osteotomy, and a biplanar osteotomy of the ilium ensuring that the posterior column remains intact.
- For the authors, the intraoperative fluoroscopy is critical throughout the entire procedure and makes the operation safe, teachable, and reproducible.
- An anterior-posterior (AP) image is used to ensure proper medial-lateral placement of the curved osteotome on the ischium as well as proper orientation (Fig. 4.4).
- An oblique 55°–65° (65° preferred except in heavy-set patients) image is used while making the ischial osteotomy to determine the appropriate depth of the osteotomy (Fig. 4.5).

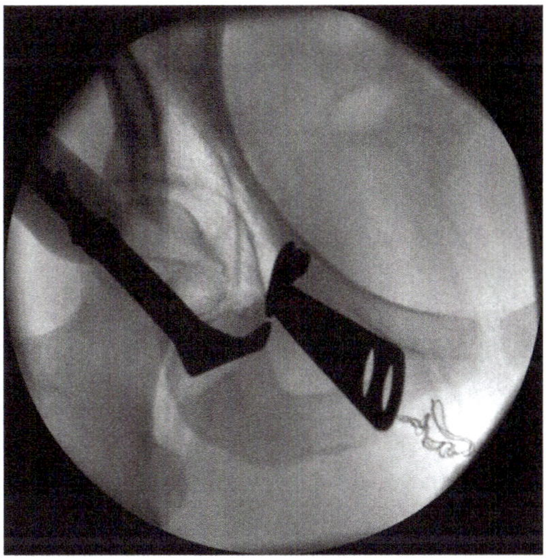

Fig. 4.4 Intraoperative AP fluoroscopic image demonstrating the appropriate placement of the ischial osteotome. A Hohmann retractor is in the medial aspect of the pubis

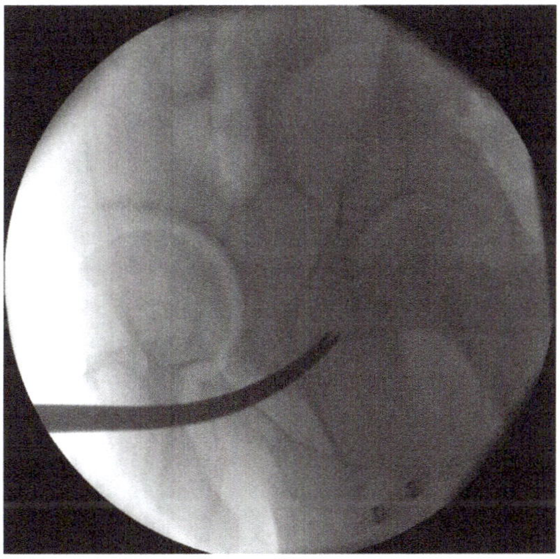

Fig. 4.5 Intraoperative oblique fluoroscopic image demonstrating the appropriate depth of the ischial osteotome

- Once the ischial osteotomy is completed, the osteotome can be left in place to serve as a guide while the posterior iliac osteotomy is performed as the medial aspect of the osteotome can often be palpated over the quadrilateral surface. However leaving this osteotome in place can cause increased tension on the femoral nerve, and as such the leg should remain flexed as long as the osteotome is in place (Fig. 4.6).

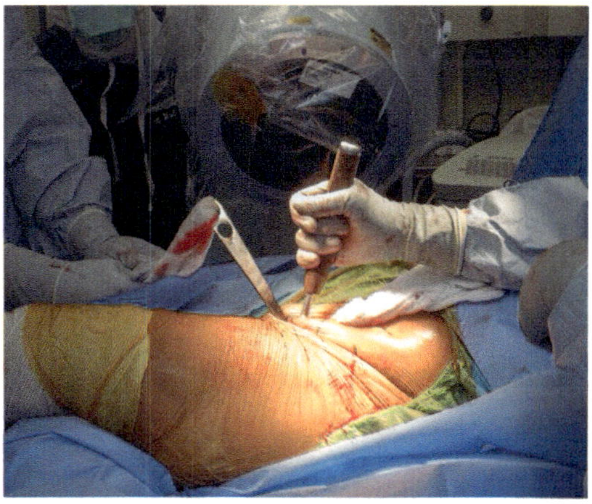

Fig. 4.6 Intraoperative photograph of the ischial osteotome in place with a Hohmann retractor in the pubis and the image intensifier in the background

- If a rectus-sparing PAO is performed then we would always recommend removing the osteotome from the ischium.
- The pubic bone can now be fully exposed and if needed another sharp Hohmann retractor can be placed more medially in the pubis if needed. Blunt retractors should be placed around the superior and inferior aspect of the pubis to protect the obturator neurovascular structures while making this osteotomy.
- The proper orientation of the pubic cut is critical to allow mobilization of the acetabular fragment. The osteotomy should be oriented from proximal-medial to distal-lateral away from the joint.
- An AP image is used to determine the level of the iliac cut which is typically just distal to the ASIS. This osteotomy must be proximal enough to allow for satisfactory fixation of the acetabular fragment. In cases of severe dysplasia the cut may sometimes be above the ASIS.
- Once the level of the iliac cut is determined with an AP image, the oblique 55°–65° image is used to determine the depth of the cut. The oblique image may need to be adjusted depending on the patient's bony morphology and habitus to ensure that the posterior column and articular surface are clearly visible.

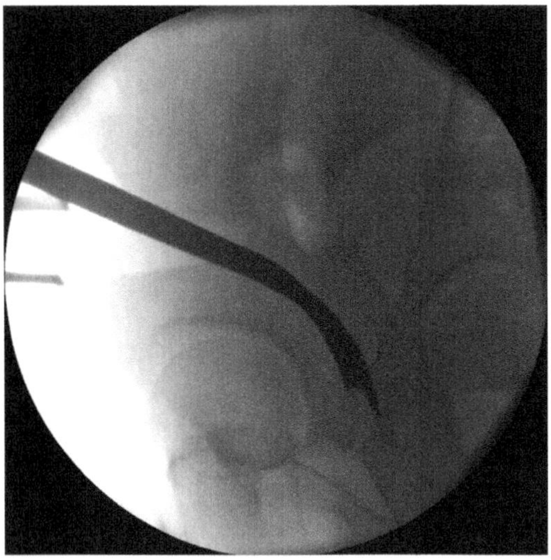

Fig. 4.7 Intraoperative oblique fluoroscopic image demonstrating the posterior iliac cut as it joins the ischial cut. Both the articular surface and posterior column are intact and clearly visible

- With clear radiographic visualization of the posterior column and articular surface, the posterior iliac osteotomy can be safely performed. Often several passes are required to complete this osteotomy (Fig. 4.7).

4.3.5 Mobilization and Correction of the Acetabular Fragment

- After completion of the osteotomies the posterior column should remain intact, and the acetabular fragment must now be freely mobilized.
- The two most common sites where the fragment is restricted are the pubic osteotomy and the junction of the posterior column and ischial osteotomy.
- A 4 mm Schanz pin is placed in the acetabular fragment to assist in mobilization. The 4 mm Schanz pin can be exchanged for a 6 mm one if fixation is lost.
- Obtaining the proper correction is the most challenging aspect of the procedure. For a typical correction in a dysplastic patient, the acetabular fragment is displaced medially, rotated anteriorly and laterally (with care taken to maintain proper anteversion), and provisionally fixed with two smooth 3.2 mm Steinmann pins.
- After provisional fixation an intraoperative AP radiograph of the pelvis is obtained to assess the correction. Care must be taken to ensure that the pelvis is not tilted in any direction as this will alter the assessment of acetabular correction.
- A satisfactory correction is obtained when the weight-bearing surface of the acetabulum is between 0° and 10° off horizontal, the femoral head is congruous, and the anterior wall covers less of the femoral head than the posterior wall; they meet at the lateral edge of the sourcil ensuring proper acetabular version, and the femoral head is medialized within 5 mm of the ilioischial line (Fig. 4.8).
- Care must be taken to ensure that the fragment is not overcorrected laterally as this can lead to impingement and the fovea coming into the weight-bearing surface.
- The hip should be taken through a complete range of motion. The hip should be able to flex up to 110°–115° without impingement of the head-neck junction on the acetabular rim. If there is impingement, we ensure that the fragment has not been inadvertently retroverted. If the socket is not retroverted the head-neck junction ratio can be improved by performing an osteochondroplasty.
- Once the correction is satisfactory, the acetabular fragment is fixed with fully threaded

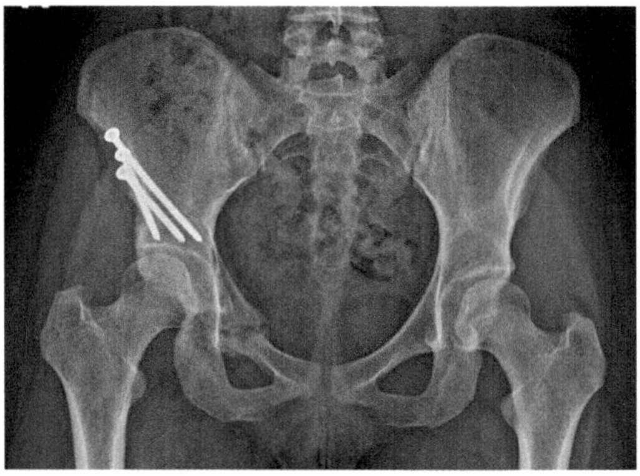

Fig. 4.8 Postoperative AP pelvic radiograph demonstrating satisfactory correction of classic hip dysplasia on the right side

4.5 mm cortical screws. In some patients with smaller bony anatomy, 3.5 mm screws can be utilized. The screws may be countersunk to decrease their prominence, but in our experience this has not resulted in a lower rate of hardware removal.
- Due to the morbidity associated with taking down the rectus to address intra-articular pathology, the central compartment is only evaluated if there is a high index of suspicion for symptomatic intra-articular pathology. Hip arthroscopy prior to the PAO is a safe aid to evaluate and treat the central compartment.

4.3.6 Wound Closure

- After correction there is often a prominent AIIS which may be trimmed and used as bone graft in the anterior gap of the iliac osteotomy.
- If a capsulotomy was performed the capsule is repaired with resorbable suture while the rectus femoris is reattached to the AIIS with nonresorbable suture.
- With the hip flexed the sartorius muscle is repaired to the ASIS through a bone tunnel using the tag suture as a guide.
- A deep drain is placed intrapelvic and removed on postoperative day 1. The deep fascia is closed with buried interrupted sutures, and skin closure is performed in a routing fashion with resorbable suture and glue.

4.4 Postoperative Regimen

Postoperatively patient mobilization with ambulatory aids begins on the day of surgery. Most patients receive scheduled acetaminophen and oral narcotics as needed for pain in conjunction with their intraoperative periarticular injection. For venous thromboembolism (VTE) prophylaxis in low-risk patients, low-dose aspirin twice daily is used for 6 weeks. A structured physical therapy regimen typically starts 2 weeks after surgery, while full weight bearing is not permitted until 6 weeks. Abduction exercises, water therapy, and stationary bike exercises are started after 4 weeks.

4.5 Avoiding Pitfalls and Complications

Pelvic osteotomies, particularly a PAO, are complex procedures with significant potential complications. The overall experience of the surgeon performing the procedure is a major factor as the learning curve for this procedure is steep with a high risk of complications early on [14, 22]. These procedures should be performed by surgeons that have had dedicated training in the technique by surgeons who routinely perform the procedure. Additionally, we have found that utilization of cadaveric lab is extremely helpful for surgeons prior to independently performing a PAO.

Complications after PAO include but are not limited to neurovascular injuries, intra-articular extension of the osteotomies, infection, nonunion, heterotopic ossification, and VTEs. A body mass index (BMI) greater than 30 kg/m^2 is a known risk factor for complications after a PAO with a 22% rate of major complication reported in the literature compared to a 3% rate in patients with a BMI under 30 kg/m^2 [23].

While major nerve injuries after PAOs are rare with one study reporting a complication rate of 2.1% for major femoral or sciatic nerve dysfunction, it is a devastating complication [21]. Because of this risk, the use of intraoperative EMG is standard in our practice. Minor nerve-related injuries on the other hand are common with up to 75% of patients reporting paresthesia in the lateral aspect of the thigh after surgery related to either direct injury or traction to branches of the lateral femoral cutaneous nerve [21, 22]. Most of these patients do not require further treatment, but patients should be made aware of this complication prior to the procedure due to the high incidence.

The incidence of stress fractures after PAOs is controversial. Previous reports have placed the incidence between 2 and 3%, but more recent literature has reported the rate to be much higher at 18% [24]. Although most stress fractures heal uneventfully, nonunion of the pubic osteotomy is much more common in these patients. Fortunately most nonunions of the pubis are an asymptomatic radiographic finding. Bone grafting or plate fixation of stress fractures and nonunions is rarely required.

Although much less common with the use of intraoperative fluoroscopy, inadvertent extension of an osteotomy into an undesired location can occur. Intra-articular extension of the ischial osteotomy can occur particularly in patients with cephalad migration of the femoral head. While this intra-articular extension does not cause a joint incongruity, it can interrupt the blood supply to the acetabular fragment [25]. Intra-articular extension of the vertical limb of the iliac osteotomy on the other hand can create a joint incongruity after correction leading to secondary arthrosis. The iliac osteotomy can also be inadvertently extended through the posterior column which can destabilize the pelvic ring.

By far the most common complication after PAO remains poor positioning of the acetabular fragment with both overcorrection and retroversion being common. Overcorrection of the acetabular fragment can result in impingement symptoms or posterior subluxation of the femoral head. Anterior impingement can be a sign of excessive anterior correction or retroversion of the acetabular fragment. Obtaining a true AP pelvic radiograph and taking the hip through a range of motion intraoperatively can help the surgeon recognize these problems. If recognized intraoperatively, the acetabular fragment can be repositioned, and extra-articular impingement can be addressed. Although the learning curve is steep and potential complications for this procedure are high, in our hands a well-done osteotomy in properly selected patients is a relatively reliable and successful procedure for patients with symptomatic hip dysplasia.

References

1. Leunig M, Siebenrock KA, Ganz R. Rationale of periacetabular osteotomy and background work. Instr Course Lect. 2001;50:229–38.
2. Ganz R, Klaue K, Vinh TS, Mast JW. A new periacetabular osteotomy for the treatment of hip dysplasias. Technique and preliminary results. Clin Orthop. 1988;232:26–36.
3. Smith-Petersen MN. Approach to and exposure of the hip joint for mold arthroplasty. J Bone Joint Surg Am. 1949;31A:40–6.
4. Heyworth BE, Novais EN, Murray K, Cvetanovich G, Zurakowski D, Millis MB, Kim Y-J. Return to play after periacetabular osteotomy for treatment of acetabular dysplasia in adolescent and young adult athletes. Am J Sports Med. 2016;44:1573–81.
5. Clohisy JC, Carlisle JC, Beaulé PE, Kim Y-J, Trousdale RT, Sierra RJ, Leunig M, Schoenecker PL, Millis MB. A systematic approach to the plain radiographic evaluation of the young adult hip. J Bone Joint Surg Am. 2008;90:47–66.
6. Ezoe M, Naito M, Inoue T. The prevalence of acetabular retroversion among various disorders of the hip. J Bone Joint Surg Am. 2006;88:372–9.
7. Maquet P. Biomechanics of hip dysplasia. Acta Orthop Belg. 1999;65:302–14.
8. Peters CL, Erickson JA, Hines JL. Early results of the Bernese periacetabular osteotomy: the learning curve at an academic medical center. J Bone Joint Surg Am. 2006;88:1920–6.
9. Clohisy JC, Barrett SE, Gordon JE, Delgado ED, Schoenecker PL. Periacetabular osteotomy for the treatment of severe acetabular dysplasia. J Bone Joint Surg Am. 2005;87:254–9.
10. Steppacher SD, Tannast M, Ganz R, Siebenrock KA. Mean 20-year follow-up of Bernese periacetabular osteotomy. Clin Orthop. 2008;466:1633–44.
11. Trousdale RT, Ekkernkamp A, Ganz R, Wallrichs SL. Periacetabular and intertrochanteric osteotomy for the treatment of osteoarthrosis in dysplastic hips. J Bone Joint Surg Am. 1995;77:73–85.
12. Siebenrock KA, Schöll E, Lottenbach M, Ganz R. Bernese periacetabular osteotomy. Clin Orthop. 1999;363:9–20.
13. Cunningham T, Jessel R, Zurakowski D, Millis MB, Kim Y-J. Delayed gadolinium-enhanced magnetic resonance imaging of cartilage to predict early failure of Bernese periacetabular osteotomy for hip dysplasia. J Bone Joint Surg Am. 2006;88:1540–8.
14. Zaltz I, Baca G, Kim Y-J, et al. Complications associated with the periacetabular osteotomy: a prospective multicenter study. J Bone Joint Surg Am. 2014;96:1967–74.

15. Hussell JG, Rodriguez JA, Ganz R. Technical complications of the Bernese periacetabular osteotomy. Clin Orthop. 1999;363:81–92.
16. Kalhor M, Collado D, Leunig M, Rego P, Ganz R. Recommendations to reduce risk of nerve injury during Bernese periacetabular osteotomy (PAO). JBJS Essent Surg Tech. 2017;7:e34.
17. Kamada S, Naito M, Shiramizu K, Nakamura Y, Kinoshita K. Is the obturator artery safe when performing ischial osteotomy during periacetabular osteotomy? Int Orthop. 2011;35:503–6.
18. Gautier E, Ganz K, Krügel N, Gill T, Ganz R. Anatomy of the medial femoral circumflex artery and its surgical implications. J Bone Joint Surg Br. 2000;82:679–83.
19. Myers SR, Eijer H, Ganz R. Anterior femoroacetabular impingement after periacetabular osteotomy. Clin Orthop. 1999;363:93–9.
20. Beaulé PE, Dowding C, Parker G, Ryu J-J. What factors predict improvements in outcomes scores and reoperations after the Bernese periacetabular osteotomy? Clin Orthop. 2015;473:615–22.
21. Sierra RJ, Beaule P, Zaltz I, Millis MB, Clohisy JC, Trousdale RT. Prevention of nerve injury after periacetabular osteotomy. Clin Orthop. 2012;470:2209–19.
22. Davey JP, Santore RF. Complications of periacetabular osteotomy. Clin Orthop. 1999;363:33–7.
23. Novais EN, Potter GD, Clohisy JC, Millis MB, Kim YJ, Trousdale RT, Carry PM, Sierra RJ. Obesity is a major risk factor for the development of complications after peri-acetabular osteotomy. Bone Joint J. 2015;97-B:29–34.
24. Malviya A, Dandachli W, Beech Z, Bankes MJ, Witt JD. The incidence of stress fracture following periacetabular osteotomy: an under-reported complication. Bone Joint J. 2015;97-B:24–8.
25. Beck M, Leunig M, Ellis T, Sledge JB, Ganz R. The acetabular blood supply: implications for periacetabular osteotomies. Surg Radiol Anat. 2003;25:361–7.

Navigated Rotational Acetabular Osteotomy

5

Nobuhiko Sugano, Hidetoshi Hamada, and Masaki Takao

5.1 Introduction

Acetabular redirection osteotomy has been established as one of the most effective joint-preserving surgeries in the early stages of hip disorder secondary to hip dysplasia. It allows the reorientation of the acetabulum along with hyaline articular cartilage to a more relevant weight-bearing position over the femoral head while maintaining the integrity of pelvic ring structure. Several types of periacetabular osteotomies have yielded satisfactory long-term clinical results, including Eppright's dial osteotomy [1], Wagner's spherical acetabular osteotomy [2], and Ganz Bernese periacetabular osteotomy (PAO) [3]. Rotational acetabular osteotomy (RAO), which was first introduced into the English literature by Ninomiya and Tagawa in 1984 [4], is currently used widely in Japan at the early stages of osteoarthritis with hip dysplasia [5]. In RAO, the periacetabular fragment is osteotomized spherically around the center of the acetabular dome using a curved osteotome, and is rotated laterally and anteriorly, as well as transferred medially. Due to the spherical shape of the acetabular fragment, RAO has the advantage of allowing rotation of the fragment in any direction readily to enhance the contact area between the acetabular bone surface and the residual pelvic bone surface. On the other hand, there is a risk of intra-articular penetration of the osteotome and necrosis of the fragment because the osteotomy line is close to the joint [6–8]. For successful RAO, therefore, surgeons need to understand the three-dimensional morphology of hip dysplasia of the individual acetabulum and to be skillful in the accurate cutting of bone and rotating of the acetabulum.

To perform this complicated and technically demanding procedure safely and accurately, we started to use CT-based planning and navigation for RAO in 1999 [9–11]. Since there have been still few clinical reports on navigation for RAO [12–15], it would be interesting for readers to describe our CT-based navigation techniques for RAO and its outcomes.

5.2 Indication and Preoperative Planning

Young and middle-aged symptomatic patients with congenital dysplasia of the hip are candidates for RAO (Fig. 5.1). Preferable indications which permit expectation of satisfactory outcomes are (1) expectation of good joint congruity and acetabular coverage by RAO; (2) pre- or early stage of osteoarthritis on preoperative radiographs; (3) younger age at operation (less

N. Sugano (✉) · H. Hamada · M. Takao
Departments of Orthopaedic Medical Engineering and Orthopaedic Surgery, Osaka University Graduate School of Medicine, Osaka, Japan
e-mail: n-sugano@umin.net; hide-hamada@umin.ac.jp; masaki-tko@umin.ac.jp

W. R. Drescher et al. (eds.), *Advances in Specialist Hip Surgery*,
https://doi.org/10.1007/978-3-030-61830-8_5

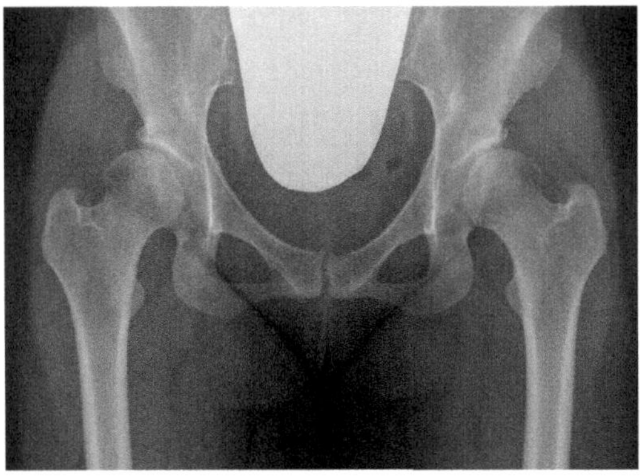

Fig. 5.1 An AP radiograph of the pelvis of a 34-year-old female with bilateral hip dysplasia

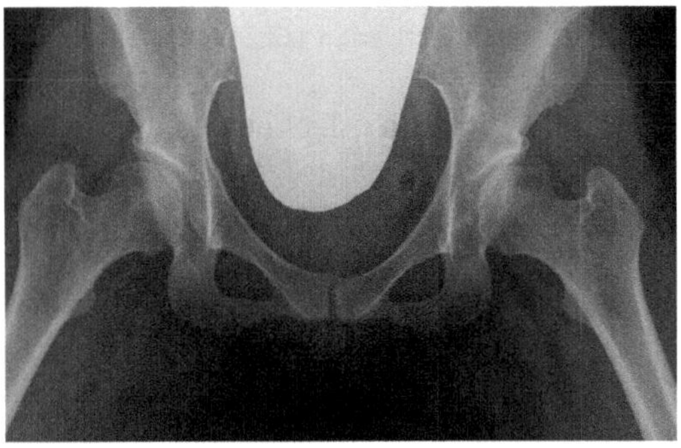

Fig. 5.2 An AP radiograph of the pelvis in hip abduction. According to the Shenton lines, hip subluxation in Fig. 5.1 is improved

than 50); and (4) little deformity of the femoral head. Poor joint congruity on postoperative radiographs is likely to result in inferior clinical and radiological outcomes. Preoperatively, postoperative joint congruity and acetabular coverage can be simulated on anteroposterior radiographs with the hip in abduction (Fig. 5.2).

Preoperatively, transverse CT images from the level of the superior anterior iliac spine to the bottom of the ischium are obtained using a helical CT scanner. The slice thickness is 3 mm, and the pitch is 3 mm. The radiation dose of this protocol is calculated to be less than 3 mSV. Three-dimensional acetabular and femoral bone surface models are reconstructed from the CT data of each patient. In the preoperative planning on the 3D surface models, a sphere is fitted to the femoral head to determine the hip center. The diameter of the sphere is increased by 20–25 mm for osteotomy design (Fig. 5.3). This sphere size keeps a minimum thickness of the acetabulum (15 mm) and the sphere is moved antero-medially to avoid thinning of the posterior column and to medialize the hip center. The acetabular fragment is rotated laterally (20°–30°) with the goal of reorienting the acetabulum to 30° of CE angle (Fig. 5.4). Overcorrection of anterior acetabular coverage may reportedly cause reduced range of motion (ROM) and postoperative femoral acetabular impingement [16]. We analyzed acetabular and femoral morphologies on 3D CT images and found that the anterior and lateral acetabular coverage of both normal and dysplastic hips showed wide variations [17, 18]. In normal hips, the mean lateral 3D CE angle was 35.6° (range 21.4°–59.2°), and the mean anterior 3D CE angle was 58.6° (34.6°–73.9°). The hip ROM simulation of 52 DDH-affected hips after RAO with several patterns of femoral head coverage was compared with that of 73 normal hips using computer models reconstructed from CT images. After RAO with a lateral 3D CE angle of 30° and an anterior 3D CE angle of 55° producing a coverage similar to that of normal hips, the maximal flexion and maximal internal rotation at 110° flexion with 20° adduction were significantly smaller than those of the normal group [16]. The location and morphology of the anterior inferior iliac spine are major factors to influence the postoperative bony ROM [19]. Therefore, the acetabulum is rotated only laterally nowadays.

5.3 Surgical Technique

The patient is positioned in a lateral position on the operating table. A pelvic dynamic reference frame with LEDs is fixed to the pelvic rim using two percutaneous apex pins and a Hoffmann external fixation system. The skin incision is made laterally over the proximal femur extending about 6 cm above and below the greater trochanter. Although a combination of anterior iliofemoral and posterior approaches was used in the original procedure by Ninomiya and Tagawa [4], we use a lateral transtrochanteric approach to expose the entire periacetabular bone surface and

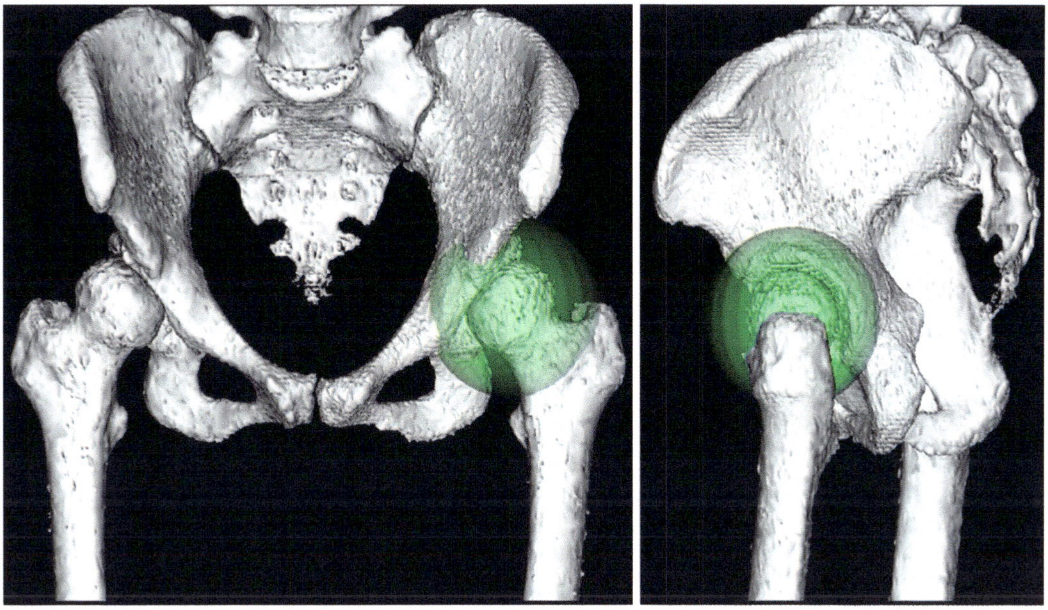

Fig. 5.3 CT-based preoperative planning. An osteotomy sphere with a minimum 15 mm thickness of acetabular fragment is shown (green)

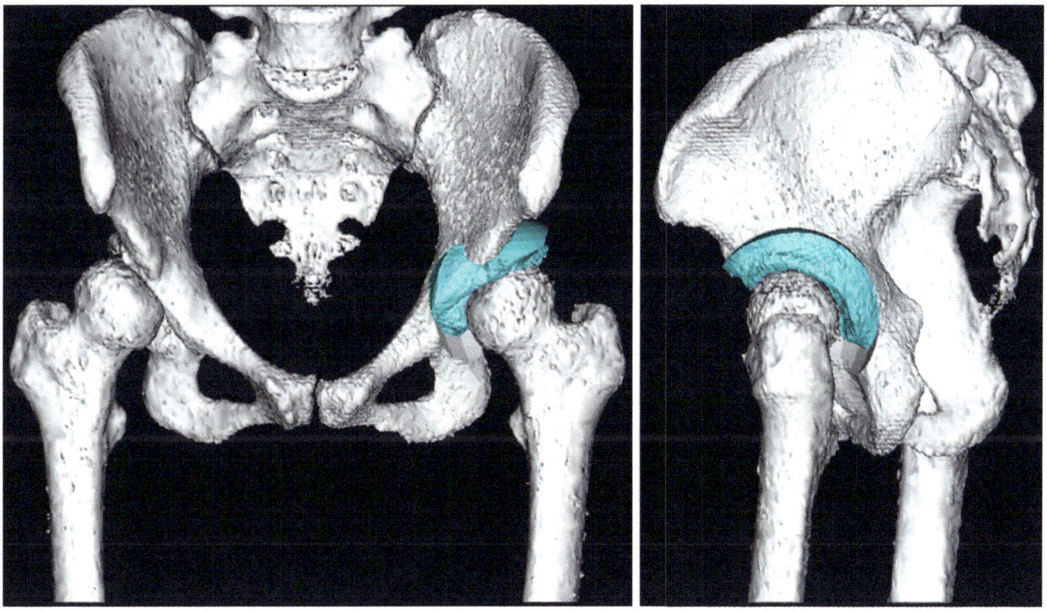

Fig. 5.4 CT-based preoperative planning. The acetabular fragment (blue) is rotated 25° laterally

to preserve the strength of the hip abductor muscles. The posterior short rotators from the piriformis to the obturator externus are released and retracted posteriorly. The greater trochanter is osteotomized and is retracted proximally along with the gluteus medius and minimus muscles, and then the upper and posterior aspects of the capsule of the hip joint and surrounding iliac bone are exposed. Recently, we found that it is not necessary to release external rotator muscles

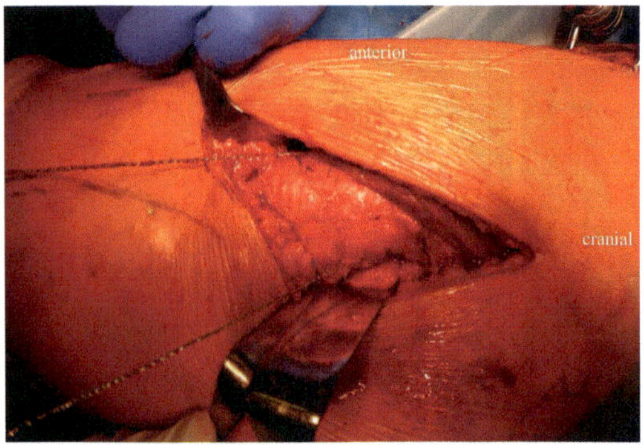

Fig. 5.5 A Gigli saw was introduced from the cranial side of the greater trochanter under the gluteus medius, gluteus minimus, and piriformis to cut the greater trochanter and to expose the ilium around the acetabulum

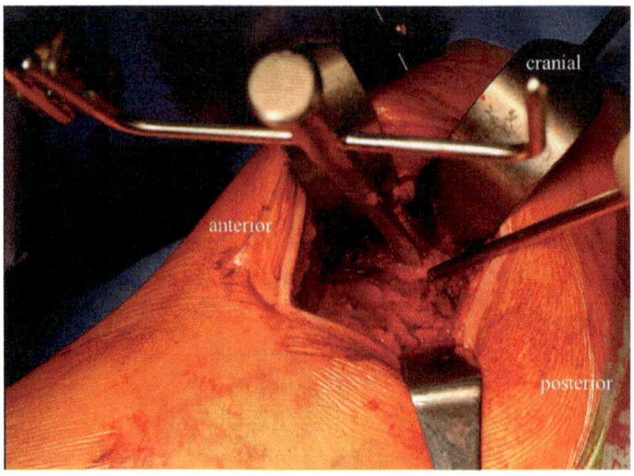

Fig. 5.6 An osteotome with a navigation tracker is introduced into the pelvis by locating the tip on the monitor (Fig. 5.7)

by keeping the piriformis attached to the greater trochanter and the other external rotator muscles are only separated from the capsule and periacetabulum (Fig. 5.5).

Shape-based surface registration of the patient's pelvis to the previously constructed bone model of the pelvis is performed using 30 surface points [20]. The accuracy of registration is verified by touching bony landmarks. The first version of our in-house-developed navigation system consisted of an optical 3D localizer (OPTOTRAK3020, Northern Digital, Waterloo, Canada), a custom-made dynamic reference frame with active light-emitting diodes (LEDs), custom-made surgical tools designed to work with a dynamic reference frame, an OPTOTRAK pen probe, and a UNIX-based Sun Ultra-SPARK workstation (Sun Microsystems, Santa Clara, California). The navigation software was developed using an open-source software system (Visualization Toolkit, Kitware, Clifton Park, New York). We introduced a commercially available CT-based navigation system (OrthoMap 3D Navigation System; Stryker Orthopaedics, Mahwah, NJ, USA) for RAO in 2011 [11].

The navigation system allowed surgeons to confirm the position and direction of the osteotome three-dimensionally and interactively in relation to preoperative computer planning (Figs. 5.6 and 5.7). Therefore, neither image intensification nor X-ray was used. After completing the osteotomy of the ilium, ischium, and pubis, the periacetabular fragment is rotated laterally, so as to match the acetabular fragment's new position to the preoperative planning. The position of the acetabular fragment is estimated by touching the edge points of the rim and osteotomy line with a probe (Fig. 5.8). After deciding on the position of the periacetabular fragment, two 2.4 mm diameter Kirschner wires were used for fixation of the fragment in the initial nine hips. The K-wires were removed 6 weeks after operation. Although the fragment could be easily and reliably secured by Kirschner wires, this fixation method had disadvantages of interference with postoperative exercise and the necessity of a second surgery to remove the wires. Therefore, 3–5 resorbable screws made from a composite of poly-L-lactic acid and hydroxyapatite granules are used now for ease of rehabilitation (Fig. 5.9). No bone grafting is needed although a calcium phosphate block is sometimes used to fill small gaps between the fragments. Using two AO large cancellous screws with washers, the greater trochanter is reattached to the femur in its original position (Figs. 5.10 and 5.11). Partial weight bearing was started at 4 weeks and full weight bearing at 12 weeks postoperatively. Good bone remodeling of the osteotomy site is observed at 6–12 months (Fig. 5.12).

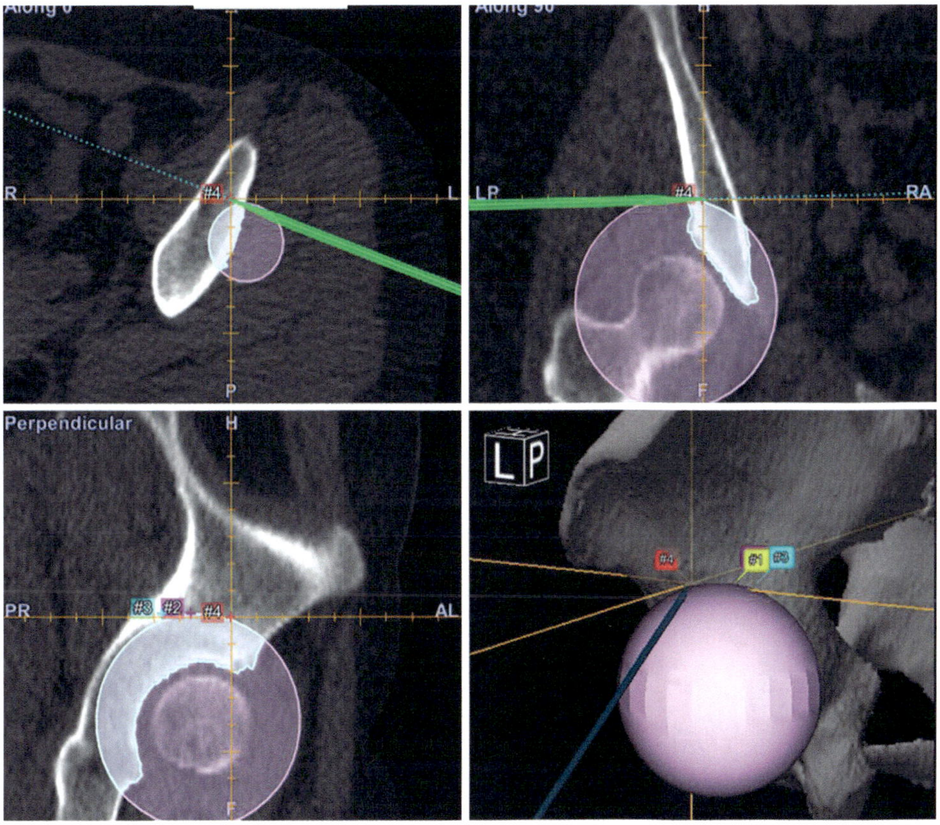

Fig. 5.7 The navigation monitor displays the position and direction of the osteotome tip on the three orthogonal CT reconstructed views and 3D view with the osteotomy plan

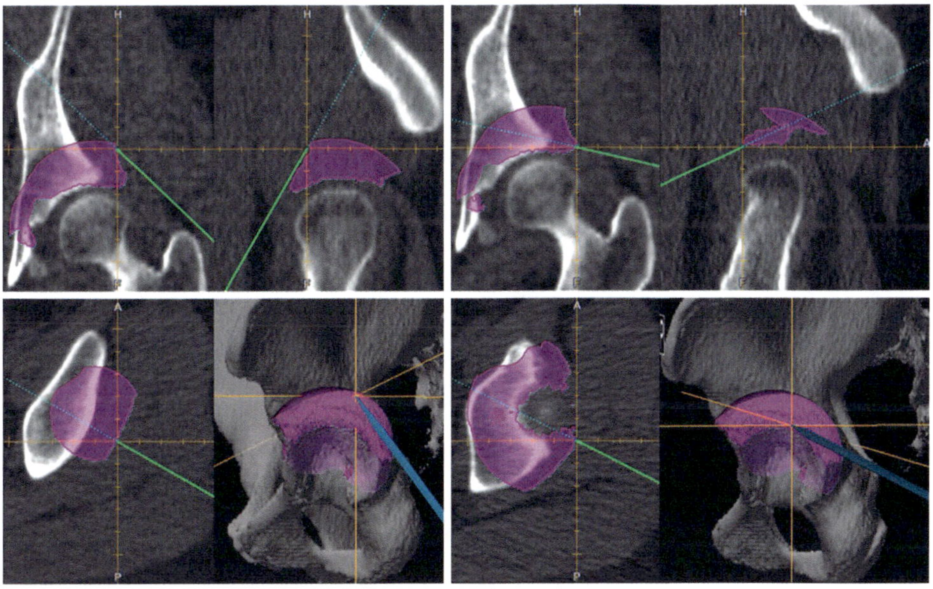

Fig. 5.8 The position of the rotated acetabulum is confirmed with a pointer by touching multiple surface points around the acetabulum

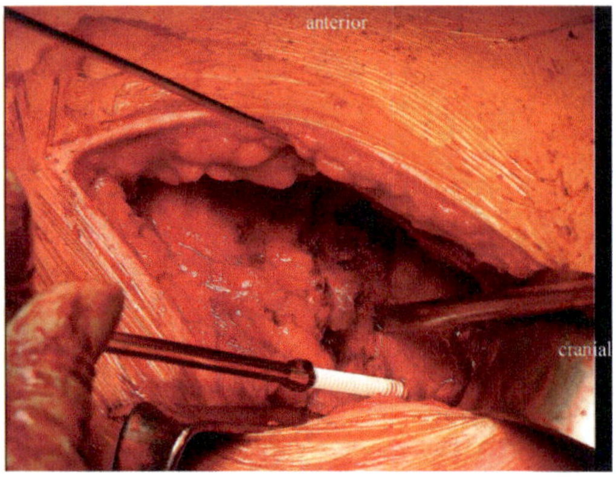

Fig. 5.9 After temporal fixation of the fragment with a Kirschner wire, the acetabular fragment is rigidly fixed with resorbable screws made from a composite of poly-L-lactic acid and hydroxyapatite granules

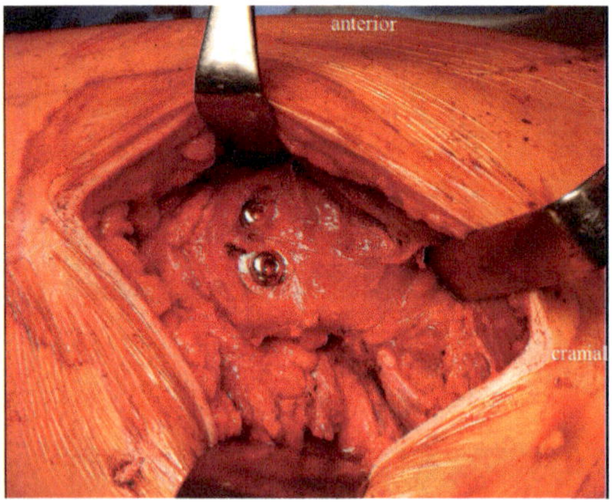

Fig. 5.10 The greater trochanter is relocated and rigidly fixed with two AO large cancellous screws with washers

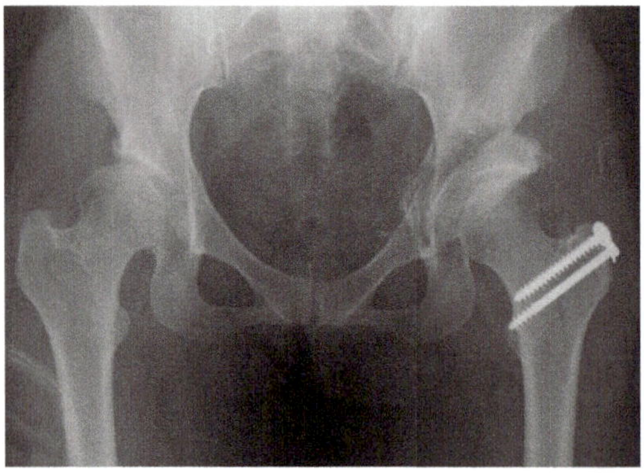

Fig. 5.11 An AP radiograph of the pelvis immediately after RAO

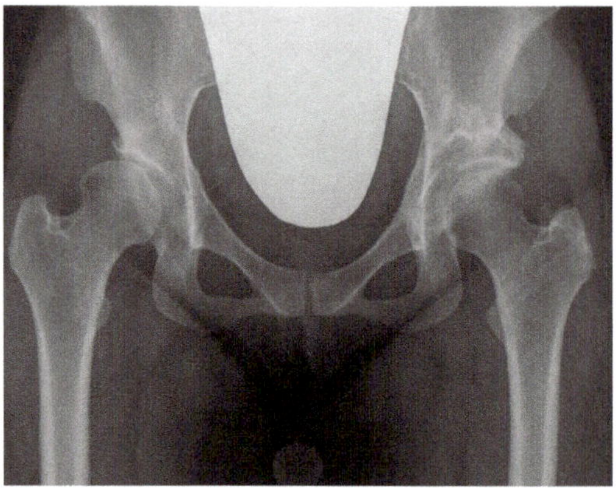

Fig. 5.12 An AP radiograph of the pelvis 2 years after RAO. The cancellous screws have been removed and good remodeling of the osteotomy site is seen

5.4 Outcomes of Our Initial Case Series

Radiographic measurements in the initial 36 hips in 29 cases with symptomatic hip dysplasia who underwent RAO showed that the level of the osteotomy from the articular surface ranged from 15 to 20 mm with an average of 16 mm ± 1.3 mm (SD). No fragmentation or cracking of the acetabulum due to intra-articular osteotome perforation was identified. The average center-edge angle improved significantly from 1° on preoperative radiographs to 34° on the immediate postoperative radiographs ($p < 0.001$). There was one hip which showed less than 20° of postoperative CE angle. The average acetabular roof angle and the head lateralization index also improved significantly ($p < 0.001$ and $p = 0.046$, respectively).

All patients were followed up for a minimum of 2 years with a mean follow-up of 8 years. There were no complications such as infection, nonunion, avascular necrosis, nor neurovascular injuries. The Merle d'Aubigné and Postel hip score [21] improved from 13.7 preoperatively to 16.9 at the latest follow-up. Radiographically, progression of joint space narrowing was found in one hip. The remaining cases showed no progression of osteoarthritis. No hip was converted to total hip arthroplasty at 10 years.

5.5 Discussion

Langlotz et al. first developed navigation for PAO [12] and their visualization aids worked well in a series of 14 hips [13]. They suggested that the system was able to help reduce potential risk and thus increase safety and accuracy for this difficult class of surgical interventions. On the other hand, a randomized control study of 18 hips in each group which compared navigation and conventional techniques of periacetabular osteotomy showed no significant differences in radiological parameters nor clinical scores [15]. They concluded that the use of this image-guided technique in periacetabular osteotomy is often unnecessary when an experienced surgeon performs the surgery. However, their navigation system did not show preoperative planning superimposed on the bone model data and only the tip of the osteotome was shown as a line on the monitor. Therefore, the small number of cases and navigation with a primitive user interface without preoperative planning may have failed to show the benefits. Preoperative planning is a major benefit of CT-based navigation and RAO could be undergone safely and accurately even by surgeons who seldom perform pelvic osteotomies [11].

Our initial experience confirms that CT-based navigation for RAO achieves a high level of precision in cutting the periacetabulum with a minimum thickness of 15 mm without intraoperative X-rays. Moreover, navigation helps surgeons to intraoperatively evaluate the position of the reorientated acetabulum by landmark point matching, leading to significant postoperative improvements in the CE angle, the acetabular roof angle, and the head lateralization index. However, there is still a variation in the postoperative CE angle, even though preoperative planning is aimed at a CE angle of 30°. This means the landmark matching technique to evaluate the position of the reorientated acetabulum is not as accurate as real-time tracking of the navigated osteotome. An additional tool to track the acetabular fragment such as a fiducial marker or a tracker should improve the accuracy of reorientation.

In conclusion, CT-based navigation for RAO is safe and accurate showing substantial clinical improvements in patients with symptomatic hip dysplasia. The cutting of the periacetabulum under CT-based navigation maintains a 15 mm minimum thickness of the acetabular fragment which prevents ischemic necrosis of the fragment while eliminating intra-articular penetration by the osteotome so that it can reduce the risk for reoperation.

References

1. Eppright RH. Dial osteotomy of the acetabulum in the treatment of dysplasia of the hip. J Bone Joint Surg. 1975;57-A:1172.
2. Wagner H. Osteotomies for congenital hip dislocation. In: The hip. Proceedings of the Fourth Open Scientific Meeting of the Hip Society. St Louis: CV Mosby; 1976. p. 45–66.
3. Ganz R, Klaue K, Vinh TS, Mast JW. A new periacetabular osteotomy for the treatment of hip dysplasias. Technique and preliminary results. Clin Orthop. 1988;232:26–36.
4. Ninomiya S, Tagawa H. Rotational acetabular osteotomy for the dysplastic hip. J Bone Joint Surg Am. 1984;66:430–6.
5. Yasunaga Y, Ochi M, Yamasaki T, Shoji T, Izumi S. Rotational acetabular osteotomy for pre- and early osteoarthritis secondary to dysplasia provides durable results at 20 years. Clin Orthop Relat Res. 2016;474(10):2145–53.
6. Ninomiya S. Rotational acetabular osteotomy for the severely dysplastic hip in the adolescent and adult. Clin Orthop. 1989;247:127–37.
7. Matsui M, Masuhara K, Nakata K, Nishii T, Sugano N, Ochi T. Early deterioration after modified rotational acetabular osteotomy for the dysplastic hip. J Bone Joint Surg Br. 1997;79:220–4.
8. Nakamura S, Ninomiya S, Takatori Y, Morimoto S, Umeyama T. Long-term outcome of rotational acetabular osteotomy: 145 hips followed for 10-23 years. Acta Orthop. 1998;69:259–65.
9. Nakahodo K, Sasama T, Sato Y, Sugano N, Ohzono K, Nishii T, Nishihara S, Yonenobu K, Ochi T, Tamura S. Intraoperative update of 3D bone model during computer navigation of pelvic osteotomies using real-time 3D position data. In: Lemke H, Vannier M, Inamura K, Farman A, Doi K, editors. Computer assisted radiology and surgery. 14th International Symposium and Exhibition (CARS 2000), San Francisco, CA. Amsterdam: Elsevier; 2000. p. 252–6.
10. Koyama T, Sugano N, Nishii T, Miki H, Sato Y, Yoshikawa H, Tamura S. Computer-assisted spherical

osteotomy with a curved-bladed Tuke Saw. Comput Aided Surg. 2006;11(4):202–8.
11. Takao M, Nishii T, Sakai T, Sugano N. Comparison of rotational acetabular osteotomy performed with navigation by surgeons with different levels of experience of osteotomies. Int J Comput Assist Radiol Surg. 2017;12(5):841–53.
12. Langlotz F, Stucki M, Bachler R, Scheer C, Ganz R, Berlemann U, Nolte LP. The first twelve cases of computer assisted periacetabular osteotomy. Comput Aided Surg. 1997;2(6):317–26.
13. Langlotz F, Bachler R, Berlemann U, Nolte LP, Ganz R. Computer assistance for pelvic osteotomies. Clin Orthop Relat Res. 1998;354:92–102.
14. Mayman DJ, Rudan J, Yach J, Ellis R. The Kingston periacetabular osteotomy utilizing computer enhancement: a new technique. Comput Aided Surg. 2002;7(3):179–86.
15. Hsieh PH, Chang YH, Shih CH. Image-guided periacetabular osteotomy: computer-assisted navigation compared with the conventional technique: a randomized study of 36 patients followed for 2 years. Acta Orthop. 2006;77(4):591–7.
16. Hamada H, Takao M, Nakahara I, Sakai T, Nishii T, Sugano N. Hip range-of-motion (ROM) is less than normal after rotational acetabular osteotomy for developmental dysplasia of the hip: a simulated ROM analysis. J Orthop Res. 2016;34(2):217–23.
17. Nakahara I, Takao M, Sakai T, Nishii T, Yoshikawa H, Sugano N. Gender differences in 3D morphology and bony impingement of human hips. J Orthop Res. 2011;29(3):333–9.
18. Nakahara I, Takao M, Sakai T, Miki H, Nishii T, Sugano N. Three-dimensional morphology and bony range of movement in hip joints in patients with hip dysplasia. Bone Joint J. 2014;96-B(5):580–9.
19. Hamada H, Takao M, Sakai T, Sugano N. Morphological variation of the anterior inferior iliac spine affects hip range of motion in flexion after rotational acetabular osteotomy. Int Orthop. 2018;42(6):1247–52.
20. Sugano N, Sasama T, Sato Y, Nakajima Y, Nishii T, Yonenobu K, Tamura S, Ochi T. Accuracy evaluation of surface-based registration methods in a computer navigation system for hip surgery performed through a posterolateral approach. Comput Aided Surg. 2001;6:195–203.
21. Merle d'Aubigné R, Postel M. Functional results of hip arthroplasty with acrylic prosthesis. J Bone Joint Surg Am. 1954;36:451–75.

Part III

Arthroscopy of the Hip

Hip Arthroscopy and Impingement

6

Jin-Woo Kim, Tae-Young Kim, Yong-Chan Ha,
and Taek-Rim Yoon

Hip arthroscopy was initially described in 1931, and then it has been gaining popularity in the medical field only since the 1980s [1]. There was a significant increase in the number of cases reported by ABOS (American Board of Orthopaedic Surgery) candidates from 2003 to 2009 and a larger increase between 2006 and 2010. There has also been a sharp increase in the number of reports of hip arthroscopy in the literature in this period as well.

The use of hip arthroscopy was initially limited due to the technical difficulties presented by the anatomy of the hip joint, which, compared with other joints, presents additional challenges due to the thick soft-tissue envelope, the constrained bony anatomy, the proximity of neurovascular structures, and a lack of instrumentation capable of handling the depth of the joint. Several papers have described a learning curve for hip arthroscopy, and a recent review showed that complications and operating time decrease after about 30 cases of arthroscopic surgery [2].

The development of specific instrumentation, improved techniques in exposure, and patient positioning have allowed for greater accessibility to the joint and have expanded the indications for the procedure.

Indications for hip arthroscopy with intra-articular pathology include labral tears, removal of loose bodies, femoroacetabular impingement (FAI), chondral lesions, synovial diseases, ligamentum teres injuries, adhesive capsulitis [3], capsular laxity and instability, septic arthritis, and osteoarthritis. Indications for hip arthroscopy with extra-articular pathology include greater trochanteric pain syndrome, snapping hip syndrome, extra-articular femoroacetabular impingement such as ischiofemoral impingement, or subspine impingement.

A successful outcome from arthroscopic surgery of the hip requires careful patient selection and recognition of technical factors that may preclude the procedure or compromise clinical outcomes.

The relative contraindications that surgeons should be cautious include moderate osteoarthritis, dysplasia, inflammatory arthritis, neurological injury, chronic proximal hamstring avulsion, chronic abductor avulsion with severe retraction and fatty atrophy, and internal snapping hip with

J.-W. Kim
Department of Orthopaedic Surgery, Eulji Medical Center, Eulji University College of Medicine, Seoul, South Korea

T.-Y. Kim
Department of Orthopaedic Surgery, Konkuk University Medical Center, School of Medicine, Konkuk University, Seoul, South Korea

Y.-C. Ha
Department of Orthopaedic Surgery, Chung-Ang University College of Medicine, Seoul, South Korea

T.-R. Yoon (✉)
Center for Joint Disease, Chonnam National University Hwasun Hospital, Jeonnam, South Korea

W. R. Drescher et al. (eds.), *Advances in Specialist Hip Surgery*,
https://doi.org/10.1007/978-3-030-61830-8_6

severe femoral neck anteversion. The absolute contraindications of hip arthroscopy include advanced osteoarthritis, severe proximal femoral deformity (Legg-Calvé-Perthes disease, slipped capital femoral epiphysis) necessitating an osteotomy, ankylosis, dysplasia with femoral head migration, greater trochanteric impingement, and severe acetabular retroversion.

There is also good evidence demonstrating inferior outcomes and a higher rate of conversion to total hip arthroplasty when radiographic joint space is less than 2 mm [4, 5]. Therefore, care should be taken to evaluate the radiographic degree of osteoarthritis within the affected hip. Studies have shown worse results in patients with preexisting osteoarthritis of the hip [6]. Severe ankylosis of the joint is an important absolute contraindication because arthroscopic instruments cannot be safely used if the hip cannot be distracted or distended, although many of the hip joint problems are associated with some degree of ankylosis and it can be distracted enough for arthroscopic procedure. Dysplastic features with femoral head migration (>1 cm lateral or break in Shenton's line) indicate more global structural instability, and arthroscopic treatment alone should be avoided. Symptomatic greater trochanteric impingement is best treated via open approaches that include relative femoral neck lengthening and/or greater trochanter distalization. Finally, anterior rim resection in the presence of severe acetabular retroversion may exacerbate instability (from a posteriorly deficient acetabulum); thus, an anteverting periacetabular osteotomy (PAO) will be a better choice.

6.1 Operative Setup

The preferred position of patients for hip arthroscopy is either supine or lateral. Each surgeon has their preferences.

The supine position is more frequently used because of surgeon's familiarity of the anatomy and easier usage of the fracture table. In obese patients, the lateral position is usually recommended. However, the lateral position needs special distraction devices in addition to the operating table. In patients with large anterolateral bone spurs, the joint can be easily entered through the posterior peritrochanteric portal.

Proper traction is important for access to the joint, as well as for procedures involving the intra-articular portion or central compartment of the hip. The placement of 4.5 or 5.5 mm cannulas needs 10–12 mm of distraction (Fig. 6.1). Time for traction should not exceed 2 h to decrease the

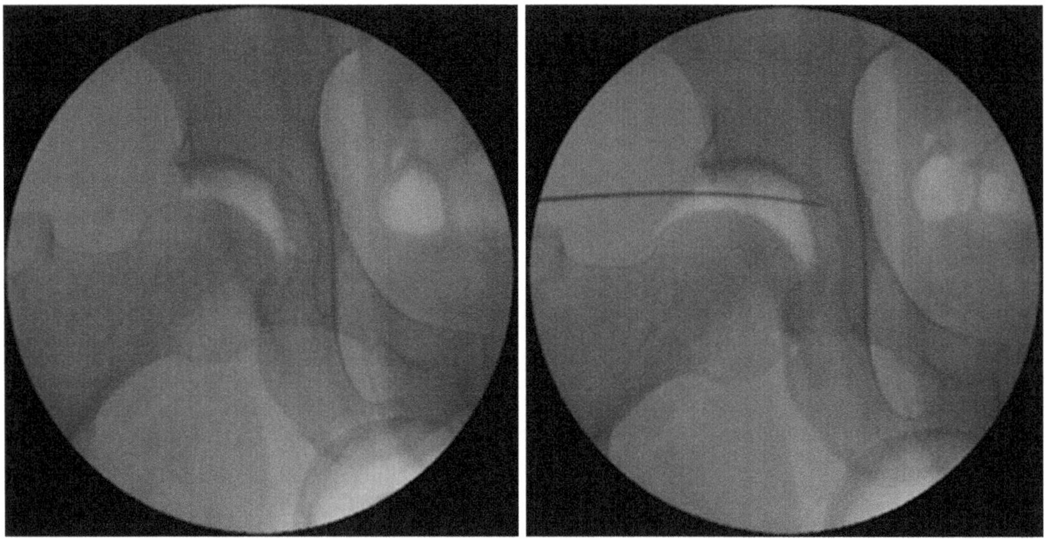

Fig. 6.1 Fluoroscopic images after joint traction and air arthrogram using a spinal needle placed into the hip joint

chance of traction neurapraxia. A well-padded, usually oversized perineal post is also helpful. The laterally placed perineal post improves the vector of the traction force and decreases the risk of neurapraxia.

The 70-degree arthroscope is used for most central compartment procedures and the 30-degree arthroscope is used for labral repair and peripheral compartment procedures.

Three standard portals (anterolateral, anterior, and posterolateral) have been used for most hip arthroscopy. Some surgeons prefer modified portals or two portals depending on their experiences (Fig. 6.2).

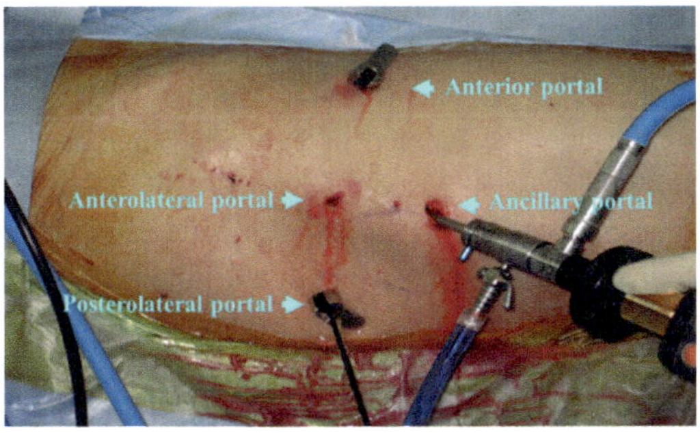

Fig. 6.2 Intraoperative photograph showing the portals which are anterior, anterolateral, posterolateral, and ancillary

The anterolateral portal is usually placed first under the fluoroscopic guidance. This portal is made approximately 1 cm superior and anterior to the anterior edge of the greater trochanter. The posterolateral and anterior portals are made under direct visualization with the camera in the anterolateral portal. The posterolateral portal is made 1 cm posterior and superior to the greater trochanter. The anterior portal is placed by the intersection of a line drawn from the tip of the greater trochanter and a line extending inferiorly from the anterior superior iliac spine.

Some resisted feeling to place an anterolateral portal requires to be inspected to be sure that there has not been inadvertent penetration of the labrum because the anterolateral portal is made without direct visualization (Fig. 6.3). Several additional accessory portals can be made depending on the procedure.

When two portals are used, it is better to make a midlateral portal and anterior portal. Midlateral portal is made just above the tip of the greater trochanter. Anterior portal is made 1.5–2 cm distal and lateral to the anterosuperior iliac spine. Viewing portal and working portal can be used interchangeably (Fig. 6.4).

The anatomy of neurovascular structures around each portal should be understood. The

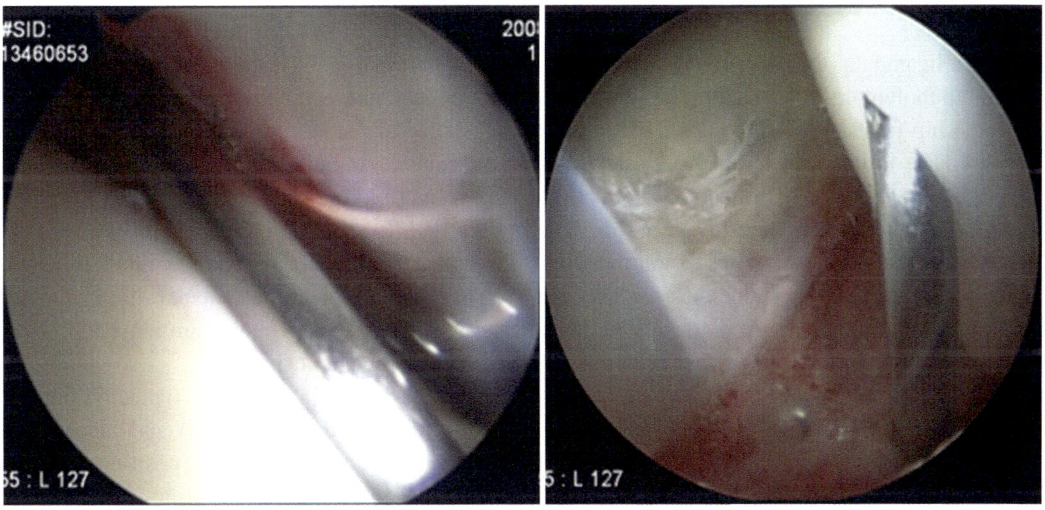

Fig. 6.3 Arthroscopic image of the initial view through the anterolateral portal showing the anterior triangle and placing anterior portal using spinal needle and arthroscopic image from the anterolateral portal demonstrating spinal needle localization of the posterolateral portal

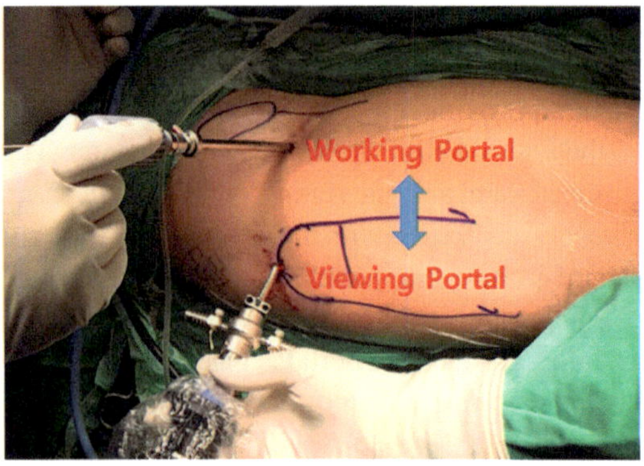

Fig. 6.4 Intraoperative photograph showing the viewing and working portal

nearest neurovascular structure for the anterolateral and midlateral portal is the superior gluteal nerve. The anterior portal passes close to the lateral femoral cutaneous nerve and ascending branch of the lateral femoral circumflex artery. The closest neurovascular structure around the posterolateral portal is the sciatic nerve. A cadaver study determined the distances of the arthroscopic portals to neurovascular structures: the anterolateral portal is 6 cm from the superior gluteal nerve and 4 cm from the sciatic nerve, the posterolateral portal lies 2.2 cm from the sciatic nerve, and the anterior portal is 1.5 cm from the lateral femoral cutaneous nerve, although several branches of this nerve may be closer [7].

Three ligaments (the iliofemoral, ischiofemoral, and pubofemoral) around the hip joint compose the hip joint capsule and contribute to hip stability. The iliofemoral ligament resists external rotation of the hip. The ischiofemoral ligament is a restraint to internal rotation. The pubofemoral ligament also helps to control external rotation. Because of the thickness of this ligament, capsulotomy is usually performed to allow increased maneuverability and increased visualization of certain pathologies. There was controversy about the repair of capsulotomy. However, the entire capsulotomy should be repaired if instability of hip joint is suspected. Several studies have shown an increase in external rotation after capsulotomy, which returns to normal with repair. Another recent study showed improved patient outcomes when the entire T-capsulotomy was repaired compared with partial repair with only the vertical limb repaired [8].

6.2 Labral Tears

The acetabular labrum is a ring of fibrocartilage that acts as a suction seal to ensure continuous lubrication of the hip joint and improve joint stability and kinematics by distributing contact forces and deepening the hip joint.

In the presence of a labral tear, this latter function is lost and may lead to increased contact pressure, which is thought to have a role in the development of degenerative disease. In a study of 436 patients, 73% of those with labral tears or fraying had articular damage, with most of the damage located in the same zone as the labral damage. Also, the severity of chondral damage was greater in patients with labral tears than in patients who had an intact labrum. During surgical treatment of labral tears, the labrum is typically debrided or repaired based on tear pattern and healing potential. Labral pathology most commonly occurs along the anterior and superior acetabular margins, but the location typically reflects the areas of mechanical conflict between femoral and acetabular pathomorphology [9].

Two types of labral injuries were suggested as a separation of the labrum from its articular attachment and tears in various planes within the substance of the labrum. Morphologies of labral tear include radial flap tears, radial fibrillated tears, longitudinal peripheral tears, and unstable tears [10] (Fig. 6.5).

Labral-chondral separation is more common with cam-type femoroacetabular impingement, whereas intrasubstance tears are more typical of pincer impingement (Fig. 6.6).

Patients with labral tears typically present with pain (usually groin pain) and mechanical symptoms. Pain may be positional, with symptoms increasing with sitting, driving, putting on shoes, or crossing the legs.

The typical test for labrum is the impingement test. The patient lies down on the examination

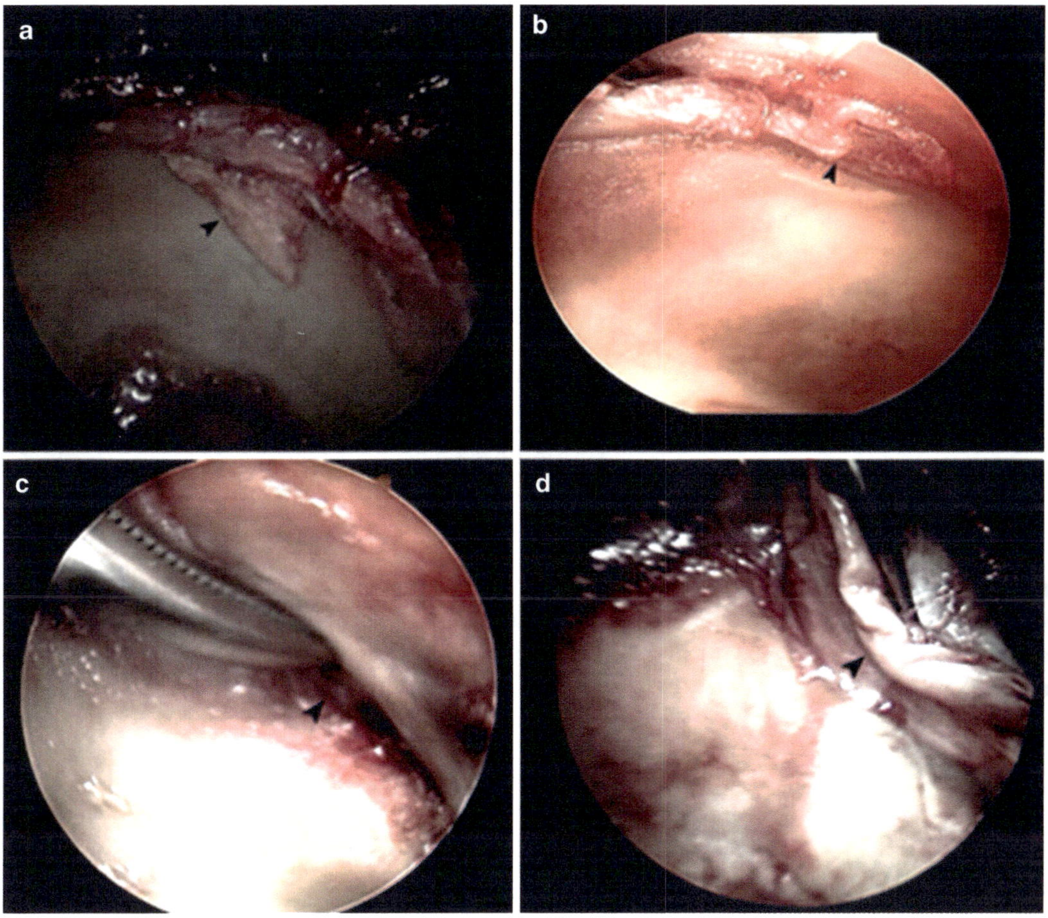

Fig. 6.5 Labral tear classification. (**a**) Type 1: radial flap tear, with disruption of the free margin of the labrum with the consequent formation of a discrete flap, in the 1- to 2-o'clock area (arrowhead). (**b**) Type 2: radial fibrillated tear, with a hairy appearance at the free margin of the labrum, in the 11- to 1-o'clock area (arrowhead). (**c**) Type 3: longitudinal peripheral tear, along the acetabular insertion of the labrum, in the 12- to 3-o'clock area (arrowhead). (**d**) Type 4: unstable tear, with subluxating labra, in the 1- to 3-o'clock area (arrowhead)

table. The examiner bends the hip fully and provokes the contact between labrum and proximal femur. Pain or discomfort provoked with this examination strongly suggests labral tear. Patrick's test is another sign for labral tear. Limitation of range of motion (ROM) is a sign for labral tear that has been undiagnosed for a longer time.

Radiographs of the pelvis and hip should be taken for diagnosis of the labral tear. Sometimes radiographs for the lumbar spine may be necessary to differentiate the spinal diseases.

CT (computed tomography) offers greater detail in bony architecture. Magnetic resonance imaging (MRI) can be used for diagnosing labral tear and some other soft-tissue diseases. The best diagnostic tool for labral tear is MR arthrography (MRA).

Initial management is usually conservative, with rest, anti-inflammatory agents, and physical therapy. Persistent pain after conservative treatment is treated with labral debridement or repair.

The objectives of labral preservation are to treat the resultant symptoms and restore the hip seal and stability. In addition, labral repair is performed with the goal of preventing the premature development of arthritis, which has been shown to correlate with labral tears [11].

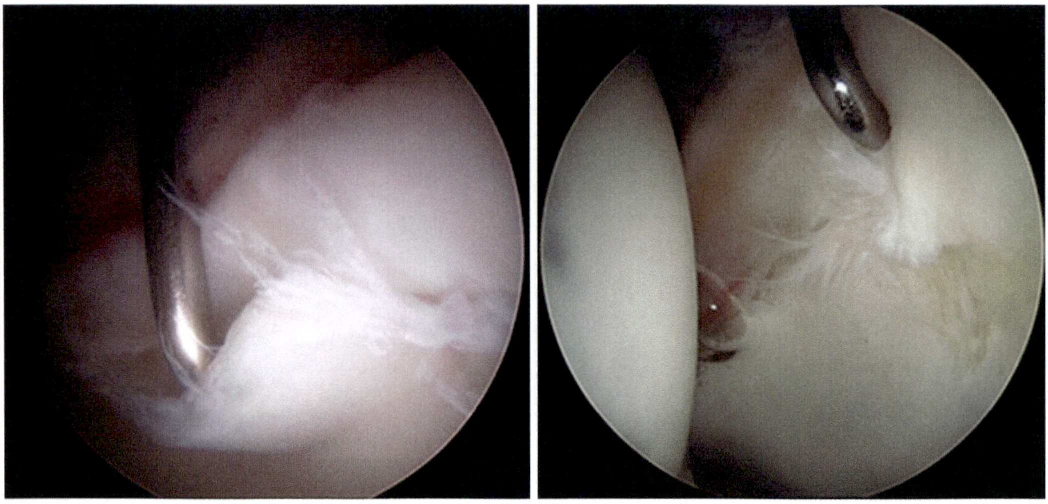

Fig. 6.6 Labral-chondral in cam-type and intrasubstance tears in pincer-type FAI

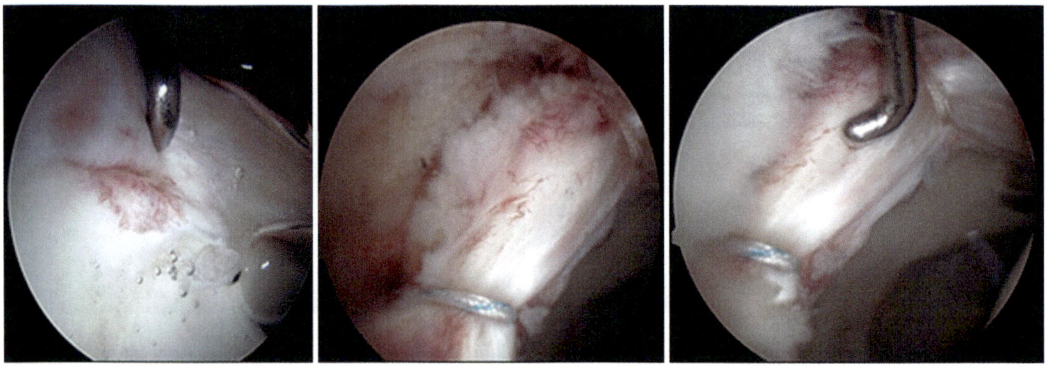

Fig. 6.7 Arthroscopic images of labral tear and suture configuration after labral repair

Konan et al. [12] analyzed 1631 hips in 1609 patients in a review of 28 studies. Among them, 12 studies reported good results of 82% (67–100%) for labral debridement. Five studies reported a comparison between reattachment and debridement. Four studies reported better results with reattachment and one study reported no difference. In this review, they were not able to draw accurate conclusions because of selection bias, use of historical controls, and high rates of follow-up loss.

It is logical to debride the degenerative labrum because torn labrum is a source of discomfort and pain, and to repair good-quality labrum with good potential to heal because physiological function can be preserved.

The choice of suture configuration during labral repair is based on the quality of the labral tissue remaining (Fig. 6.7). In patients with robust labral tissue, a labral base repair is recommended. When the labrum is significantly frayed, a circumferential repair is considered to avoid laceration of the remaining labrum by the suture. In either type of repair, it is important to maintain the labral contact with the femoral head, reestablishing the suction seal. It should be remembered that anchors placed too far from the acetabular rim or sutures that are overtightened may evert the labral edge.

6.3 Femoroacetabular Impingement

Femoroacetabular impingement (FAI) is a form of abnormal bony morphology in which the proximal femur contacts the acetabulum with abnormal contact to the labrum during terminal motion. This abnormal contact leads to damage of the acetabular labrum and articular cartilage and may lead to what was previously thought of as idiopathic osteoarthritis of the hip.

FAI is classified as the following three types: cam impingement in which the abnormal contact is due to an aspherical femoral head, pincer impingement from acetabular overcoverage or retroversion, and combined impingement, which has elements of pincer and cam. Cam impingement is most common in young males, but pincer impingement is most common in middle-aged women.

Cam impingement results from a nonspherical femoral head, with decreased head-neck offset, abutting against the acetabulum. The impingement usually occurs in flexion and results in a shearing of the articular surface and avulsion of the labrum (Fig. 6.8).

Pincer impingement results from abnormal contact between the acetabular rim and the femoral head-neck junction caused by acetabular overcoverage, which may be global (in coxa profunda), or more focal in the anterosuperior acetabulum (in acetabular retroversion). This

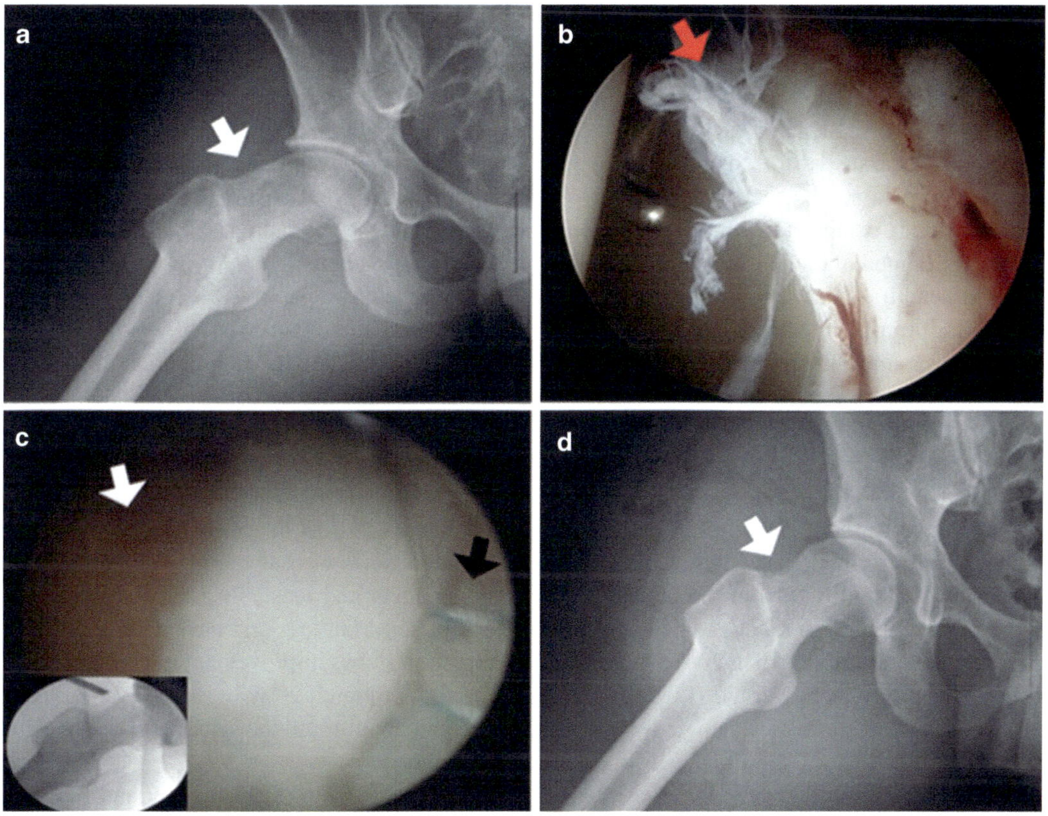

Fig. 6.8 Cam lesion and labral tear in a 20-year-old man. (**a**) The cam lesion (white arrow) was seen on the preoperative modified Dunn view. (**b**) The labral tear lesion was seen through the arthroscope (red arrow). (**c**) Arthroscopic labral repair (black arrow) and femoroplasty (white arrow) were done under C-arm image intensifier guidance. (**d**) Postoperative plain film in modified Dunn view showing proper correction (white arrow) of the cam lesion

abnormal contact causes intrasubstance tears of the labrum. In worsening pincer impingement, the femoral head can be levered from the acetabular socket, causing chondral damage in the posteroinferior acetabulum (contrecoup injury). Cam and pincer impingement usually exist together in most cases.

Patients with femoroacetabular impingement often complain of groin pain with an insidious onset. Pain is usually positional: for example the patients may complain of pain while sitting, driving, or putting on socks and shoes.

Posture and gait of the patients are first examined. An impingement test may reproduce the patient's pain: with the patient supine and the hip flexed as much as possible, the hip is adducted and internally rotated or the hip is abducted and externally rotated.

Radiographic evaluation begins with plain radiographs, which may include anteroposterior pelvic, false profile, cross-table lateral, frog-leg lateral, and Dunn views of the hip. The acetabulum is assessed for coxa profunda, acetabular protrusion, or acetabular retroversion. Coxa profunda is indicated when the acetabular teardrop lies medial to the ilioischial line. If the femoral head lies medial to the ilioischial line, acetabular protrusion is indicated. With acetabular retroversion, the anterior wall crosses lateral to the posterior wall, creating a "crossover sign." Certain measurements can be used to assess acetabular coverage. The center-edge angle is the angle formed between a line that is perpendicular to the transverse axis of the pelvis that passes through the center of the femoral head and a second line from the center of the femoral head to the lateral edge of the acetabular sourcil. Values of less than 20–25° may indicate acetabular undercoverage (Fig. 6.9). Any preoperative osteoarthritic changes of the hip are noted. On all views, femoral head sphericity and femoral head-neck offset are evaluated. The alpha angle is determined on lateral radiographs. This angle is formed by a line through the center of the femoral head and neck and a second line from the center of the femoral head to the point where the femoral head radius exits a concentric circle drawn around the femoral head. An alpha angle of more than 50° is typical in hips with loss of sphericity (Fig. 6.10).

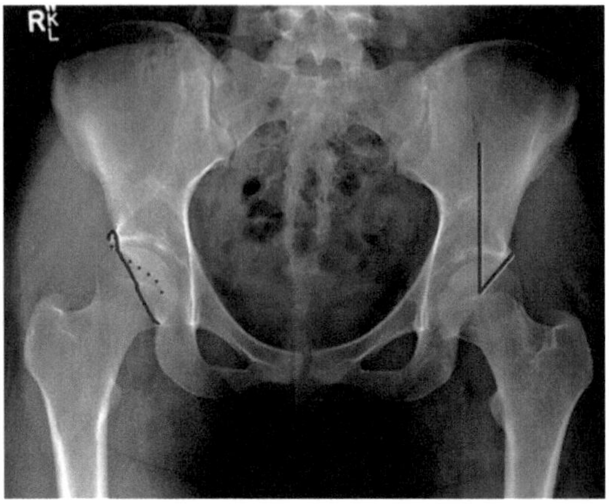

Fig. 6.9 AP pelvis X-ray demonstrating acetabular retroversion creating crossover sign (right hip) and center-edge angle (left hip)

CT may help further define bony anatomy. MRI is used to assess labral and chondral injuries.

All existing FAI is not associated with the groin pain. A review by Frank et al. documented a 37% incidence of radiographic FAI in asymptomatic individuals [13]. Asymptomatic FAI is not indicated for operative treatment. Treatment of symptomatic FAI is initially conservative, which includes activity modification, nonsteroidal anti-inflammatory drugs (NSAIDs), and physical therapy. Patients who do not respond to conservative treatment may be the indication for surgical treatment. The goal of arthroscopic treatment is to treat labral pathology and chondral damage, as well as to remove sites of bony impingement and reestablish the femoral head-neck offset. Many reports have shown that FAI correction shows improvement in pain and function [14–16] and 90% of high-level athletes were able to return to the same level of competition [17].

After surgery, physical therapy and range of motion are begun in the first 24–48 h and a stationary bike can be used immediately. Patients are encouraged to tolerable weight bearing in pincer removal or are limited to touchdown weight bearing for 2–4 weeks in cases with cam removal depending on the degree of removal.

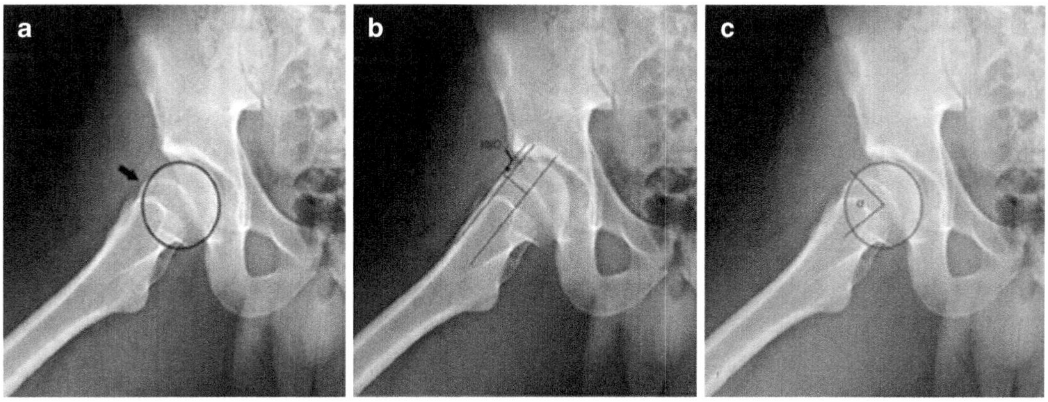

Fig. 6.10 Modified Dunn 45-degree lateral views of the right hip demonstrating (**a**) bony bump of femoral head, (**b**) femoral head-neck offset, and (**c**) an alpha angle

Aggressive range of motion is avoided for several weeks and impact activities are not recommended for 2–3 months. Return to sports may take 4–6 months.

6.4 Labral Reconstruction

Sometimes the labrum is too damaged to repair or may be absent which may be seen in a primary or a revision setting. A cadaver study demonstrated an increase in joint contact forces with decreased contact areas after resection of the labrum [18]. Reconstructing the labrum did reverse some of these changes.

Allografts and autografts can be used. The source of grafts includes iliotibial band (ITB), gracilis tendon [19], semitendinosus [20], quadriceps tendon [21], and ligamentum teres [22], among others. Allograft techniques using tibialis anterior [23] and ITB and hamstring tendon [24] have also been described.

In young and active patients, labral reconstruction may help to provide some protection to the hip joint. The choices of graft include the iliotibial band, gracilis, and ligamentum teres. The technique involves side-to-side repair with the native labrum and repair of the graft to the acetabular rim with anchors placed 1 cm apart. Labral reconstruction has shown increased patient satisfaction and improved hip scores [25].

Physical therapy is necessary to restore passive followed by active motion and then strength. It is essential for patients to perform passive circumduction motions of the hip as soon after arthroscopy as possible to prevent capsular adhesions. When labral resection was compared to labral reconstruction in similarly matched groups, in some categories patient-reported outcomes in the reconstruction group were significantly better than those in the resection group even though both groups showed improvement [20].

6.5 Greater Trochanteric Pain Syndrome

Greater trochanteric pain syndrome (GTPS) is a regional pain syndrome characterized by chronic, intermittent pain accompanied by tenderness of the lateral proximal thigh, involving the greater trochanter (GT) area and the buttock [26, 27].

Causes of greater trochanteric pain syndrome range from bursitis to partial- or full-thickness tears of the abductor tendon. It was higher in women and patients with coexisting low back pain, osteoarthritis, ITB tenderness, and obesity [28].

Weakness may also be present in patients with abductor tendon pathology. Initial treatments are activity modification, physical therapy, nonsteroidal anti-inflammatory medication, and trochanteric steroidal injections. An MRI can be useful to determine the integrity of the abductor tendon in patients with persistent pain or weakness. Arthroscopic tendon repair may be indicated in these patients. Short-term follow-up studies demonstrate improvement in symptoms, strength, and patient satisfaction after tendon repair [29–31].

6.6 Snapping Hip

There are various causes of snapping hip. Intra-articular pathology (labral tears, FAI, or loose bodies) may cause a sensation of snapping or popping in the hip. External snapping hip occurs when the iliotibial band snaps over the greater trochanter when the hip moves between flexion and extension. The snapping may be painless and no treatment is usually needed. Internal snapping hip occurs when the psoas tendon snaps over the iliopectineal eminence, femoral head, or a prominent acetabular component after total hip arthroplasty. Internal snapping typically is reproduced when the flexed, externally rotated hip is brought into extension and internal rotation.

Initial treatment typically is nonsurgical and consists of physical therapy, anti-inflammatory medication, and steroid injection for painful external or internal snapping hips. Surgical release may be indicated if conservative treatment fails. For external snapping hips, an arthroscopic release of the iliotibial band is performed. For internal snapping hips, an arthroscopic release of the psoas tendon at the lesser trochanter or at the level of the hip joint is also performed (Fig. 6.11).

The psoas tendon typically is released at the end of the surgical procedure to prevent fluid extravasation into the retroperitoneal space.

Continued pain and hip flexor weakness are some of the most worrisome potential complications.

Risk of hip flexor weakness may be less in the central approach; however, in contrast to the peripheral approach, there is a greater risk of anterior thigh paresthesia due to femoral nerve branches lying directly over the iliopsoas muscle and a branch of the lateral femoral cutaneous nerve, which lies in close proximity to the location of the anterior portal [32–35].

A recent review showed that there were fewer complications and less postoperative pain associated with arthroscopic release compared with open procedures [36, 37].

6.7 Complications of Hip Arthroscopy

Hip arthroscopy, although less invasive, presents significant challenges to the arthroscopist and has a complication rate that ranges from 0.41 to 7.5% [38–40]. Most common complications are traction neurapraxia which affects the femoral, sciatic, pudendal, or lateral femoral cutaneous nerves. Injury to the femoral nerve and common peroneal nerve may also occur from traction, and in the case of the femoral nerve, iatrogenic injury

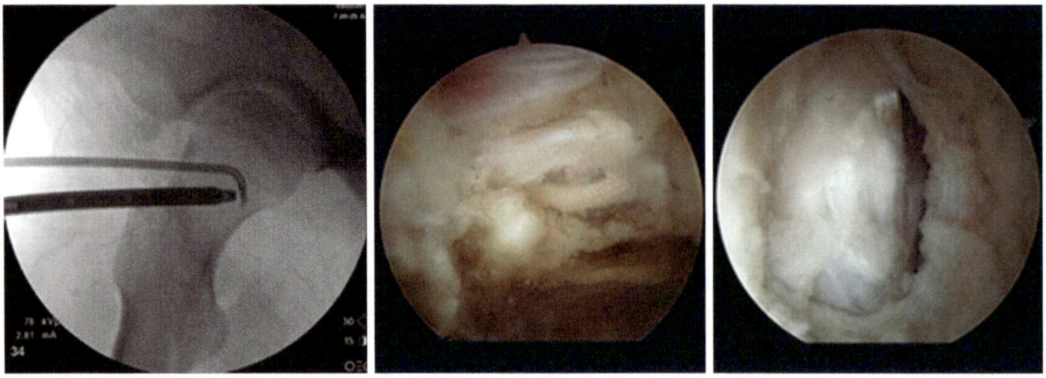

Fig. 6.11 Fluoroscopic and arthroscopic images of psoas tendon release for internal snapping hip

can occur from excessive medial portal placement or during repair of a torn labrum and/or pincer resection. The lateral femoral cutaneous nerve may be damaged if the anterior portal is placed too far medially. Excessive traction may also cause pressure damage to the perineal areas. The risk of permanent nerve injury is low after hip arthroscopy and may be limited to 1% of cases [40].

Vascular injury, although rare, may occur after hip arthroscopy. Injury to the inferior gluteal artery from laceration or pseudoaneurysm and occlusion at the ankle from a traction boot have been reported in the literature [40]. Injury to the lateral epiphyseal branch of the medial femoral circumflex artery can occur with femoral osteoplasty and may result in avascular necrosis (AVN) of the femoral head, requiring hip replacement. To avoid the neurovascular complication, traction time should be documented and limited whenever possible and the least amount of traction necessary to adequately distract the joint should be applied. Newer perineal posts have abundant padding and should be used against the perineum during traction. Surgeon should avoid femoral osteoplasty beyond the lateral synovial fold without directly visualizing and protecting the superior retinacular vessels and also avoid high intra-articular pump pressures during arthroscopy (50 mmHg pump pressure is typically adequate for visualization).

Scuffing of the articular surfaces and iatrogenic damage to the labrum may occur during placement of the initial anterolateral portal, as this portal is not made under direct visualization. Patients with difficult distraction, osteoarthritis, and profunda or protrusio deformity have been shown to be at higher risk of iatrogenic cartilage injury during hip arthroscopy [41].

Iatrogenic labral penetration may occur during initial portal placement in up to 20% of patients [42]. Damage to the labrum may compromise the ability to perform a repair, impair the stabilizing effect of the labrum, and result in the loss of suction-seal phenomenon in the hip joint. During labral repair, medialization of the labrum can occur as a result of improper anchor placement and can also impair the ability of the labrum to dissipate force. Anchor penetration into the articular cartilage can occur during anchor insertion and result in damage to the acetabular cartilage. This can result in a compromised joint with inadequate repair of the acetabular labrum. Pointing the bevel of the spinal needle toward the femoral head and placing the initial needle anterior to the superior femoral head are helpful to avoid iatrogenic scuffing of articular cartilage and labral penetration.

Inadequate resection of femoroacetabular impingement such as bony overresection or underresection may be one of the complications after hip arthroscopy. In a recent investigation of 37 patients undergoing revision hip arthroscopy, the authors found that 95% of patients had residual FAI, and 97% had radiographic evidence of persistent impingement [43].

Hip instability may occur if too much of the acetabular rim is resected. Underresection of pincer or cam deformities can lead to incomplete relief and a need for further surgery. Overresection of a femoral neck cam lesion places the femoral neck at risk for fracture. In a cadaveric study, it was shown that 30% of the anterolateral quadrant of the femoral head-neck junction could be safely resected without affecting the load-bearing capacity of the proximal femur [44].

To avoid the inadequate resection of femoroacetabular impingement, surgeons should carefully plan for the resection of any cam or pincer lesion with preoperative X-rays, sometimes in addition with 3-dimensional imaging. Appropriate capsulotomies should be performed for exposure because lack of visualization is a common cause of underresection of FAI, especially cam. Cortical notching greater than 4 or 6 mm depths and resection of more than 30% of the femoral head-neck junction should be avoided.

Although the majority of these complications are minor in nature, they may be catastrophic for the patient in rare instances and may require repeated surgery or result in life-threatening illness.

References

1. Burman MS. Arthroscopy or the direct visualization of joints: an experimental cadaver study. J Bone Joint Surg Am. 1931;13:669–95.
2. Lee YK, Ha YC, Hwang DS, et al. Learning curve of basic hip arthroscopy technique: CUSUM analysis. Knee Surg Sports Traumatol Arthrosc. 2013;21:1940–4.
3. Byrd JW, Jones KS. Adhesive capsulitis of the hip. Arthroscopy. 2006;22:89–94.
4. Domb BG, Gui C, Lodhia P. How much arthritis is too much for hip arthroscopy: a systematic review. Arthroscopy. 2015;31:520–9.
5. Philippon MJ, Briggs KK, Carlisle JC, et al. Joint space predicts THA after hip arthroscopy in patients 50 years and older. Clin Orthop Relat Res. 2013;471:2492–6.
6. Larson CM, Giveans MR, Taylor M. Does arthroscopic FAI correction improve function with radiographic arthritis? Clin Orthop Relat Res. 2011;469:1667–76.
7. Robertson WJ, Kelly BT. The safe zone for hip arthroscopy: a cadaveric assessment of central, peripheral, and lateral compartment portal placement. Arthroscopy. 2008;24:1019–26.
8. Ekhtiari S, de Sa D, Haldane CE, et al. Hip arthroscopic capsulotomy techniques and capsular management strategies: a systematic review. Knee Surg Sports Traumatol Arthrosc. 2017;25:9–23.
9. Khanduja V, Villar RN. Arthroscopic surgery of the hip: current concepts and recent advances. J Bone Joint Surg Br. 2006;88:1557–66.
10. Lage LA, Patel JV, Villar RN. The acetabular labral tear: an arthroscopic classification. Arthroscopy. 1996;12:269–72.
11. McCarthy JC, Noble PC, Schuck MR, et al. The watershed labral lesion: its relationship to early arthritis of the hip. J Arthroplast. 2001;16:81–7.
12. Haddad B, Konan S, Haddad FS. Debridement versus re-attachment of acetabular labral tears: a review of the literature and quantitative analysis. Bone Joint J. 2014;96-b:24–30.
13. Frank JM, Harris JD, Erickson BJ, et al. Prevalence of femoroacetabular impingement imaging findings in asymptomatic volunteers: a systematic review. Arthroscopy. 2015;31:1199–204.
14. Philippon MJ, Ejnisman L, Ellis HB, et al. Outcomes 2 to 5 years following hip arthroscopy for femoroacetabular impingement in the patient aged 11 to 16 years. Arthroscopy. 2012;28:1255–61.
15. Philippon MJ, Weiss DR, Kuppersmith DA, et al. Arthroscopic labral repair and treatment of femoroacetabular impingement in professional hockey players. Am J Sports Med. 2010;38:99–104.
16. Philippon MJ, Yen YM, Briggs KK, et al. Early outcomes after hip arthroscopy for femoroacetabular impingement in the athletic adolescent patient: a preliminary report. J Pediatr Orthop. 2008;28:705–10.
17. Nho SJ, Magennis EM, Singh CK, et al. Outcomes after the arthroscopic treatment of femoroacetabular impingement in a mixed group of high-level athletes. Am J Sports Med. 2011;39(Suppl):14S–9S.
18. Lee S, Wuerz TH, Shewman E, et al. Labral reconstruction with iliotibial band autografts and semitendinosus allografts improves hip joint contact area and contact pressure: an in vitro analysis. Am J Sports Med. 2015;43:98–104.
19. Matsuda DK. Arthroscopic labral reconstruction with gracilis autograft. Arthrosc Tech. 2012;1:e15–21.
20. Domb BG, El Bitar YF, Stake CE, et al. Arthroscopic labral reconstruction is superior to segmental resection for irreparable labral tears in the hip: a matched-pair controlled study with minimum 2-year follow-up. Am J Sports Med. 2014;42:122–30.
21. Park SE, Ko Y. Use of the quadriceps tendon in arthroscopic acetabular labral reconstruction: potential and benefits as an autograft option. Arthrosc Tech. 2013;2:e217–9.
22. Sierra RJ, Trousdale RT. Labral reconstruction using the ligamentum teres capitis: report of a new technique. Clin Orthop Relat Res. 2009;467:753–9.
23. Larson CM, Giveans MR, Samuelson KM, et al. Arthroscopic hip revision surgery for residual femoroacetabular impingement (FAI): surgical outcomes compared with a matched cohort after primary arthroscopic FAI correction. Am J Sports Med. 2014;42:1785–90.
24. Costa Rocha P, Klingenstein G, Ganz R, et al. Circumferential reconstruction of severe acetabular labral damage using hamstring allograft: surgical technique and case series. Hip Int. 2013;23(Suppl 9):S42–53.
25. Boykin RE, Patterson D, Briggs KK, et al. Results of arthroscopic labral reconstruction of the hip in elite athletes. Am J Sports Med. 2013;41:2296–301.
26. Tortolani PJ, Carbone JJ, Quartararo LG. Greater trochanteric pain syndrome in patients referred to orthopedic spine specialists. Spine J. 2002;2:251–4.
27. Williams BS, Cohen SP. Greater trochanteric pain syndrome: a review of anatomy, diagnosis and treatment. Anesth Analg. 2009;108:1662–70.
28. Segal NA, Felson DT, Torner JC, et al. Greater trochanteric pain syndrome: epidemiology and associated factors. Arch Phys Med Rehabil. 2007;88:988–92.
29. Alpaugh K, Chilelli BJ, Xu S, et al. Outcomes after primary open or endoscopic abductor tendon repair in the hip: a systematic review of the literature. Arthroscopy. 2015;31:530–40.
30. Chandrasekaran S, Lodhia P, Gui C, et al. Outcomes of open versus endoscopic repair of abductor muscle tears of the hip: a systematic review. Arthroscopy. 2015;31:2057–67.e2.
31. McCormick F, Alpaugh K, Nwachukwu BU, et al. Endoscopic repair of full-thickness abductor tendon tears: surgical technique and outcome at minimum of 1-year follow-up. Arthroscopy. 2013;29:1941–7.

32. Ilizaliturri VM Jr, Buganza-Tepole M, Olivos-Meza A, et al. Central compartment release versus lesser trochanter release of the iliopsoas tendon for the treatment of internal snapping hip: a comparative study. Arthroscopy. 2014;30:790–5.
33. Kelly BT, Williams RJ 3rd, Philippon MJ. Hip arthroscopy: current indications, treatment options, and management issues. Am J Sports Med. 2003;31:1020–37.
34. Wettstein M, Jung J, Dienst M. Arthroscopic psoas tenotomy. Arthroscopy. 2006;22:907 e1–4.
35. Jani S, Safran MR. Internal snapping hip syndrome. In: Byrd JW, Guanche CA, editors. AANA advanced arthroscopy: The Hip 1st Edition, ELSEVIER; 2010. p. 125–32.
36. Ilizaliturri VM Jr, Camacho-Galindo J. Endoscopic treatment of snapping hips, iliotibial band, and iliopsoas tendon. Sports Med Arthrosc Rev. 2010;18:120–7.
37. Khan M, Adamich J, Simunovic N, et al. Surgical management of internal snapping hip syndrome: a systematic review evaluating open and arthroscopic approaches. Arthroscopy. 2013;29:942–8.
38. Bozic KJ, Chan V, Valone FH 3rd, et al. Trends in hip arthroscopy utilization in the United States. J Arthroplast. 2013;28:140–3.
39. Gupta A, Redmond JM, Hammarstedt JE, et al. Safety measures in hip arthroscopy and their efficacy in minimizing complications: a systematic review of the evidence. Arthroscopy. 2014;30:1342–8.
40. Harris JD, McCormick FM, Abrams GD, et al. Complications and reoperations during and after hip arthroscopy: a systematic review of 92 studies and more than 6,000 patients. Arthroscopy. 2013;29:589–95.
41. McCarthy JC, Lee JA. Hip arthroscopy: indications, outcomes, and complications. Instr Course Lect. 2006;55:301–8.
42. Badylak JS, Keene JS. Do iatrogenic punctures of the labrum affect the clinical results of hip arthroscopy? Arthroscopy. 2011;27:761–7.
43. Philippon MJ, Schenker ML, Briggs KK, et al. Revision hip arthroscopy. Am J Sports Med. 2007;35:1918–21.
44. Mardones RM, Gonzalez C, Chen Q, et al. Surgical treatment of femoroacetabular impingement: evaluation of the effect of the size of the resection. J Bone Joint Surg Am. 2005;87:273–9.

7 Evolution, Current Concepts, and Future Developments in Arthroscopic Surgery of the Hip

Ori Weiss, Andrew Lim, Jessica Kamal, and Vikas Khanduja

7.1 Introduction

With the advent of the videoscope, keyhole surgery was possible. This revolutionized the surgical landscape and opened doors to procedures that were more efficient and effective from the perspective of both health economics and more importantly patient outcomes.

The use of arthroscopic procedures have been widespread in the surgery of the knee and the shoulder for many years; however, the hip until relatively recently had been largely neglected. Only since the 1980s, and more intensely since the 1990s, has it been gaining popularity. Over the past 30 years, indications for hip arthroscopy have grown immensely. Minimally invasive arthroscopic procedures are one of the fastest growing areas of orthopedics, witnessed by the exponentially increasing numbers of publications in the literature. Studies have demonstrated considerable increases in the number of hip arthroscopies, worldwide; between 2007 and 2011 there was a 475% increase in the total number of hip arthroscopies in the USA [1]. In Korea, the number of hip arthroscopies doubled from 596 to 1262 [2]. These numbers are also reflected in the UK where a 727% increase is seen between 2002 and 2013. The projection of the trend foresees there to be a 1388% increase in the number of procedures until 2023 [3]. These increases are a testament to the positive outcomes that are achieved and its low complication rates.

As indications and contraindications for hip arthroscopy have not been universally defined, successful outcomes following hip arthroscopy require careful patient selection as well as a keen awareness of factors that may technically preclude the procedure or compromise clinical outcomes.

The aim of this chapter is to bring the reader up-to-date with the evolution, current concepts, and future development of hip arthroscopy.

7.2 Impact and Scalability of Hip Arthroscopy

Musculoskeletal diseases have had such an impact on the world's health economy that the WHO proclaimed the last decade to be the Bone and Joint Decade (2000–2010). Musculoskeletal conditions such as femoroacetabular impingement (FAI) and labral tears are being diagnosed more than ever before with the improvement in imaging technology such as magnetic resonance imaging [4–7]. Recent studies on the prevalence of FAI and labral tears demonstrated that 14% and 36% of each study population, who were asymptomatic, had these conditions, respectively

O. Weiss · A. Lim · J. Kamal · V. Khanduja (✉)
Young Adult Hip Service, Department of Trauma and Orthopaedics, Addenbrooke's—Cambridge University Hospital, Cambridge, UK
e-mail: jk677@cam.ac.uk; vk279@cam.ac.uk

W. R. Drescher et al. (eds.), *Advances in Specialist Hip Surgery*,
https://doi.org/10.1007/978-3-030-61830-8_7

[6, 8]. The main concern of FAI and labral tears is that it is mainly affecting younger patients and increases the patient's predisposition to osteoarthritis [9]. Evidently, FAI and labral tears are conditions that will have substantial economic impact on the society and will affect the quality of life of the greater population.

7.2.1 Cost-Effectiveness

7.2.1.1 Arthroscopic Management of FAI

Multiple studies have demonstrated the positive impact that hip arthroscopy can have on the economy. A study in 2012 by Shearer et al. utilized the incremental cost-effectiveness ratio (ICER) to demonstrate a means to quantify the cost-effectiveness of hip arthroscopy for FAI. The finding was that the ICER per quality-affected life years (QALY) for hip arthroscopy was 3.5 times less than those who have preoperative arthritis [10]. A more recent study by Mather et al. compared the cost-effectiveness of hip arthroscopy versus nonoperative treatment. Alongside a gain of 2.03 quality-adjusted life years of the study period, there was a 10-year saving of $67,418 per patient from hip arthroscopy as opposed to nonoperative treatment. It is evident that FAI, which is a significant economic burden on the society may be alleviated by hip arthroscopy and is cost effective [11].

7.2.2 Arthroscopic Management of Labral Tears

Similarly, for labral tears, a study by Kahlenberg et al. [12] in 2014 demonstrated that by simply diagnosing labral tears associated with FAI, the Medicare system in the USA is saving $1766.35 per patient. Labral tears, on their own, were found to be cost effective for 94.5% of patients in a study completed in 2016, with its cost-effectiveness increasing for those who present younger, reflecting the importance of early prevention of deterioration. The ICER, in this study, was determined to be $745 per QALY for those who had hip arthroscopy. The widely accepted willingness-to-pay value is approximately 100,000 to 150,000 dollars [13, 14]. Hence, the ICER per QALY is well under the accepted threshold. Whether it be for FAI or labral tears, the ability of hip arthroscopies to prevent substantial long-term pathology and improve quality of life ensures that it is a worthy investment for the governing funding bodies.

7.3 The History of Arthroscopy

7.3.1 Development of the Endoscope

Curiosity and the desire to examine the body cavities can be traced back to ancient times, as long ago as 400 B.C. Hippocrates searched for a method to look inside the organs, and created the first endoscopic instrument in history: a rectal speculum. However, "closed" cavities posed a specific problem, with the necessity to introduce light in the cavity to be able to visualize structures.

The earliest known instrument designed to look into the bladder was called a "Lichtleiter" and was presented to the Rome Academy of Science in 1806 by Philipp Bozzini, a young German army surgeon who was frustrated with trying to locate bullets in his patients [15, 16]. In Bozzini's instrument the light of a candle was used by means of a mirror in a two-tube device, thus providing sufficient light to explore these cavities (Fig. 7.1).

Almost 50 years later, Desormeaux developed his "gasogene cystoscope," which provided light by the combustion of gasoline and turpentine that was reflected into the bladder by a mirror [15]. The next significant advance in endoscopic instrumentation came in 1879, when Edison developed the incandescent light bulb. A few years later, in 1886, the first cystoscope with an incandescent bulb for illumination was developed by Leiter and Nitze in Germany.

Two major subsequent improvements in endoscopes were the development of fiber or "cold" light in 1955 to provide illumination [17] and, in 1960, the rod lens optical system for viewing

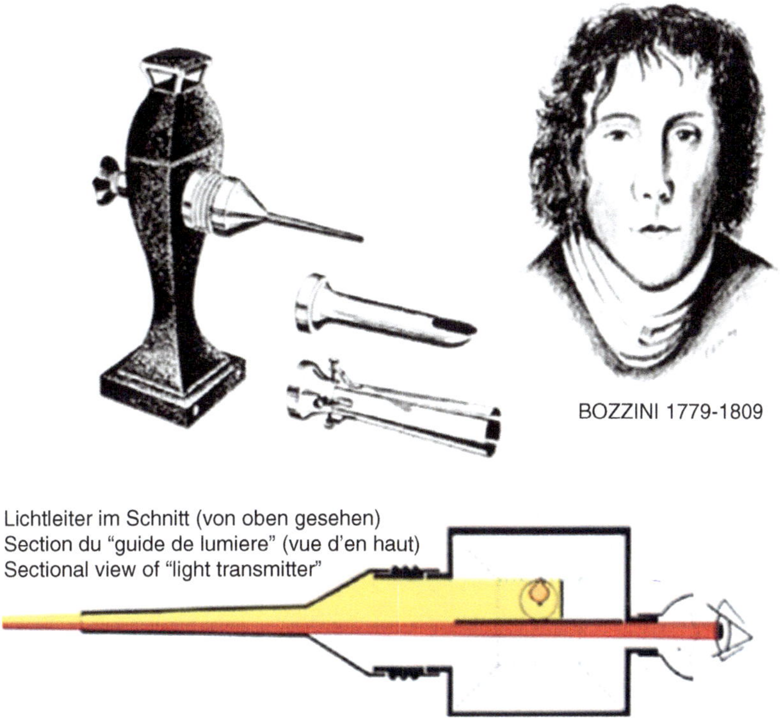

Fig. 7.1 Magrill ACL, Nakano N, Khanduja V. Historical review of arthroscopic surgery of the hip. Int Orthop. 2017;41(10):1983–94. Source is your publication: "Magrill ACL, Nakano N, Khanduja V. Historical review of arthroscopic surgery of the hip. Int Orthop. 2017;41(10):1983–94." (Originally published at: Doral MN, Tandogan RN, Mann G, Verdonk R. Sports injuries: prevention, diagnosis, treatment and rehabilitation. 2012)

[18]. Both of these were developed by an English physicist named Hopkins and are now used in almost all endoscopes.

Cameras with photographic film recorded the early images seen during endoscopic procedures. Then, a major breakthrough in imaging occurred when television became a reality. In the latter half of the century, colour television cameras became so small that they could be incorporated into the lens system of an arthroscope which is where modern arthroscopy is currently.

7.3.2 Early Evolution of Arthroscopy

Hip arthroscopy is often thought of as a relatively new procedure but the first to perform a true arthroscopy was Severin Nordentoft (1866–1922). In 1912, in Berlin, at the 41st Congress of the German Society of Surgery, this Danish surgeon and radiologist presented a paper in which he, first, suggested the use of an endoscope to diagnose a meniscal tear. He was the first to call this technique arthroscopy [19].

A few years later in 1918, Professor Kenji Takagi (1888–1963) of Tokyo applied the endoscopic principles of cystoscopy to the examination of cadaveric knees [20].

Parallel developments were made in the west. The first writings appeared in the American literature in 1925, when Philip Heinrich Kreuscher (1883–1943) reported on the use of the arthroscope in diagnosing meniscal pathology [16, 20].

In 1931 Michael Burman (1896–1974) published a comprehensive article on arthroscopy that detailed his many experiments on cadaveric joints, including the hip joint. This is the first time hip arthroscopy was mentioned in the literature [21, 22].

7.3.3 Early Hip Arthroscopists

After the pioneering work of Burman in describing hip arthroscopy, there were more who helped develop hip arthroscopy to its present stage. Takagi continued to work on arthroscopy and published a paper reporting the first clinical application of hip arthroscopy in 1939 [23].

Masaki Watanabe (1911–1994), the protégé of Takagi, continued to develop much more sophisticated endoscopes using electronics and optics, which became popular in the post-World War II era in both Japan and America. He was able to obtain the first colour photographs of the inside of a knee joint which was presented at the SICOT Congress in Barcelona in 1957 [15].

Despite this growth of arthroscopy in general, clinical applications of arthroscopy of the hip were largely ignored from Takagi's paper of 1939 until the 1970s.

The International Arthroscopy Association was founded in 1974, and Watanabe was elected as its first President. At its first meeting in Copenhagen, in 1975, a French surgeon Aignan opened a new chapter in hip arthroscopy with his presentation of attempted diagnostic arthroscopy and biopsy of 51 hips [16].

James Glick in San Francisco began performing hip arthroscopy in 1977, and along with his partner **Thomas Sampson**, he developed the new technique of performimg hip arthroscopy in the lateral decubitus position.

In the UK, in the mid-1980s, **Richard Villar** from Cambridge corresponded with both **James Glick** and **Richard Hawkins** and began to pioneer hip arthroscopy on the British side of the Atlantic and trained a number of surgeons including the senior author.

7.3.4 Technical Aspects

7.3.4.1 Irrigation System

Irrigation and distention of the joint are essential in all arthroscopic procedures. The inflow may pass directly through the arthroscopic sheath or through a separate portal by means of a cannula. Arthroscopic pumps should be used carefully, and the tightness of muscle compartments and soft-tissue spaces should be monitored closely. Joint distention pressures in the hip generally should be 45–50 mmHg which usually provides safe distention and clear vision. Because of the increased likelihood of extravasation, pressure should be kept as minimal as possible [24, 25].

7.3.4.2 Patient Positioning

The position of the patient is dependent on the surgeon's preference; however, there are advantages and disadvantages to both the supine and lateral positions.

The supine position—offers a familiar orientation of the joint to all orthopedic surgeons [26, 27]. It can be used on any standard fracture table with no necessary modifications. Drawbacks to the supine position include its use in obese patients because the pannus can interfere with maneuverability of instruments, difficulty in gaining access to the joint in patients with a large anterolateral osteophyte, and potentially decreased posterior access [28, 29].

The lateral position—is considered to have superior maneuverability in obese patients because the abdominal pannus and buttock drop away from the operative field. In addition, it provides superior access to the posterior and inferior joint spaces compared with the supine position [29, 30]. Disadvantages include the extra time required to position the patient, having to make adjustments to the perineal and traction posts of the fracture table, and having to use special traction devices attached to a standard operating table [30–32].

7.3.4.3 Operating Room Setup

Supine

The patient is placed in the supine position on the fracture table. The perineal post is positioned laterally against the medial thigh of the hip to be operated upon. The foot of the surgical side is then well padded with cast padding and placed in the foot holder in neutral rotation. The hip is then extended and slightly abducted [22, 30, 32, 33].

Lateral

The patient is positioned in the lateral decubitus position with the operative hip superior. The perineal post is pushed up against the medial thigh of the operative leg, and the hip is then slightly abducted and flexed to relax the capsule.

Anesthesia

General anesthesia is commonly used for hip arthroscopy. Epidural anesthesia can potentially be used; however, neuromuscular blockade is required to ensure complete muscle relaxation. Antibiotic prophylaxis is warranted using one of the cephalosporins. Deep Vein Thrombosis (DVT) prophylaxis is accomplished using compression stockings and a sequential pump [22].

Distraction

Between 10 and 12 mm of distraction is needed for placement of a 4.5–5.5 mm cannula into the joint. With devices that have tensiometers, approximately 50 lb. of force is required (for patients who are of smaller habitus and flexible, it is advised to commence with 25–50 lb. of force and with patients with a larger body habitus and stiff joints a force of 50–75 lb. may be required). Traction time should be limited to less than 2 h to decrease the possibility of traction neurapraxias [29, 34]. The post should be placed laterally. This improves the vector of the traction force and decreases the risk of neurapraxia. Often less traction is required after the joint has been accessed, relieving the negative pressure.

Portals

A number of portals can be utilized to access the hip joint; however, there are three standard portals utilized by most surgeons: the anterolateral, anterior, and posterolateral. The relevant landmarks for portal placement are the anterior superior iliac spine, anterior, superior and posterior border of the greater trochanter, and the femoral pulse.

Anterolateral portal: In both approaches the anterolateral portal is usually the first portal to be established; this portal is made approximately 1 cm superior and anterior to the anterior edge of the greater trochanter. The anterolateral portal pierces the gluteus medius muscle and then the hip capsule. The nearest neurovascular structure is the superior gluteal nerve.

Posterolateral portal: It is made 1 cm posterior and superior to the greater trochanter.

The posterolateral portal passes through the gluteus medius and minimus muscles. The closest neurovascular structure is the sciatic nerve.

Anterior portal is determined by the intersection of a line drawn from the tip of the greater trochanter and a line extending inferiorly from the anterior superior iliac spine. The anterior portal passes through the sartorius and the rectus femoris muscles and then the hip capsule. This portal passes close to the lateral femoral cutaneous nerve and ascending branch of the lateral femoral circumflex artery.

Numerous additional accessory portals can be placed under direct visualization depending on the procedure.

7.3.5 Indications

Various techniques are being developed to help perform procedures in and around the hip joint that were previously performed by conventional, open methods. Today, the indications for hip arthroscopy have greatly expanded and continue to evolve [35] (Table 7.1).

7.3.6 Intra-articular Pathologies

7.3.6.1 Labral Tears

Labral pathology commonly occurs in the form of a tear or intra-substance degeneration with or

Table 7.1 Indications for hip arthroscopy divided into extra-articular and intra-articular hip pathologies

Extra-articular	Intra-articular
Extra-articular hip impingement	FAI (cam and pincer type)
Greater trochanteric pain syndrome	Chondral lesions
Snapping hip syndromes	Labral pathology
Proximal hamstring disorders	Ligamentum teres injuries
Sciatic nerve entrapment	Synovial based disorders
Abductor muscle tears	Loose bodies/synovial chondromatosis
	Adhesive capsulitis
	Capsular laxity and instability
	Septic arthritis

without a cyst and can be secondary to FAI, dysplasia, SCFE, Perthes' disease, any morphological abnormality of the hip, or trauma. Labral pathology most commonly occurs along the anterior and superior acetabular margins [36]. Labral tears do not have the capacity to heal and the philosophy of management has been to address the disrupted suction seal in the hip which the labrum is responsible for. Therefore, although debridement has historically been the mainstay of treatment and has demonstrated good results [37], the move is towards repairing the labrum especially if there is detachment from the acetabular rim. Recent evidence also demonstrates superior results of repair when compared with debridement [38–40].

7.3.6.2 Chondral Lesions

Chondral pathology can occur secondary to trauma, both acute and chronic, from repetitive mechanical impingement (FAI) or as a result of acetabular rim overload that occurs as a result of acetabular dysplasia. Chondral injuries may occur on either the articular surface of the femoral head (more common with acute trauma) or the acetabulum (typical with FAI) and dysplasia. These defects have limited healing capacity and are reported to have inferior outcomes after arthroscopy in comparison to those without articular cartilage defects [41–43]. However, advances in arthroscopic treatment now allow for visualization of the entire articular surface of the hip, debridement, marrow stimulation techniques (i.e., drilling, microfracture), gluing the articular surface with fibrin and even techniques like autologous chondrocyte implantation to treat these chondral lesions [27].

7.3.6.3 Femoroacetabular Impingement

Surgical intervention for femoroacetabular impingement (FAI) is one of the commonest indications for hip arthroscopy currently. FAI consists of a pathomorphological variation of the hip which leads to impingement between the femoral head-neck junction and the acetabular rim during functional range of motion [38]. Two basic types of impingement have been described:

Cam impingement occurs when the anterosuperior femoral head-neck junction is prominent or the femoral neck has a diminished offset from the adjacent femoral head and this asphericity then leads to the femoral head-neck junction abuting against the acetabular labro-chondral junction leading to damage.

Pincer impingement on the other hand occurs when the acetabular rim has an area of overcoverage (focal or global) which leads to the femoral neck abutting against the excessive rim in flexion leading to impingement.

Arthroscopic intervention, like the open technique, allows for excision of the bony impingement lesion on the femoral or the acetabular side and then deals with the resultant effects of impingement on the articular cartilage and labrum as described in the previous section.

7.3.6.4 Ligamentum Teres Injuries

Lesions of the ligamentum teres include partial or complete traumatic tears, degenerative tears, and avulsion fractures at the foveal insertion of the femoral head [44]. Partial tears can lead to mechanical symptoms of clicking and also pain and complete tears can lead to symptoms of instability especially in dancers and gymnasts. Arthroscopy allows for debridement and radiofrequency shrinkage of partial tears. Isolated cases of ligamentum teres reconstruction have also been reported with good short-term outcomes in patients with a complete rupture [45–49].

7.3.6.5 Synovial Based Pathology

The synovial lining of the hip can degenerate over time secondary to trauma, repetitive stress to the joint, and/or inflammatory arthropathies. Pigmented villonodular synovitis, rheumatoid arthritis, and synovial chondromatosis are examples of synovial based diseases. Arthroscopy in the setting of synovial based disease not only allows for treatment but can also confirm the underlying diagnosis by synovial biopsies in a minimally invasive fashion.

7.3.6.6 Osteonecrosis

The role of hip arthroscopy in the diagnosis and management of osteonecrosis is controversial.

Some even consider that it is a contraindication [50, 51]. However, the procedure allows staging of the disease and management of associated chondral flaps. It also enables treatment of patients with mechanical symptoms such as locking, giving way, or clicking secondary to an aspherical femoral head, a chondral lesion, or a loose body. Retrograde drilling of avascular lesions is also possible arthroscopically with accurate placement of the tip of the drill.

7.3.6.7 Loose Bodies

Loose bodies may develop secondary to a traumatic event or result from degenerative changes and reactive bone formation. Patients with loose bodies often present with mechanical symptoms, such as popping, catching, and locking [52]. Numerous loose bodies may be the product of primary or secondary synovial chondromatosis/osteochondromatosis. Removal of the fragments and treatment of associated chondral pathology can readily be performed arthroscopically with good outcomes [53].

7.3.6.8 Capsular Disorders (Adhesive Capsulitis, Capsular Laxity, and Instability)

Adhesive capsulitis—is a more recent indication for hip arthroscopy, as it was first clinically recognized in 1999 [54]. Adhesive capsulitis of the hip is thought to be more prevalent than previously recorded in the literature. Arthroscopy can effectively treat these patients in a minimally invasive fashion, allowing for a capsulotomy or capsulectomy of the pathologically thickened capsule and intra-articular synovectomy.

Laxity and instability—Capsular laxity may be caused by traumatic injuries, atraumatic hip injuries (repetitive external rotation with axial loading), or other predisposing conditions such as acetabular dysplasia, generalized ligamentous laxity, or connective tissue disorders. Capsular repair has become more common in lieu of integrity of the iliofemoral ligament being reported more readily on MRI as well as reports of iatrogenic capsular laxity secondary to large capsulotomies at hip arthroscopy leading to dislocation [55–57].

7.3.6.9 Septic Arthritis

Infection can cause rapid chondrolysis and irreversible damage to the articular surfaces of the joint. Arthroscopic drainage for acute septic arthritis has been reported with favorable short-term outcomes, including irrigation, lavage, and debridement of the infected tissue. This approach is sometimes favorable over a conventional open exposure and arthrotomy, which is associated with potentially increased morbidity, greater pain, and an extended hospital stay [58]. However, arthroscopy is not a definitive treatment for sepsis associated with abscess formation, extra-articular involvement, or osteomyelitis.

7.3.7 Extra-articular Hip Pathology

7.3.7.1 Extra-articular Hip Impingement

The common extra-articular hip impingement syndromes are described below:

(a) **Ischiofemoral impingement**: Quadratus femoris muscle becomes compressed between the lesser trochanter and the ischial tuberosity.
(b) **Subspine impingement**: Mechanical conflict occurs between an enlarged or malori-ented anterior inferior iliac spine (AIIS) and the distal anterior femoral neck.
(c) **Pectineo-foveal impingement**—rare condition. Pectineo-foveal impingement may be symptomatic when medial synovial fold impinges against overlying soft tissue, primarily the zona orbicularis [59, 60].
(d) **Iliopsoas impingement**—as discussed in the next section. See internal snapping hip.
(e) **Deep gluteal syndrome**—as discussed in the next section.

7.3.7.2 Greater Trochanteric Pain Syndrome (GTPS)

Greater trochanteric pain syndrome (GTPS) is a term used to describe chronic pain over the lateral aspect of the hip in the region of the greater trochanter. It encompasses several pathologies and it is relatively common affecting 10–25%

of the population [36]. The most common form of GTPS is trochanteric bursitis, which is an inflammatory condition of the bursa between the trochanteric facets and the gluteus medius, gluteus minimus, and iliotibial band caused by repetitive trauma. Pain can also be a result of tendonitis or tearing of the abductor musculature [61]. Trochanteric bursitis and focal tears of the gluteus medius and minimus tendon can be effectively treated with arthroscopic bursectomy, iliotibial band release, and/or tendon repair to the greater trochanter [62].

7.3.7.3 Snapping Hip Syndrome (Coxa Saltans)

Snapping hip syndrome is characterized by an audible (internal coxa saltans) or visible (external coxa saltans):

Internal snapping hip (also known as iliopsoas impingement)—most common type, caused by iliopsoas tendon sliding over the iliopectineal eminence, AIIS, acetabular rim, or femoral head. Asymptomatic snapping requires no treatment [22]. However, arthroscopic procedures for recalcitrant symptoms include the removal of osseous impingement and/or the release or lengthening of the iliopsoas and also addressing the underlying labral tear to alleviate symptoms [54].

External snapping hip is associated with a thickening of the iliotibial band as the iliotibial band slides over/catches on the greater trochanter during hip extension from a flexed position. Patients can often reproduce the visible snapping. Additionally, palpation of the greater trochanter with hip flexion and extension may allow the identification of abnormal motion and friction of the iliotibial band. On occasion, the insertion of the gluteus maximus may be involved as well and endoscopy of the hip allows for release of the iliotibial band and partial release of the gluteus maximus as well along with a trochanteric bursectomy.

7.3.7.4 Proximal Hamstring Disorders

The proximal hamstrings' origin lies close to the sciatic nerve and the lesser trochanter, which can all be involved in the cause of posterior hip pain. Avulsion of the hamstring from the ischial tuberosity is a rare injury that occurs during forceful hip flexion and knee extension [63]. Chronic ruptures, which may require reconstruction with allograft material, may be best treated via an open surgical approach [64] but fresh tears with no retraction of the hamstrings are treated endoscopically with good outcomes.

7.3.7.5 Sciatic Nerve Entrapment (Deep Gluteal Syndrome)

The sciatic nerve passes through the sciatic notch intimately in association with the piriformis muscle, which can compress the nerve and lead to symptoms. Pain can also be secondary to nerve entrapment by the hamstring, quadratus femoris/gemellus inferior, obturator internus/gemellus superior, or scar tissue [65]. Sciatic nerve decompression is a relatively new indication for hip endoscopy and has been described well with good outcomes. It requires careful attention to detail and familiarity with the anatomy of the subgluteal space [36].

7.3.8 Contraindications of Hip Arthroscopy

Hip arthroscopy is a relatively new technique and appropriate indications continue to be refined. Successful outcomes require careful patient selection as well as a keen awareness of factors that may technically preclude the procedure or compromise clinical outcomes.

Anything that precludes entry into the hip joint, i.e., severe osteoarthritis [66, 67] or ankylosis [28], is an absolute contraindication. It is also well known that outcomes for hip arthroscopy in patients with a joint space of less than 2 mm or more than 50% joint space narrowing on plain radiographs are poor with a higher rate of conversion to THR and should therefore be avoided [67, 68]. Arthroscopy should also be performed in the case of a septic joint with osteomyelitis [69]. Additionally, skin ulceration and acute inflammation in the vicinity of the proposed arthroscopy portals remain absolute contraindications [70].

Hip arthroscopy should also not be the sole treatment in the setting of acetabular and/or femoral dysplasia. Dysplastic features include femoral head migration (>1 cm lateral or break in the Shenton line), lateral and anterior center-edge angle less than 20°, and a Tönnis angle greater than 15°. Also severe patterns of FAI, such as slipped capital femoral epiphysis or Perthes deformities, indicate a more global structural instability that is not amendable to hip arthroscopy alone and are better treated with open surgical hip dislocation. Additionally, rim resection in the presence of severe acetabular retroversion can further destabilize a posteriorly deficient acetabulum. Anteversion/reverse PAO should be considered in these situations. However, hip arthroscopy in these settings may be used as an adjunct to pelvic or femoral osteotomy to treat intra-articular pathology.

Relative contraindications include obesity [27, 71]; known neurological injury/disorders, such as pudendal neuralgia or peroneal or sciatic nerve palsy, as hip traction may risk further neurologic impairment [72, 73]; borderline acetabular dysplasia to avoid iatrogenic instability [74–76]; and severe femoral neck anteversion [1].

7.3.9 Complications of Hip Arthroscopy

The number of hip arthroscopies is increasing around the world and so are the number and type of complications related to this technique [77]. The complication rate varies greatly from 1.34 to 15% according to previous studies [31, 78–81]. Today, with improvement of technology and experience of the surgeons, the complication rate ranges from 0.5 to 5% [27, 82]. In a recent systematic review of 36,761 cases of hip arthroscopies, the overall complication rate was 3.3% [79].

The application of longitudinal traction and secondary counterpressure are the most frequent causes of complications [83–85]. Direct compression between the post and perianal soft tissues can lead to ischemic injuries and wounds. There are reports of the perineal post causing a small vaginal tear, partial skin necrosis of the scrotum, hematoma at the labia majora, and vulvar edema [80, 83, 86]. In a recent systematic review, only 28 cases (0.08%) of perineal skin damage were reported [79].

Positioning and traction can place tension on the soft tissues, stretching the nerve, injuring its myelin sheath [83, 87], and leading to tissue damage and ischemia. These injuries are typically neurapraxias, and recovery should be expected. Neurapraxias are the most commonly reported complications in hip arthroscopy. The overall rate of neurapraxia has been reported as between 0.48 and 20% [84]. The common nerves involved are lateral femoral cutaneous nerve, sciatic nerve, pudendal nerve, and rarely obturator nerve. In a recent systematic review of 36,761 cases of hip arthroscopies, the incidence of neurapraxia was 0.9%; all were temporary and resolved spontaneously [88].

To prevent these traction-type injuries, minimizing the duration of traction and positioning the hip in slight flexion can help relax the anterior capsule and anterior structures. It is generally recommended that traction time should not exceed 2 h, and that intermittent traction be used if a longer time is necessary [72, 79].

Chondral scuffing and labral puncture can occur during hip arthroscopy [88] and insufficient traction has usually been reported to be the main cause of these injuries [31, 84]. A minimum distraction of 10 mm followed by an intra-articular injection of 20–40 mL of normal saline for distension of the joint is recommended at the time of creating the first portal in order to prevent damage to the femoral head and labrum.

Other complications include but are not limited to AVN of the femoral head [89], inadequate reshaping of the cam deformity [88], instrument breakage necessitating foreign body removal [88, 90, 91], fluid extravasation and compartment syndrome [92–96], and heterotrophic ossification (HO) secondary to trauma during portal placement and the creation and distribution of bone debris following cam or rim osteoplasty [97]. HO is found to be the third most common complication after nerve injures and iatrogenic injuries [88]. Prevention of this complication requires the hip joint to be lavaged carefully at the end of procedure to ensure that all the bony debris from the osteoplasty has been cleared [98]. Secondly prophylaxis with indomethacin or naproxen [99] should be considered for 4–6 weeks and the surgeon should ensure that large capsulotomies are sutured following the procedure [100].

Although infection and thromboembolic disease have been reported following hip arthroscopy, their incidence is relatively low [27, 88].

Overzealous resection of the femoral neck can lead to a femoral neck fracture and present as a complication when treating cam deformities [101]. Khanduja et al. in a large systematic review reported ten femoral neck fracture cases post-hip arthroscopy out of 36,761 subjects (0.03%) [27, 88]. Careful and calibrated resection of the deformity and partial weight bearing for 6–8 weeks following treatment of a cam lesion is recommended to minimize the fracture risk [90, 101, 102].

Hip instability following hip arthroscopy could occur because of soft tissue laxity or inadequate bony cover and is difficult to diagnose [103]. This is a rare complication, and the few reported cases share several risk factors, including female, age from 39 to 52 years, early occurrence, and anterior instability [56, 57, 91, 104, 105]. Additionally, center-edge angle <25°, primary hyper laxity, and previous episodes of traumatic instability must be identified preoperatively. Rim resection should be avoided in patients who have a lateral center-edge angle of 20° or less and large capsulotomies should also be avoided in these patients; if carried out then a capsular repair should be undertaken (Table 7.2).

Table 7.2 Complications during and after arthroscopy [88]

Complication	*n* (% of all complications)	Percentage of all cases
Nerve injury	339 (27.7)	0.9
Temporary (all)	338 (27.7)	0.9
Temporary (pudendal nerve)	110 (9.0)	0.3
Temporary (lateral femoral cutaneous nerve)	95 (7.8)	0.3
Temporary (sciatic nerve)	56 (4.6)	0.2
Temporary (common peroneal nerve)	19 (1.6)	0.05
Temporary (femoral nerve)	7 (0.6)	0.02
Temporary (unclear)	51 (4.2)	0.1
Permanent (all)	1 (0.1)	0.00
Permanent (unclear)	1 (0.1)	0.00
Iatrogenic injury	254 (20.8)	0.7
Chondral injury	140 (11.5)	0.4
Labral injury	114 (9.3)	0.3
Heterotopic ossification	219 (17.9)	0.6
Adhesion	89 (7.3)	0.2
Infection	79(6.4)	0.2
Superficial	70 (5.7)	0.2
Deep	9 (0.7)	0.02
Other complications		
Deep vein thrombosis	34 (2.8)	0.09
Perineal skin damage	28 (2.3)	0.08
Vascular injury (hematoma)	21 (1.7)	0.06
Broken instrumentation	20 (1.6)	0.05
Muscle pain	20 (1.6)	0.05
Intra-abdominal fluid extravasation	13 (1.1)	0.04
Anchor problem	11 (0.9)	0.03
Incomplete reshaping	11 (0.9)	0.03
Femoral neck fracture	10 (0.8)	0.03
Hip instability	9 (0.7)	0.02
Iliopsoas tendinitis	9 (0.7)	0.02
Avascular necrosis of the femoral head	7 (0.6)	0.02
Ankle pain	6 (0.5)	0.02
Arthrofibrosis	6 (0.5)	0.02
Bursitis	5 (0.4)	0.01
Hypothermia	5 (0.4)	0.01
Reflex sympathetic dystrophy	5 (0.4)	0.01
Pulmonary embolism	4 (0.3)	0.01
Snapping sound	4 (0.3)	0.01
Death	3 (0.2)	0.01
Gluteus medius tear	3 (0.2)	0.01
Hip dislocation	3 (0.2)	0.01
Dehiscence of suture	2 (0.2)	0.01
Pneumonia	2 (0.2)	0.01
Skin burn	1 (0.1)	<0.005
Total	1222	3.3

7.4 The Future of Hip Arthroscopy

Minimally invasive arthroscopic procedures are one of the fastest growing areas of orthopedics, witnessed by the exponentially increasing numbers worldwide and also the number of publications in the literature. Future developments in hip surgery will be multifaceted in nature and will be expedited by advances in technology, biomaterials, and analysis of outcomes. Essential to this evolutionary process will be advances in radiological imaging, particularly visualizing dynamic joint motion and allowing functional patho-analysis. This will allow much better understanding of genetic, traumatic, and pathologic hip morphological abnormalities [22].

7.4.1 Computer Navigation in Hip Arthroscopy

The recent integration of computer-assisted surgery (CAS) as a resource for both preoperative planning and intraoperative assistance in orthopedic procedures has paved the way for more accurate surgical execution and associated potential for more favorable postoperative outcomes with more consistent and reproducible correction of deformity.

By integrating patient-specific information with dynamized imaging studies (CT or MRI) into computer software, CAS allows for more precise, definitive characterization of the pathomorphology and provides more accurate preoperative planning [106]. The goals of utilizing CAS are not only to improve patient outcomes, but also to lower the rates of revision surgery. An ideal system also allows for intraoperative real-time feedback of an individual's anatomy in relation to surgical instrumentation to allow for increased surgical accuracy.

7.4.2 Tissue Engineering and Regeneration

As the field of hip arthroscopy continues to evolve, the biological understanding of orthopedic tissues, namely articular cartilage, labrum, and ligamentum teres, continues to expand.

The field as a whole can be broadly divided into tissue engineering, diagnostic platforms, cellular therapies, healing therapies, and supporting technologies.

Possibilities include biological resurfacings in the form of either stem cell implantation, matrix associated autologous chondrocyte implantation, or mosaic plasties to fill defects in the articular cartilage. When faced with a clinical dilemma as to which tissue-engineered solution may be of value, the surgeon can think of varying degrees of regenerative medicine complexity based upon the theory of the "reconstructive ladder" (Fig. 7.2). As one moves up the ranks of the reconstructive ladder, the complexity of the regenerative medicine solution increases as well [107].

Although biological and tissue engineering solutions for hip arthroscopy are presently limited, the use of tissue engineering, as well as regenerative medicine technology, does represent an exciting paradigm for addressing orthopedic sports medicine problems.

7.4.3 Imaging Techniques

The field of hip arthroscopy has also seen advances in preoperative planning techniques and imaging, with 3-D models of the hip, based on patients' CT scans. Recent software advances also facilitate decision-making by enabling better imaging diagnostics, preoperative planning, and prognostic imaging.

7.4.4 Dynamic Diagnostic Imaging

The fundamental weakness of present imaging studies for diagnosing hip pathology is that many patient complaints arise during dynamic loading, often in specific positions. However, conventional imaging is only performed with the patient in a standing or supine position with the hip oriented near neutral which rarely portrays the specific site of impingement or the morphologic features of hip involved.

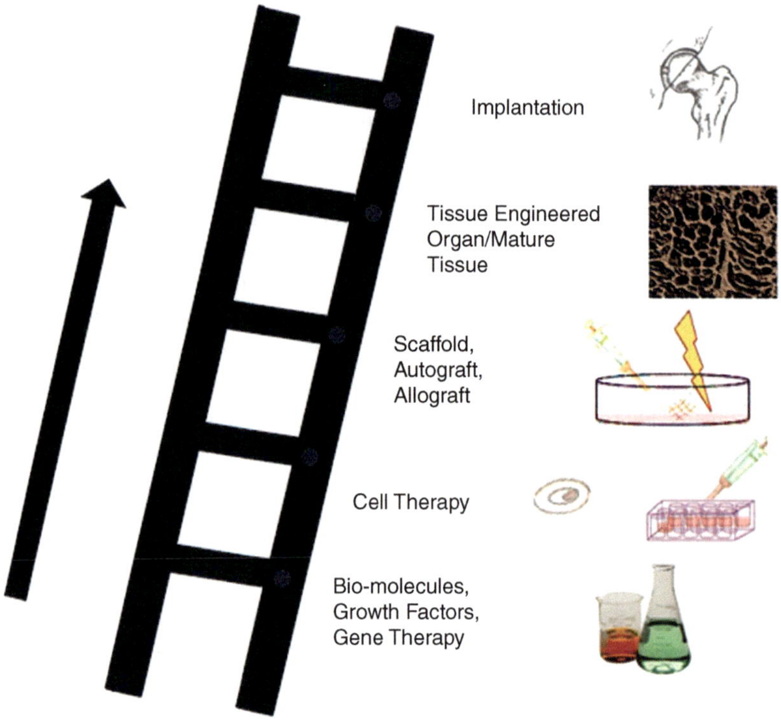

Fig. 7.2 Schematic diagram demonstrating the concept of the reconstructive ladder of tissue engineering and regenerative medicine. As one proceeds up the rungs of the reconstructive ladder, the regenerative medicine construct becomes more complex and structured. Based upon the clinical scenario, one can easily attain a tissue-engineered solution from any rung of reconstructive ladder. Source: Stubbs AJ, Howse EA, Mannava S. Tissue engineering and the future of hip cartilage, labrum and ligamentum teres. J Hip Preserv Surg. 2016;3(1):23–9. Copyrights: Source Of Figure 7.2 - A free, Creative Commons license-attribution 4.0 international (cc by 4.0): https://creativecommons.org/licenses/by/4.0/

Today, new technologies and software enable us to simulate a three-dimensional model of the hip joint kinematics—another fundamental step in developing a personalized diagnosis and treatment plan for hip preservation.

7.4.5 Prognostic Imaging

The health of cartilaginous tissue dominates the prognosis of all interventions for hip preservation. Consequently, the future of hip preservation surgery is inextricably linked to the ability of radiologists and imaging modalities to predict the long-term viability of cartilage within the hip. It is expected that advances in technology will lead to greater accuracy and sensitivity of modalities for imaging cartilage as well as the subchondral bone, capsule, and labrum—which enable diagnostic and prognostic criteria to be refined.

7.4.6 Surgical Training

Pioneers of hip arthroscopy unanimously agree that the learning curve of arthroscopic procedures is steep and fraught with dangers that may befall the inexperienced enthusiast. While the model of apprenticeship training in surgery remains relevant, the emergence of technically demanding disciplines such as arthroscopy, combined with a reduction in operating opportunities for trainees, has resulted in steep learning curves [108].

Over the last decade, there has been increasing investigation of the potential role of virtual reality (VR) simulation in solving this problem.

Advances in this field have prompted a rapid expansion in the number of commercially marketed low and high fidelity surgical simulators, with more than 400 models currently available [109]. The demonstration of "real-world" benefits to orthopedic surgical training of two previously validated simulators for knee and shoulder arthroscopy is highly promising and certinaly seems to be the way forward.

References

1. Truntzer JN, Shapiro LM, Hoppe DJ, Abrams GD, Safran MR. Hip arthroscopy in the United States: an update following coding changes in 2011. J Hip Preserv Surg. 2017;4(3):250–7.
2. Lee YK, Ha YC, Yoon BH, Koo KH. National trends of hip arthroscopy in Korea. J Korean Med Sci. 2014;29(2):277–80.
3. Palmer AJ, Malak TT, Broomfield J, Holton J, Majkowski L, Thomas GE, et al. Past and projected temporal trends in arthroscopic hip surgery in England between 2002 and 2013. BMJ Open Sport Exerc Med. 2016;2(1):e000082.
4. Roling MA, Mathijssen NM, Bloem RM. Incidence of symptomatic femoroacetabular impingement in the general population: a prospective registration study. J Hip Preserv Surg. 2016;3(3):203–7.
5. Lee WY, Kang C, Hwang DS, Jeon JH, Zheng L. Descriptive epidemiology of symptomatic femoroacetabular impingement in young athlete: single center study. Hip Pelvis. 2016;28(1):29–34.
6. Lee AJ, Armour P, Thind D, Coates MH, Kang AC. The prevalence of acetabular labral tears and associated pathology in a young asymptomatic population. Bone Joint J. 2015;97-B(5):623–7.
7. Groh MM, Herrera J. A comprehensive review of hip labral tears. Curr Rev Musculoskelet Med. 2009;2(2):105–17.
8. Hack K, Di Primio G, Rakhra K, Beaulé PE. Prevalence of cam-type femoroacetabular impingement morphology in asymptomatic volunteers. JBJS. 2010;92(14):2436–44.
9. Imam S, Khanduja V. Current concepts in the diagnosis and management of femoroacetabular impingement. Int Orthop. 2011;35(10):1427–35.
10. Shearer DW, Kramer J, Bozic KJ, Feeley BT. Is hip arthroscopy cost-effective for femoroacetabular impingement? Clin Orthop Relat Res. 2012;470(4):1079–89.
11. Mather RC 3rd, Nho SJ, Federer A, Demiralp B, Nguyen J, Saavoss A, et al. Effects of arthroscopy for femoroacetabular impingement syndrome on quality of life and economic outcomes. Am J Sports Med. 2018;46(5):1205–13.
12. Kahlenberg CA, Han B, Patel RM, Deshmane PP, Terry MA. Time and cost of diagnosis for symptomatic femoroacetabular impingement. Orthop J Sports Med. 2014;2(3):2325967114523916.
13. Grosse SD. Assessing cost-effectiveness in healthcare: history of the $50,000 per QALY threshold. Expert Rev Pharmacoecon Outcomes Res. 2008;8(2):165–78.
14. Neumann PJ, Cohen JT, Weinstein MC. Updating cost-effectiveness—the curious resilience of the $50,000-per-QALY threshold. N Engl J Med. 2014;371(9):796–7.
15. Jackson RW. A history of arthroscopy. Arthroscopy. 2010;26(1):91–103.
16. Magrill ACL, Nakano N, Khanduja V. Historical review of arthroscopic surgery of the hip. Int Orthop. 2017;41(10):1983–94.
17. Hopkins HH, Kapany NS. Transparent fibres for the transmission of optical images. Optica Acta Int J Opt. 2010;1(4):164–70.
18. Hopkins HH. Improvements in or relating to optical systems. British patent. 1960(July 15):954–629.
19. David P, Luigi M. History of arthroscopy. Can Open Orthop Traumatol J. 2016;3:23–7.
20. O'Connor RL, Shahriaree H. O'Connor's textbook of arthroscopic surgery. Philadelphia: Lippincott Williams & Wilkins; 1984.
21. Byrd JWT. Overview and history of hip arthroscopy. In: JWT B, editor. Operative hip arthroscopy. 3rd ed. New York: Springer; 2013. p. 1–7.
22. McCarthy JC, Noble PC, Villar RN. Hip joint restoration. New York: Springer; 2017.
23. Orthop TK, Tatsr JJ. The arthroscope: the second report. J Jpn Orthop Assoc. 1939;14:441–66.
24. Smart LR, Oetgen M, Noonan B, Medvecky M. Beginning hip arthroscopy: indications, positioning, portals, basic techniques, and complications. Arthroscopy. 2007;23(12):1348–53.
25. Burrus MT, Cowan JB, Bedi A. Avoiding failure in hip arthroscopy: complications, pearls, and pitfalls. Clin Sports Med. 2016;35(3):487–501.
26. Awan N, Murray P. Role of hip arthroscopy in the diagnosis and treatment of hip joint pathology. Arthroscopy. 2006;22(2):215–8.
27. Khanduja V, Villar RN. Arthroscopic surgery of the hip: current concepts and recent advances. J Bone Joint Surg Br. 2006;88(12):1557–66.
28. Byrd JW. Hip arthroscopy. J Am Acad Orthop Surg. 2006;14(7):433–44.
29. Glick JM. Hip arthroscopy by the lateral approach. Instr Course Lect. 2006;55:317–23.
30. Mason JB, McCarthy JC, O'Donnell J, Barsoum W, Mayor MB, Busconi BD, et al. Hip arthroscopy: surgical approach, positioning, and distraction. Clin Orthop Relat Res. 2003;406:29–37.
31. McCarthy JC, Lee JA. Hip arthroscopy: indications, outcomes, and complications. Instr Course Lect. 2006;55:301–8.
32. Byrd JW. Hip arthroscopy: surgical indications. Arthroscopy. 2006;22(12):1260–2.

33. Byrd JW. Hip arthroscopy by the supine approach. Instr Course Lect. 2006;55:325–36.
34. Glick JM, Sampson TG, Gordon RB, Behr JT, Schmidt E. Hip arthroscopy by the lateral approach. Arthroscopy. 1987;3(1):4–12.
35. Rath E, Tsvieli O, Levy O. Hip arthroscopy: an emerging technique and indications. Isr Med Assoc J. 2012;14(3):170–4.
36. Ross JR, Larson CM, Bedi A. Indications for hip arthroscopy. Sports Health. 2017;9(5):402–13.
37. Byrd JW, Jones KS. Hip arthroscopy for labral pathology: prospective analysis with 10-year follow-up. Arthroscopy. 2009;25(4):365–8.
38. Larson CM, Giveans MR. Arthroscopic management of femoroacetabular impingement: early outcomes measures. Arthroscopy. 2008;24(5):540–6.
39. Larson CM, Giveans MR, Stone RM. Arthroscopic debridement versus refixation of the acetabular labrum associated with femoroacetabular impingement: mean 3.5-year follow-up. Am J Sports Med. 2012;40(5):1015–21.
40. Schilders E, Dimitrakopoulou A, Bismil Q, Marchant P, Cooke C. Arthroscopic treatment of labral tears in femoroacetabular impingement: a comparative study of refixation and resection with a minimum two-year follow-up. J Bone Joint Surg Br. 2011;93(8):1027–32.
41. Byrd JW, Jones KS. Prospective analysis of hip arthroscopy with 2-year follow-up. Arthroscopy. 2000;16(6):578–87.
42. Streich NA, Gotterbarm T, Barie A, Schmitt H. Prognostic value of chondral defects on the outcome after arthroscopic treatment of acetabular labral tears. Knee Surg Sports Traumatol Arthrosc. 2009;17(10):1257–63.
43. Ward JP, Rogers P, Youm T. Failed hip arthroscopy: causes and treatment options. Orthopedics. 2012;35(7):612–7.
44. Cerezal L, Kassarjian A, Canga A, Dobado MC, Montero JA, Llopis E, et al. Anatomy, biomechanics, imaging, and management of ligamentum teres injuries. Radiographics. 2010;30(6):1637–51.
45. Amenabar T, O'Donnell J. Arthroscopic ligamentum teres reconstruction using semitendinosus tendon: surgical technique and an unusual outcome. Arthrosc Tech. 2012;1(2):e169–74.
46. Haviv B, O'Donnell J. Arthroscopic debridement of the isolated Ligamentum Teres rupture. Knee Surg Sports Traumatol Arthrosc. 2011;19(9):1510–3.
47. Menge TJ, Mitchell JJ, Briggs KK, Philippon MJ. Anatomic arthroscopic Ligamentum Teres reconstruction for hip instability. Arthrosc Tech. 2016;5(4):e737–e42.
48. Philippon MJ, Pennock A, Gaskill TR. Arthroscopic reconstruction of the ligamentum teres: technique and early outcomes. J Bone Joint Surg Br. 2012;94(11):1494–8.
49. Simpson JM, Field RE, Villar RN. Arthroscopic reconstruction of the ligamentum teres. Arthroscopy. 2011;27(3):436–41.
50. Byrd JW. Hip arthroscopy: patient assessment and indications. Instr Course Lect. 2003;52:711–9.
51. McCarthy J, Puri L, Barsoum W, Lee JA, Laker M, Cooke P. Articular cartilage changes in avascular necrosis: an arthroscopic evaluation. Clin Orthop Relat Res. 2003;406:64–70.
52. Diulus CA, Krebs VE, Hanna G, Barsoum WK. Hip arthroscopy technique and indications. J Arthroplast. 2006;21(4 Suppl 1):68–73.
53. Helms CA, Major N, Anderson MW, Kaplan P, Dussault R. Musculoskeletal MRI. 2nd ed. Philadelphia: Saunders Elsevier; 2009.
54. Kelly BT, Williams RJ 3rd, Philippon MJ. Hip arthroscopy: current indications, treatment options, and management issues. Am J Sports Med. 2003;31(6):1020–37.
55. Matsuda DK. Fluoroscopic templating technique for precision arthroscopic rim trimming. Arthroscopy. 2009;25(10):1175–82.
56. Mei-Dan O, McConkey MO, Brick M. Catastrophic failure of hip arthroscopy due to iatrogenic instability: can partial division of the ligamentum teres and iliofemoral ligament cause subluxation? Arthroscopy. 2012;28(3):440–5.
57. Ranawat AS, McClincy M, Sekiya JK. Anterior dislocation of the hip after arthroscopy in a patient with capsular laxity of the hip. A case report. J Bone Joint Surg Am. 2009;91(1):192–7.
58. Rutz E, Brunner R. Septic arthritis of the hip—current concepts. Hip Int. 2009;19(Suppl 6):S9–12.
59. Dienst M, Godde S, Seil R, Hammer D, Kohn D. Hip arthroscopy without traction: in vivo anatomy of the peripheral hip joint cavity. Arthroscopy. 2001;17(9):924–31.
60. Bardakos NV. Hip impingement: beyond femoroacetabular. J Hip Preserv Surg. 2015;2(3):206–23.
61. Benzel EC. Techniques, complication avoidance, and management. New York: Churchill Livingstone; 2005. 1600 p.
62. Voos JE, Rudzki JR, Shindle MK, Martin H, Kelly BT. Arthroscopic anatomy and surgical techniques for peritrochanteric space disorders in the hip. Arthroscopy. 2007;23(11):1246.e1–5.
63. Beltran L, Ghazikhanian V, Padron M, Beltran J. The proximal hamstring muscle-tendon-bone unit: a review of the normal anatomy, biomechanics, and pathophysiology. Eur J Radiol. 2012;81(12):3772–9.
64. Benazzo F, Marullo M, Zanon G, Indino C, Pelillo F. Surgical management of chronic proximal hamstring tendinopathy in athletes: a 2 to 11 years of follow-up. J Orthop Traumatol. 2013;14(2):83–9.
65. Martin HD, Shears SA, Johnson JC, Smathers AM, Palmer IJ. The endoscopic treatment of sciatic nerve entrapment/deep gluteal syndrome. Arthroscopy. 2011;27(2):172–81.

66. Farjo LA, Glick JM, Sampson TG. Hip arthroscopy for acetabular labral tears. Arthroscopy. 1999;15(2):132–7.
67. Larson CM, Giveans MR, Taylor M. Does arthroscopic FAI correction improve function with radiographic arthritis? Clin Orthop Relat Res. 2011;469(6):1667–76.
68. Philippon MJ, Briggs KK, Carlisle JC, Patterson DC. Joint space predicts THA after hip arthroscopy in patients 50 years and older. Clin Orthop Relat Res. 2013;471(8):2492–6.
69. Kaminski A, Muhr G, Kutscha-Lissberg F. Modified open arthroscopy in the treatment of septic arthritis of the hip. Ortop Traumatol Rehabil. 2007;9(6):599–603.
70. McCarthy JC. Hip arthroscopy: when it is and when it is not indicated. Instr Course Lect. 2004;53:615–21.
71. Krebs VE. The role of hip arthroscopy in the treatment of synovial disorders and loose bodies. Clin Orthop Relat Res. 2003;406:48–59.
72. Flierl MA, Stahel PF, Hak DJ, Morgan SJ, Smith WR. Traction table-related complications in orthopaedic surgery. J Am Acad Orthop Surg. 2010;18(11):668–75.
73. Frontera WR, Micheli LJ, Herring SA, SIlver JK. Clinical sports medicine medical management and rehabilitation. Philadelphia: Saunders/Elsevier; 2007.
74. Nawabi DH, Degen RM, Fields KG, McLawhorn A, Ranawat AS, Sink EL, et al. Outcomes after arthroscopic treatment of femoroacetabular impingement for patients with borderline hip dysplasia. Am J Sports Med. 2016;44(4):1017–23.
75. Larson CM, Ross JR, Stone RM, Samuelson KM, Schelling EF, Giveans MR, et al. Arthroscopic management of dysplastic hip deformities: predictors of success and failures with comparison to an arthroscopic FAI cohort. Am J Sports Med. 2016;44(2):447–53.
76. Domb BG, Stake CE, Lindner D, El-Bitar Y, Jackson TJ. Arthroscopic capsular plication and labral preservation in borderline hip dysplasia: two-year clinical outcomes of a surgical approach to a challenging problem. Am J Sports Med. 2013;41(11):2591–8.
77. Bozic KJ, Chan V, Valone FH 3rd, Feeley BT, Vail TP. Trends in hip arthroscopy utilization in the United States. J Arthroplast. 2013;28(8 Suppl):140–3.
78. Oak N, Mendez-Zfass M, Lesniak BP, Larson CM, Kelly BT, Bedi A. Complications in hip arthroscopy. Sports Med Arthrosc Rev. 2013;21(2):97–105.
79. Sampson TG. Complications of hip arthroscopy. Clin Sports Med. 2001;20(4):831–5.
80. Griffin DR, Villar RN. Complications of arthroscopy of the hip. J Bone Joint Surg Br. 1999;81(4):604–6.
81. Funke EL, Munzinger U. Complications in hip arthroscopy. Arthroscopy. 1996;12(2):156–9.
82. Shetty VD, Villar RN. Hip arthroscopy: current concepts and review of literature. Br J Sports Med. 2007;41(2):64–8.
83. Byrd JWT. Operative hip arthroscopy. 3rd ed. New York: Springer; 2013.
84. Clarke MT, Arora A, Villar RN. Hip arthroscopy: complications in 1054 cases. Clin Orthop Relat Res. 2003;406:84–8.
85. Ilizaliturri VM Jr, Gonzalez-Gutierrez B, Gonzalez-Ugalde H, Camacho-Galindo J. Hip arthroscopy after traumatic hip dislocation. Am J Sports Med. 2011;39(Suppl):50S–7S.
86. Souza BGS, Dani WS, Honda EK, Ricioli W, Guimarães RP, Ono NK, et al. Do complications in hip arthroscopy change with experience? Arthroscopy. 2010;26(8):1053–7.
87. Elsaidi GA, Ruch DS, Schaefer WD, Kuzma K, Smith BP. Complications associated with traction on the hip during arthroscopy. J Bone Joint Surg Br. 2004;86(6):793–6.
88. Nakano N, Lisenda L, Jones TL, Loveday DT, Khanduja V. Complications following arthroscopic surgery of the hip: a systematic review of 36 761 cases. Bone Joint J. 2017;99-b(12):1577–83.
89. Sener N, Gogus A, Akman S, Hamzaoglu A. Avascular necrosis of the femoral head after hip arthroscopy. Hip Int. 2011;21(5):623–6.
90. Guanche CA, Bare AA. Arthroscopic treatment of femoroacetabular impingement. Arthroscopy. 2006;22(1):95–106.
91. Matsuda DK. Acute iatrogenic dislocation following hip impingement arthroscopic surgery. Arthroscopy. 2009;25(4):400–4.
92. Fowler J, Owens BD. Abdominal compartment syndrome after hip arthroscopy. Arthroscopy. 2010;26(1):128–30.
93. Verma M, Sekiya JK. Intrathoracic fluid extravasation after hip arthroscopy. Arthroscopy. 2010;26(9 Suppl):S90–4.
94. Sharma A, Sachdev H, Gomillion M. Abdominal compartment syndrome during hip arthroscopy. Anaesthesia. 2009;64(5):567–9.
95. Haupt U, Volkle D, Waldherr C, Beck M. Intra- and retroperitoneal irrigation liquid after arthroscopy of the hip joint. Arthroscopy. 2008;24(8):966–8.
96. Ladner B, Nester K, Cascio B. Abdominal fluid extravasation during hip arthroscopy. Arthroscopy. 2010;26(1):131–5.
97. Fabricant PDMT, Cross MB, et al. Avoiding complications in hip arthroscopy. Oper Tech Sports Med. 2011;19:108–13.
98. Matsuda DK, Calipusan CP. Adolescent femoroacetabular impingement from malunion of the anteroinferior iliac spine apophysis treated with arthroscopic spinoplasty. Orthopedics. 2012;35(3):e460–3.
99. Beckmann JT, Wylie JD, Potter MQ, Maak TG, Greene TH, Aoki SK. Effect of naproxen prophy-

laxis on heterotopic ossification following hip arthroscopy: a double-blind randomized placebo-controlled trial. J Bone Joint Surg Am. 2015;97(24):2032–7.
100. Bedi A, Zbeda RM, Bueno VF, Downie B, Dolan M, Kelly BT. The incidence of heterotopic ossification after hip arthroscopy. Am J Sports Med. 2012;40(4):854–63.
101. Ilizaliturri VM Jr. Complications of arthroscopic femoroacetabular impingement treatment: a review. Clin Orthop Relat Res. 2009;467(3):760–8.
102. Byrd JW. Hip arthroscopy in athletes. Instr Course Lect. 2003;52:701–9.
103. Braly BA, Beall DP, Martin HD. Clinical examination of the athletic hip. Clin Sports Med. 2006;25(2):199–210, vii.
104. Souza BG, Dani WS, Honda EK, Ricioli W Jr, Guimaraes RP, Ono NK, et al. Do complications in hip arthroscopy change with experience? Arthroscopy. 2010;26(8):1053–7.
105. Benali Y, Katthagen BD. Hip subluxation as a complication of arthroscopic debridement. Arthroscopy. 2009;25(4):405–7.
106. Pearle AD, Kendoff D, Musahl V. Perspectives on computer-assisted orthopaedic surgery: movement toward quantitative orthopaedic surgery. J Bone Joint Surg Am. 2009;91:7.
107. Stubbs AJ, Howse EA, Mannava S. Tissue engineering and the future of hip cartilage, labrum and ligamentum teres. J Hip Preserv Surg. 2016;3(1):23–9.
108. Bartlett JD, Lawrence JE, Stewart ME, Nakano N, Khanduja V. Does virtual reality simulation have a role in training trauma and orthopaedic surgeons? Bone Joint J. 2018;100-b(5):559–65.
109. Stunt J, Wulms P, Kerkhoffs G, Dankelman J, van Dijk C, Tuijthof G. How valid are commercially available medical simulators? Adv Med Educ Pract. 2014;5:385–95.

8 Current Concepts in the Management of Femoroacetabular Impingement

Yuichi Kuroda, Ankit Rai, Kenki Matsumoto, and Vikas Khanduja

8.1 Introduction

Femoroacetabular impingement (FAI) is characterised by incongruent contact between the femoral head-neck junction and the acetabulum due to bony abnormalities in one, or both, of these structures [1, 2]. This, over time, leads to progressive damage of the acetabular labrum and/or articular cartilage and is thought to be an important cause of idiopathic osteoarthritis (OA) of the hip [1]. Clinically, FAI presents with hip or groin pain along with mechanical symptoms of clicking or locking and restricted range of motion (ROM) of the hip in young adults and athletes [3, 4].

There are two distinct types of FAI: cam type and pincer type. Cam-type impingement is caused by a decreased femoral head-neck offset, often due to an osseous prominence, whereas pincer-type impingement arises from increased acetabular coverage with a normal contour of the femoral head and can be divided into general or focal overcoverage [2, 5].

Management of FAI utilises both surgical and non-surgical approaches. Surgical techniques have become an established treatment for FAI as exhibited in the United States where the proportion of patients who underwent hip arthroscopy increased by 3.65 times between 2004 and 2009 [6]. The aim of surgery is to reshape the hip joint to prevent impingement, as well as concurrently resecting, repairing or reconstructing co-morbid intra-articular injuries such as cartilage and labral damage [7]. The importance of non-surgical methods, on the other hand, is often overlooked and there are fewer publications on this topic. Non-surgical approaches such as activity modification and physiotherapy [8] predominantly target abnormal movement patterns and weakness of hip muscles found in patients with FAI [9].

Numerous studies have reported improvement in patients with FAI after surgical and non-surgical interventions [10, 11]. The aim of this chapter is to provide the reader with an evidence-based update on the management of FAI.

8.2 Surgical Treatment

The type of pathomorphology dictates the objective of surgical treatment; in pincer-type impingement, surgical treatment aims to remove the overhanging portion of the acetabular rim, whereas in cam-type impingement, the purpose is to restore the spherical shape of the femoral head [12].

Due to its minimally invasive nature, hip arthroscopy has superseded open surgery as the

Y. Kuroda · A. Rai · K. Matsumoto · V. Khanduja (✉)
Young Adult Hip Service, Department of Trauma and Orthopaedics, Addenbrooke's—Cambridge University Hospital, Cambridge, UK
e-mail: Ar798@cam.ac.uk; km640@cam.ac.uk; vk279@cam.ac.uk

W. R. Drescher et al. (eds.), *Advances in Specialist Hip Surgery*,
https://doi.org/10.1007/978-3-030-61830-8_8

preferred surgical treatment for FAI [1]. In the UK in 2013, 1908 operations for FAI were performed arthroscopically, while only 491 open operations were performed [13], and since then, the popularity of hip arthroscopy has only increased.

8.2.1 Pincer-Type FAI

Both global and focal acetabular overcoverage can be managed adequately by arthroscopic rim recession, although the former may be more dependent on the surgeon's experience [14]. The procedure seeks to eliminate the acetabular contact onto the femoral neck, but in turn it also reduces the weight-bearing area of the acetabulum. Therefore it should not be carried out on a normal or hypoplastic acetabulum and careful pre-operative planning and intra-operative execution of the plan are essential to ensure that the acetabulum is not rendered dysplastic following the procedure [15].

The gold standard technique for labral repair remains controversial. One recommendation is to detach the labrum only if the depth of rim recession is over 2–3 mm; otherwise, resection of the ossified labrum and stabilisation are sufficient [15]. A recent prospective cohort study however, has reported no difference in patient-reported outcomes between labral refixation with or without labral detachment [16]. Furthermore, in the young, healthy patients with severe labral insufficiency, labral reconstruction with a gracilis autograft achieved greater symptom improvement compared with labral refixation after acetabuloplasty [17].

The extent of centre-edge angle (CEA) reduction and target post-operative CEA also remain unknown for patients with global overcoverage. CT-based analysis of 474 asymptomatic hips showed a normal CEA value of 31°, which may represent an acceptable post-operative target for surgeons [18]; however, Sanders et al. suggest that reduction in CEA is a more important determinant of hip function than the magnitude of the preoperative or post-operative CEA [19] and therefore the jury is still out in this arena.

8.2.2 Cam-Type FAI

A greater alpha angle is associated with an increased 20-year risk of radiographic hip OA [8] and the severity of the angle corresponds to the presence of chondral defects in the acetabular rim and full-thickness delamination of the acetabular cartilage [17]. Evidently therefore, it is crucial to surgically restore the spherical shape of the femoral head for cam-type FAI; in fact, the recent multicentre randomised controlled trial, UK FASHIoN, has indicated that arthroscopy in patients with FAI with a purely cam-type deformity leads to greater clinical improvement compared with other types (mixed or pincer) [10]. The post-operative outcome after arthroscopic surgery, however, is dependent on the total volume of cam deformity, with greater volumes associated with poorer outcomes [20].

As with pincer-type FAI, the target value for arthroscopic correction is debated. A meta-analysis of 29 studies has shown that, on average, the alpha angle is decreased from 72.2° to 48.6°, with a change of 23.6° [21], but an alpha angle correction to 55° or less may be enough to obtain good clinical outcomes [22].

Two biomechanical studies, evaluating fracture risk in relation to the diameter of bone removed at the femoral head-neck junction, have also shown that bone removal of up to 30% did not significantly reduce the load-bearing capacity of the proximal femur when compared with a 10% resection [23, 24]. Mansor et al. reported however that cam over-resection of more than 5% of the diameter of the femoral head predicts inferior clinical outcomes compared with cam under-resection due to disruption of the labral seal [25]. Thus, the surgical correction of cam-type deformities, adherent to the above-advocated targets, can optimise structural integrity while preserving mobility and load-bearing capacity, as long as the integrity of the labral seal is not compromised. It is impertive to ensure an adequate surgical plan for resection of the cam lesion to ensure no over or under-correction and this can be acheieved via 3D reformatted CT scans with collision analysis.

8.2.3 Soft-Tissue Damage Concomitant with FAI

Patients who undergo hip arthroscopy for FAI frequently have labral pathology necessitating surgical intervention. Historically, labral debridement was performed as a first-line treatment; however, recent evidence suggests that debridement causes impaired sealing of the joint, which leads to the development of OA [26], and is associated with worse post-operative functional outcomes compared with labral repair [27]. Therefore, the current trend is in support of labral repair over debridement and accordingly the performance of labral repair for FAI has increased from 19% of cases in 2009 to 81% in 2017 [28].

Articular cartilage pathology in FAI is another common soft-tissue lesion found at hip arthroscopy and 88% of patients in the Danish Hip Arthroscopy Registry (DHAR) operated for symptomatic FAI had evidence of such lesions [29]. It is believed to be caused by the impaction of the cam lesion on the articular cartilage of the acetabulum [30]. Cartilage damage in FAI proceeds in the following order: bulging cartilage surface at the chondrolabral junction, full-thickness delamination and flap formation, and consequently full-thickness defects in the affected areas.

There are several methods of cartilage repair during hip arthroscopy in patients with FAI. Early changes can be managed by the debridement of bulging and loose cartilage flaps with a soft-tissue shaver or radiofrequency ablation, and this is the most common surgical method accounting for more than 81% of all cartilage procedures in patients undergoing FAI surgery [29]. More advanced changes require repair techniques including microfracture and autologous chondrocyte transplantation (ACT) or MACI [31, 32], and more recently, suturing and gluing of chondral flaps with tissel glue [33].

The majority of literature surrounding microfracture focuses on the knee joint and there are only a handful of papers describing its use in the hip [34, 35]. A recent systematic review, however, reported that it was a safe and effective treatment, especially for full-thickness, focal chondral defects [35]. Currently, the percentage of acetabular microfracture procedures was reported to be approximately 5% in both the North American group (ANCHOR study group) and DHAR [29, 36]; however given its efficacy, this figure is likely to rise in the future.

ACT is another arthroscopic technique that originated from its use in treating chondral lesions in the knee joint [37]. Recent work by Bretschneider et al. and Wilken et al. shows promising results regarding its efficacy on the hip [38, 39]. The former have shown a significant improvement in patient-reported outcomes in patients treated with autologous chondrocyte transplantation [38], and the latter have reported that chondrocytes from donors with femoral cam lesions demonstrated effective histological quality and chondrogenic potential [39].

Although many different cartilage restoration techniques are available in the hip and most of them have good short- to medium-term outcomes, current best evidence does not support any one surgical technique as a superior method due to a paucity of randomised trials [34]. To determine the superior technique for cartilage pathology, sufficient-powered long-term large-scale high-quality randomised control trials on two or three specific methods of treatment need to be conducted in the future.

8.2.4 Capsular Closure

Capsular closure has recently attracted attention due to literature suggesting that it prevents iatrogenic instability [40]. The systematic review from Riff et al. reported that the performance of patients who underwent capsular closure following hip arthroscopic surgery for FAI increased from 7 to 58% between 2009 and 2017. They also advocated that capsular closure was associated with a reduced risk of conversion to hip arthroplasty [28]. Some cadaveric studies have demonstrated that increasing capsulotomy size sequentially reduces hip joint stability, while capsular repair can restore the stability to the near-intact state [41, 42]. Furthermore, side-to-side suture repair was better able to restore capsular stability against axial stress compared with suture anchor repair [41]. Whilst there are no randomised controlled trials currently, supporting capsular closure, it seems prudent to repair the capsule especially in cases where a large capsultomy is performed to gain access and in patients with hypermobiliy or boderline dysplasia.

8.2.5 Revision Hip Arthroscopy

The British National Health Service data showed that of 6395 hip arthroscopies registered between 2005 and 2013, 286 patients (4.5%) underwent revision hip arthroscopy at a mean of 1.7 years [43]. The main indication for revision hip arthroscopy is a candidate who has symptoms due to residual cam- or pincer-type deformity that was either unaddressed or under-resected during the primary operation [44]. The literature does not support the idea that these symptoms are due to a regrowth of the deformity; Gupta et al., for example, reported no regrowth of cam deformity 2 years after femoral neck osteoplasty for FAI [45]. Therefore, a majority of the revisions were attributed to residual bony deformities.

Unfortunately, a systematic review by Sardana et al. shows that although revision hip arthroscopy is successful in improving hip functional outcomes in candidates aligning with the above-delineated criteria, these outcomes are inferior when compared with those of patients undergoing primary hip arthroscopy for FAI [44].

8.2.6 Dysplasia with FAI

Developmental dysplasia of the hip (DDH) can also lead to labral and chondral damage, and early-onset hip OA [46, 47]. Recently, Zheci et al. reviewed outcomes of hip arthroscopic surgery performed for borderline DDH (BDDH), defined by most studies as a CEA angle of 18° or 20° to 25°, and reported improvement in patient-reported outcomes. The results, however, also demonstrated an overall failure rate of 14.1% and an average reoperation rate of 8.5%. Furthermore, there was significant variation in outcomes among different studies, leading to the conclusion that efficacy is affected by multiple risk factors and patient demographics [48].

In patients with FAI and BDDH, several studies have reported favourable outcomes after hip arthroscopy with comparable outcomes to non-dysplastic patients [49, 50]. However, a higher risk of having Outerbridge grade III and IV chondral damage on the femoral head with large acetabular chondral defects than patients with non-borderline dysplastic hips was demonstrated [51]. Furthermore, Hatakeyama et al. have reported that preoperative predictors of poorer outcomes are age ≥42 years old, broken Shenton line, OA, Tönnis angle ≥15° and VCA angle ≤17° [52]. The above evidence implies therefore that when performing a hip arthroscopy on a patient with FAI and BDDH, surgical intervention should be carefully considered.

8.3 Open Surgery

In patients undergoing open surgery, several studies have reported significantly improved outcomes [53, 54]. This technique allows the surgeon to visualise the femoral head and acetabulum in its entirity, which helps to ensure complete correction of the deformity.

Surgical dislocation of the hip results in a significantly improved alpha angles in patients with cam-type impingement compared with hip arthroscopy [55]. Post-operatively however, open surgery patients had increased time off-work, longer hospital stays, worse hip function and a higher pain score compared with those undergoing arthroscopy [54]. In addition, progressive OA was demonstrated with a significant increase in Tönnis grade at the 2-year follow-up after surgical hip dislocation, despite significant improvement in symptom scores [56].

Cam osteochondroplasty with hip arthroscopy has been rapidly developing, and considering its superior clinical outcomes and minimally invasive nature, it has become the preferred option in comparison with open surgical techniques.

8.4 Post-operative Rehabilitation

Although the body of literature evaluating surgical intervention has grown, there is a paucity of evidence on the efficacy of post-operative rehabilitation programmes. One systematic review has discussed current rehabilitation protocols. It mentions that generally, immediate weight bearing is allowed if the patient can tolerate it following labral debridement, but partial weight bearing for 4–8 weeks was recommended for procedures such as labral repair, cam osteochondroplasty, pincer acetabuloplasty or microfractures for chondral lesions [57]. Several papers have advocated a rehabilitation protocol that involves four phases: Phase I (0–6 weeks) is a period of protection post-operatively with limited weight bearing, restoration of early ROM and isometric hip flexor strengthening. Phase II (4–12 weeks) advances pain-free weight bearing and ROM. Phase III (8–20 weeks) focuses more on sport-specific activity and phase IV (12 weeks) is a full recovery to an unrestricted ROM and strength [57]. This phased program with an initial period of protected weight bearing and mobility has been shown as efficacious for function, patient satisfaction and return to sport [58]. Recently, a randomised controlled trial reported that an individual physiotherapist-prescribed rehabilitation programme led to greater improvements in patient-reported outcomes, compared with patient-managed protocol, with only minor input from a physiotherapist and surgeon following arthroscopy for FAI [59]. However, since the existing reports about post-operative rehabilitation consisted of only a small number of mainly descriptive studies, it is impossible to unequivocally determine the superiority of one particular approach.

8.5 Non-surgical Treatment

Although several studies have described attempts at trials of non-surgical treatment, non-surgical protocols are rarely defined in detail and have not been standardised. However, Mansell et al. established that there was no significant difference in patient-reported outcomes between surgical and non-surgical treatments for patients with FAI syndrome using a randomised controlled trial [60]. It follows that non-surgical methods comprise an important tool in treating FAI alongside, or perhaps in certain cases, in place of surgical options.

8.6 Intra-articular Injection

Intra-articular injections of local anaesthetic and steroid are frequently performed in the routine workup and treatment of patients with FAI. Injections are generally utilised for one of the four reasons: diagnostic, prognostic, therapeutic and to buy time while the natural history of hip pain runs its course [61]. Reports have suggested that up to 50% of patients with FAI syndrome treated with an injection will not progress to surgery and non-response to injection is a strong negative predictor for surgical outcome [61, 62]. Moreover, Lynch et al. reported that while diagnostic hip injections provide substantial pain relief for patients with various hip pathologies, this relief was least for cam-type impingement [62].

The make-up of the injection is also debated; while the significant effect of corticosteroid injection in patients with symptomatic FAI and labral pathology performed by Krych et al. lasted for an average of 9.8 days, local anaesthetic injection in adults with acetabular dysplasia performed by Spruit et al. lasted for only 2.35 days [63, 64]. Notwithstanding the fact that the pathologies of the target patients were different, including corticosteroid may increase the duration of relief. In addition, a systematic review by Khan et al. presents hyaluronic acid as a viable option in providing durable therapeutic relief [65].

8.7 Physical Therapy

Improved motor control and dynamic stabilisation of the hip and pelvis provide a theoretical basis for physical therapy [66, 67]. Mansell et al. reported the protocol of physical therapy in detail [11] whereby the examiner performs a standardised clinical test comprised of six categories: anterior hip mobility (tested via the FABER position and Thomas test), hip flexion ROM, prone and seated internal rotation ROM, lumbar mobility in the quadruped rock position, gluteus medius control in the lateral step-down movement, and proprioception and lower extremity neuromuscular control in the reverse lunge. Based on the specific impairments and patients' clinical, supervised physical therapy programmes are devised, alongside a home exercise programme to address the patient's specific needs. As alluded to previously, the trial comparing outcomes following this physical therapy regimen and arthroscopic hip surgery did not find a significant difference between the groups at a 2-year follow-up [60]. On the other hand, the FAI Trial (FAIT) study led by the Oxford group in collaboration with Cambridge and other centers showed the inferior outcomes with physiotherapy than with arthroscopic hip surgery at 8-month follow-up [68]. Pennock et al. are proponents of a physical therapy plan focusing on core stability rather than flexibility, including deep hip flexion and internal rotation, achieving significant clinical improvement in a prospective cohort study [61].

Surgical bias favouring operations over conservative methods may limit evidence supporting non-surgical techniques; however as the above evidence suggests, these techniques are a viable treatment option and should be given more research attention [69].

8.8 Personalised Hip Therapy

Personal hip therapy (PHT) was proposed as a non-surgical treatment in the UK FASHIoN randomised controlled trial [70]. PHT was created from Delphi consensus, relevant literature and experiences of physiotherapists treating patients with FAI. PHT has four core components: an assessment of pain, function and range of motion; patient education; an exercise programme taught in the clinic and repeated at home; and help with pain relief, including intra-articular steroid injection [70]. PHT is believed to work by improving muscle control, strengthening musculature around the hip and appraising certain movement patterns, leading to the avoidance of hip impingement. Recently however, the UK FASHIoN group reported that although PHT improved hip-related quality of life for patients with FAI syndrome, hip arthroscopic surgery led to a greater improvement than did PHT in the shorter term [10]. Therefore, it is necessary to investigate which patients benefit most from either hip arthroscopy or PHT in future work.

8.9 The Management for FAI in Adolescents

There is paucity of literature on the treatment of FAI in adolescents. Open physes is one of the biggest challenges of managing FAI in adolescents. In the growth of the proximal femur, closure of physes is initiated at 16–18 years; 88% fusion occurs at 17–18 years and 100% fusion at 20 years [71]. A recent review of hip magnetic resonance imaging in adolescent patients undergoing hip arthroscopy demonstrated the cam pathomorphology occured at the level of the femoral physis (a mean distance of 0.07 cm). Furthermore, in skeletally immature adolescents, the cam lesion is located nearer the physis than it is in the more mature patients [72] conferring potential surgical risks such as an iatrogenic slipped capital femoral epiphysis and growth arrest of the proximal femur. Nevertheless, one systematic review has suggested that performance of hip arthroscopy and open surgical dislocation, coherent with similar surgical indications in adults, was a safe and effective means to correct symptomatic FAI deformity in adolescents. This can be attested to no cases of physeal arrest, growth disturbance or iatrogenic deformity [71]. Furthermore, Larson et al. reported that 93% of patients treated with a non-physeal-sparing arthroscopic approach for symptomatic FAI with open physes returned to their pre-injury level of sports participation without limitations [73]. Although the mean follow-up period previously reported is relatively short, future studies should be designed to evaluate outcomes in the longer term to substantiate these results.

8.10 The Future

Computer-aided technology in hip arthroplasty is constantly progressing [74]. Surgical accuracy in FAI is crucial, signified by the poorer outcomes obtained following both under- and over-resection [23–25]. Cadaver-based study has reported that an image-based navigation system achieved an acceptable level of guided femoral osteochondroplasty in the arthroscopic management of FAI [75]. In addition, robotic hip arthroscopy has been reported to enhance the level of accuracy [76].

The development of surgeons' technique is indispensable in improving post-operative outcomes. Bartlett et al. aver that virtual reality hip arthroscopy simulators have sufficient realism to promote gain of basic arthroscopic skills, supporting surgical training in orthopaedics [77].

Furthermore, a wealth of information about hip preservation surgery can be gleaned from registries such as the DHAR and Non-Arthroplasty Hip Registry (NAHR), which provide a large number of cases for review [78, 79]. Enrolment data can be used to identify patients who are suitable for surgery and to point to optimal indications in the future, which may lead to the honing of non-surgical treatments.

Thus, evolving technology and registeries will continue to bolster the management of FAI, hopefully engendering improved outcomes in the future.

8.11 Conclusion

FAI pathologically presents with hip pain and restricted ROM in young adults and athletes and can be an important aetiological factor in the development of OA. As a consequence of increasing awareness of the condition, research on the management for FAI has also been on the rise in recent years.

Regarding surgery, evidence for the target CEA for pincer-type FAI and the degree of cam resection by osteo chondroplasty has been offered by several studies, but these parameters remain controversial. The documentation of the therapeutic efficacy of labral repair compared with debridement, as well as the usefulness of hip arthroscopy compared to open surgery with hip dislocation, is substantial and is expected to increase continuously. Furthermore, arthroscopic hip surgery is also currently effective for adolescent FAI.

Non-surgical treatment modalities are also a valuable approach in treating FAI in conjunction with or instead of surgical intervention.

This chapter provides surgeons and physiotherapists with the current overview in the management of FAI. On account of inconclusive evidence in some aspects of the field, future studies would be invaluable in optimising patient outcomes in the management of FAI.

References

1. Ganz R, Parvizi J, Beck M, Leunig M, Notzli H, Siebenrock KA. Femoroacetabular impingement: a cause for osteoarthritis of the hip. Clin Orthop Relat Res. 2003;417:112–20.
2. Leunig M, Beaule PE, Ganz R. The concept of femoroacetabular impingement: current status and future perspectives. Clin Orthop Relat Res. 2009;467(3):616–22.
3. Lynch TS, Bedi A, Larson CM. Athletic hip injuries. J Am Acad Orthop Surg. 2017;25(4):269–79.
4. Wall PD, Brown JS, Parsons N, Buchbinder R, Costa ML, Griffin D. Surgery for treating hip impingement (femoroacetabular impingement). Cochrane Database Syst Rev. 2014;(9):CD010796.
5. Matsuda DK. Protrusio acetabuli: contraindication or indication for hip arthroscopy? And the case for arthroscopic treatment of global pincer impingement. Arthroscopy. 2012;28(6):882–8.
6. Montgomery SR, Ngo SS, Hobson T, Nguyen S, Alluri R, Wang JC, et al. Trends and demographics in hip arthroscopy in the United States. Arthroscopy. 2013;29(4):661–5.
7. Griffin DR, Dickenson EJ, O'Donnell J, Agricola R, Awan T, Beck M, et al. The Warwick Agreement on femoroacetabular impingement syndrome (FAI syndrome): an international consensus statement. Br J Sports Med. 2016;50(19):1169–76.
8. Nicholls AS, Kiran A, Pollard TC, Hart DJ, Arden CP, Spector T, et al. The association between hip morphology parameters and nineteen-year risk of end-stage osteoarthritis of the hip: a nested case-control study. Arthritis Rheum. 2011;63(11): 3392–400.
9. Diamond LE, Dobson FL, Bennell KL, Wrigley TV, Hodges PW, Hinman RS. Physical impairments and activity limitations in people with femoroacetabular impingement: a systematic review. Br J Sports Med. 2015;49(4):230–42.
10. Griffin DR, Dickenson EJ, Wall PDH, Achana F, Donovan JL, Griffin J, et al. Hip arthroscopy versus best conservative care for the treatment of femoroacetabular impingement syndrome (UK FASHIoN): a multicentre randomised controlled trial. Lancet. 2018;391(10136):2225–35.
11. Mansell NS, Rhon DI, Marchant BG, Slevin JM, Meyer JL. Two-year outcomes after arthroscopic surgery compared to physical therapy for femoroacetabu-

lar impingement: a protocol for a randomized clinical trial. BMC Musculoskelet Disord. 2016;17:60.
12. Larson CM, Giveans MR, Stone RM. Arthroscopic debridement versus refixation of the acetabular labrum associated with femoroacetabular impingement: mean 3.5-year follow-up. Am J Sports Med. 2012;40(5):1015–21.
13. Griffin D, Wall P, Realpe A, Adams A, Parsons N, Hobson R, et al. UK FASHIoN: feasibility study of a randomised controlled trial of arthroscopic surgery for hip impingement compared with best conservative care. Health Technol Assess. 2016;20(32):1–172.
14. Nasser R, Domb B. Hip arthroscopy for femoroacetabular impingement. EFORT Open Rev. 2018;3(4):121–9.
15. Sabetta E, Scaravella E. Treatment of pincer-type femoroacetabular impingement. Joints. 2015;3(2):78–81.
16. Redmond JM, El Bitar YF, Gupta A, Stake CE, Vemula SP, Domb BG. Arthroscopic acetabuloplasty and labral refixation without labral detachment. Am J Sports Med. 2015;43(1):105–12.
17. Matsuda DK, Burchette RJ. Arthroscopic hip labral reconstruction with a gracilis autograft versus labral refixation: 2-year minimum outcomes. Am J Sports Med. 2013;41(5):980–7.
18. Larson CM, Moreau-Gaudry A, Kelly BT, Byrd JW, Tonetti J, Lavallee S, et al. Are normal hips being labeled as pathologic? A CT-based method for defining normal acetabular coverage. Clin Orthop Relat Res. 2015;473(4):1247–54.
19. Sanders TL, Reardon P, Levy BA, Krych AJ. Arthroscopic treatment of global pincer-type femoroacetabular impingement. Knee Surg Sports Traumatol Arthrosc. 2017;25(1):31–5.
20. Ellis SH, Perriman DM, Burns AWR, Neeman TM, Lynch JT, Smith PN. Total volume of cam deformity alone predicts outcome in arthroscopy for femoroacetabular impingement. Knee Surg Sports Traumatol Arthrosc. 2020;28(4):1283–9. https://doi.org/10.1007/s00167-019-05383-9.
21. Minkara AA, Westermann RW, Rosneck J, Lynch TS. Systematic review and meta-analysis of outcomes after hip arthroscopy in femoroacetabular impingement. Am J Sports Med. 2019;47(2):488–500.
22. Fiorentino G, Fontanarosa A, Cepparulo R, Guardoli A, Berni L, Coviello G, et al. Treatment of cam-type femoroacetabular impingement. Joints. 2015;3(2):67–71.
23. Loh BW, Stokes CM, Miller BG, Page RS. Femoroacetabular impingement osteoplasty: is any resected amount safe? A laboratory based experiment with sawbones. Bone Joint J. 2015;97-B(9):1214–9.
24. Mardones RM, Gonzalez C, Chen Q, Zobitz M, Kaufman KR, Trousdale RT. Surgical treatment of femoroacetabular impingement: evaluation of the effect of the size of the resection. J Bone Joint Surg Am. 2005;87(2):273–9.
25. Mansor Y, Perets I, Close MR, Mu BH, Domb BG. In search of the spherical femoroplasty: cam overresection leads to inferior functional scores before and after revision hip arthroscopic surgery. Am J Sports Med. 2018;46(9):2061–71.
26. Song Y, Ito H, Kourtis L, Safran MR, Carter DR, Giori NJ. Articular cartilage friction increases in hip joints after the removal of acetabular labrum. J Biomech. 2012;45(3):524–30.
27. Krych AJ, Thompson M, Knutson Z, Scoon J, Coleman SH. Arthroscopic labral repair versus selective labral debridement in female patients with femoroacetabular impingement: a prospective randomized study. Arthroscopy. 2013;29(1):46–53.
28. Riff AJ, Kunze KN, Movassaghi K, Hijji F, Beck EC, Harris JD, et al. Systematic review of hip arthroscopy for femoroacetabular impingement: the importance of labral repair and capsular closure. Arthroscopy. 2019;35(2):646–56.e3.
29. Lund B, Nielsen TG, Lind M. Cartilage status in FAI patients—results from the Danish Hip Arthroscopy Registry (DHAR). SICOT J. 2017;3:44.
30. Siebenrock KA, Fiechter R, Tannast M, Mamisch TC, von Rechenberg B. Experimentally induced cam impingement in the sheep hip. J Orthop Res. 2013;31(4):580–7.
31. Korsmeier K, Classen T, Kamminga M, Rekowski J, Jager M, Landgraeber S. Arthroscopic three-dimensional autologous chondrocyte transplantation using spheroids for the treatment of full-thickness cartilage defects of the hip joint. Knee Surg Sports Traumatol Arthrosc. 2016;24(6):2032–7.
32. Mancini D, Fontana A. Five-year results of arthroscopic techniques for the treatment of acetabular chondral lesions in femoroacetabular impingement. Int Orthop. 2014;38(10):2057–64.
33. Robert H, Bowen M, Odry G, Collette M, Cassard X, Lanternier H, et al. A comparison of four tibial-fixation systems in hamstring-graft anterior ligament reconstruction. Eur J Orthop Surg Traumatol. 2015;25(2):339–47.
34. Nakano N, Gohal C, Duong A, Ayeni OR, Khanduja V. Outcomes of cartilage repair techniques for chondral injury in the hip-a systematic review. Int Orthop. 2018;42(10):2309–22.
35. MacDonald AE, Bedi A, Horner NS, de Sa D, Simunovic N, Philippon MJ, et al. Indications and outcomes for microfracture as an adjunct to hip arthroscopy for treatment of chondral defects in patients with femoroacetabular impingement: a systematic review. Arthroscopy. 2016;32(1):190–200.e2.
36. Clohisy JC, Baca G, Beaule PE, Kim YJ, Larson CM, Millis MB, et al. Descriptive epidemiology of femoroacetabular impingement: a North American cohort of patients undergoing surgery. Am J Sports Med. 2013;41(6):1348–56.
37. Fontana A, Bistolfi A, Crova M, Rosso F, Massazza G. Arthroscopic treatment of hip chondral defects: autologous chondrocyte transplantation versus simple debridement—a pilot study. Arthroscopy. 2012;28(3):322–9.
38. Bretschneider H, Trattnig S, Landgraeber S, Hartmann A, Gunther KP, Dienst M, et al. Arthroscopic matrix-

associated, injectable autologous chondrocyte transplantation of the hip: significant improvement in patient-related outcome and good transplant quality in MRI assessment. Knee Surg Sports Traumatol Arthrosc. 2020;28(4):1317–24. https://doi.org/10.1007/s00167-019-05466-7.
39. Wilken F, Slotta-Huspenina J, Laux F, Blanke F, Schauwecker J, Vogt S, et al. Autologous chondrocyte transplantation in femoroacetabular impingement syndrome: growth and redifferentiation potential of chondrocytes harvested from the femur in cam-type deformities. Cartilage. 2019. https://doi.org/10.1177/1947603519833138.
40. Smith KM, Gerrie BJ, McCulloch PC, Lewis BD, Mather RC, Van Thiel G, et al. Arthroscopic hip preservation surgery practice patterns: an international survey. J Hip Preserv Surg. 2017;4(1):18–29.
41. Khair MM, Grzybowski JS, Kuhns BD, Wuerz TH, Shewman E, Nho SJ. The effect of capsulotomy and capsular repair on hip distraction: a cadaveric investigation. Arthroscopy. 2017;33(3):559–65.
42. Wuerz TH, Song SH, Grzybowski JS, Martin HD, Mather RC 3rd, Salata MJ, et al. Capsulotomy size affects hip joint kinematic stability. Arthroscopy. 2016;32(8):1571–80.
43. Malviya A, Raza A, Jameson S, James P, Reed MR, Partington PF. Complications and survival analyses of hip arthroscopies performed in the national health service in England: a review of 6,395 cases. Arthroscopy. 2015;31(5):836–42.
44. Sardana V, Philippon MJ, de Sa D, Bedi A, Ye L, Simunovic N, et al. Revision hip arthroscopy indications and outcomes: a systematic review. Arthroscopy. 2015;31(10):2047–55.
45. Gupta A, Redmond JM, Stake CE, Finch NA, Dunne KF, Domb BG. Does the femoral cam lesion regrow after osteoplasty for femoroacetabular impingement? Two-year follow-up. Am J Sports Med. 2014;42(9):2149–55.
46. Chandrasekaran S, Darwish N, Martin TJ, Suarez-Ahedo C, Lodhia P, Domb BG. Arthroscopic capsular plication and labral seal restoration in borderline hip dysplasia: 2-year clinical outcomes in 55 cases. Arthroscopy. 2017;33(7):1332–40.
47. McCarthy JC, Lee JA. Acetabular dysplasia: a paradigm of arthroscopic examination of chondral injuries. Clin Orthop Relat Res. 2002;405:122–8.
48. Ding Z, Sun Y, Liu S, Chen J. Hip arthroscopic surgery in borderline developmental dysplastic hips: a systematic review. Am J Sports Med. 2019;47(10):2494–500. https://doi.org/10.1177/0363546518803367.
49. Cvetanovich GL, Levy DM, Weber AE, Kuhns BD, Mather RC 3rd, Salata MJ, et al. Do patients with borderline dysplasia have inferior outcomes after hip arthroscopic surgery for femoroacetabular impingement compared with patients with Normal acetabular coverage? Am J Sports Med. 2017;45(9):2116–24.
50. Nawabi DH, Degen RM, Fields KG, McLawhorn A, Ranawat AS, Sink EL, et al. Outcomes after arthroscopic treatment of femoroacetabular impingement for patients with borderline hip dysplasia. Am J Sports Med. 2016;44(4):1017–23.
51. Bolia IK, Briggs KK, Locks R, Chahla J, Utsunomiya H, Philippon MJ. Prevalence of high-grade cartilage defects in patients with borderline dysplasia with femoroacetabular impingement: a comparative cohort study. Arthroscopy. 2018;34(8):2347–52.
52. Hatakeyama A, Utsunomiya H, Nishikino S, Kanezaki S, Matsuda DK, Sakai A, et al. Predictors of poor clinical outcome after arthroscopic labral preservation, capsular plication, and cam osteoplasty in the setting of borderline hip dysplasia. Am J Sports Med. 2018;46(1):135–43.
53. Domb BG, Stake CE, Botser IB, Jackson TJ. Surgical dislocation of the hip versus arthroscopic treatment of femoroacetabular impingement: a prospective matched-pair study with average 2-year follow-up. Arthroscopy. 2013;29(9):1506–13.
54. Zingg PO, Ulbrich EJ, Buehler TC, Kalberer F, Poutawera VR, Dora C. Surgical hip dislocation versus hip arthroscopy for femoroacetabular impingement: clinical and morphological short-term results. Arch Orthop Trauma Surg. 2013;133(1):69–79.
55. Zhang D, Chen L, Wang G. Hip arthroscopy versus open surgical dislocation for femoroacetabular impingement: a systematic review and meta-analysis. Medicine (Baltimore). 2016;95(41):e5122.
56. Espinosa N, Rothenfluh DA, Beck M, Ganz R, Leunig M. Treatment of femoro-acetabular impingement: preliminary results of labral refixation. J Bone Joint Surg Am. 2006;88(5):925–35.
57. Grzybowski JS, Malloy P, Stegemann C, Bush-Joseph C, Harris JD, Nho SJ. Rehabilitation following hip arthroscopy—a systematic review. Front Surg. 2015;2:21.
58. Cheatham SW, Enseki KR, Kolber MJ. Postoperative rehabilitation after hip arthroscopy: a search for the evidence. J Sport Rehabil. 2015;24(4):413–8.
59. Bennell KL, Spiers L, Takla A, O'Donnell J, Kasza J, Hunter DJ, et al. Efficacy of adding a physiotherapy rehabilitation programme to arthroscopic management of femoroacetabular impingement syndrome: a randomised controlled trial (FAIR). BMJ Open. 2017;7(6):e014658.
60. Mansell NS, Rhon DI, Meyer J, Slevin JM, Marchant BG. Arthroscopic surgery or physical therapy for patients with femoroacetabular impingement syndrome: a randomized controlled trial with 2-year follow-up. Am J Sports Med. 2018;46(6):1306–14.
61. Pennock AT, Bomar JD, Johnson KP, Randich K, Upasani VV. Nonoperative management of femoroacetabular impingement: a prospective study. Am J Sports Med. 2018;46(14):3415–22.
62. Lynch TS, Steinhaus ME, Popkin CA, Ahmad CS, Rosneck J. Outcomes after diagnostic hip injection. Arthroscopy. 2016;32(8):1702–11.
63. Krych AJ, Griffith TB, Hudgens JL, Kuzma SA, Sierra RJ, Levy BA. Limited therapeutic benefits of intra-articular cortisone injection for patients with femoro-acetabular impingement and labral tear. Knee Surg Sports Traumatol Arthrosc. 2014;22(4):750–5.

64. Spruit M, Van Goethem CJ, Kooijman MA, Pavlov PW. Diagnostic infiltration of the hip joint with bupivacaine in adult acetabular dysplasia. Acta Orthop Belg. 1997;63(4):274–7.
65. Khan W, Khan M, Alradwan H, Williams R, Simunovic N, Ayeni OR. Utility of intra-articular hip injections for femoroacetabular impingement: a systematic review. Orthop J Sports Med. 2015;3(9):2325967115601030.
66. Casartelli NC, Maffiuletti NA, Bizzini M, Kelly BT, Naal FD, Leunig M. The management of symptomatic femoroacetabular impingement: what is the rationale for non-surgical treatment? Br J Sports Med. 2016;50(9):511–2.
67. Wright AA, Hegedus EJ, Taylor JB, Dischiavi SL, Stubbs AJ. Non-operative management of femoroacetabular impingement: a prospective, randomized controlled clinical trial pilot study. J Sci Med Sport. 2016;19(9):716–21.
68. Palmer AJR, Ayyar Gupta V, Fernquest S, Rombach I, Dutton SJ, Mansour R, et al. Arthroscopic hip surgery compared with physiotherapy and activity modification for the treatment of symptomatic femoroacetabular impingement: multicentre randomised controlled trial. BMJ. 2019;364:l185.
69. Ross JR, Bedi A, Clohisy JC, Gagnier JJ, Group AS, Larson CM. Surgeon willingness to participate in randomized controlled trials for the treatment of femoroacetabular impingement. Arthroscopy. 2016;32(1):20–4.e3.
70. Wall PD, Dickenson EJ, Robinson D, Hughes I, Realpe A, Hobson R, et al. Personalised Hip Therapy: development of a non-operative protocol to treat femoroacetabular impingement syndrome in the FASHIoN randomised controlled trial. Br J Sports Med. 2016;50(19):1217–23.
71. de Sa D, Cargnelli S, Catapano M, Bedi A, Simunovic N, Burrow S, et al. Femoroacetabular impingement in skeletally immature patients: a systematic review examining indications, outcomes, and complications of open and arthroscopic treatment. Arthroscopy. 2015;31(2):373–84.
72. Carter CW, Bixby S, Yen YM, Nasreddine AY, Kocher MS. The relationship between cam lesion and physis in skeletally immature patients. J Pediatr Orthop. 2014;34(6):579–84.
73. Larson CM, McGaver RS, Collette NR, Giveans MR, Ross JR, Bedi A, et al. Arthroscopic surgery for femoroacetabular impingement in skeletally immature athletes: radiographic and clinical analysis. Arthroscopy. 2019;35(6):1819–25.
74. Nakano N, Audenaert E, Ranawat A, Khanduja V. Review: current concepts in computer-assisted hip arthroscopy. Int J Med Robot. 2018;14(6):e1929.
75. Audenaert E, Smet B, Pattyn C, Khanduja V. Imageless versus image-based registration in navigated arthroscopy of the hip: a cadaver-based assessment. J Bone Joint Surg Br. 2012;94(5):624–9.
76. Kather J, Hagen ME, Morel P, Fasel J, Markar S, Schueler M. Robotic hip arthroscopy in human anatomy. Int J Med Robot. 2010;6(3):301–5.
77. Bartlett JD, Lawrence JE, Khanduja V. Virtual reality hip arthroscopy simulator demonstrates sufficient face validity. Knee Surg Sports Traumatol Arthrosc. 2019;27(10):3162–7. https://doi.org/10.1007/s00167-018-5038-8.
78. Maempel JF, Ting JZ, Gaston P. Assessing the outcome of hip arthroscopy for labral tears in femoroacetabular impingement using the minimum dataset of the British non-arthroplasty hip register: a single-surgeon experience. Arthroscopy. 2018;34(7):2131–9.
79. Mygind-Klavsen B, Lund B, Nielsen TG, Maagaard N, Kraemer O, Holmich P, et al. Danish Hip Arthroscopy Registry: predictors of outcome in patients with femoroacetabular impingement (FAI). Knee Surg Sports Traumatol Arthrosc. 2019;27(10):3110–20. https://doi.org/10.1007/s00167-018-4941-3.

Part IV

Osteonecrosis of the Femoral Head: Promising Hip Preservation Surgery Techniques

9 Current State of Diagnosis and Treatment of AVN of the Hip

Wolf R. Drescher, Yusuke Kubo, Thomas Pufe, and Takuaki Yamamoto

Abbreviations

ARCO	Association Research Osseous Circulation
AVN	Avascular necrosis
FSE	Fat-suppressed spin echo
GWAS	Genome-wide association study
JIC	Japanese Investigation Committee
MPSL	Methylprednisolone
MRI	Magnetic resonance imaging
ON	Osteonecrosis
ONFH	Osteonecrosis of the femoral head
ROM	Range of motion
SIF	Subchondral insufficiency fracture
STIR	Short T1 inversion recovery

W. R. Drescher (✉)
Department of Orthopedics, RWTH Aachen University Hospital, Aachen, Germany

Orthopedic Surgery of the Lower Limb and Arthroplasty, Rummelsberg Hospital, Schwarzenbruck, Germany
e-mail: wolf.drescher@sana.de

Y. Kubo · T. Pufe
Department of Anatomy and Cell Biology, RWTH Aachen University, Aachen, Germany
e-mail: ykubo@ukaachen.de; tpufe@ukaachen.de

T. Yamamoto
Faculty of Medicine, Department of Orthopaedic Surgery, Fukuoka University, Fukuoka, Japan
e-mail: yamamotot@fukuoka-u.ac.jp

9.1 Introduction

"Death of all the cellular elements of bone indicates osteonecrosis (ON)" [1], and can be of traumatic or nontraumatic origin [2].

Nontraumatic AVN of the hip affects mainly young patients and leads to secondary arthritis of the hip. Additionally, the survival of total hip arthroplasties in those young patients with AVN of the hip is inferior [3] which still nowadays makes AVN of the hip a challenge for the orthopedic surgeon.

9.2 Epidemiology

ON accounts for about 10% of more than 500,000 total joint replacements performed annually in the United States [2]. The average age of the patients receiving total hip replacement for AVN is 38 years with only 20% of patients being more than 50 years old at the time of operation [4]. In our three-decade experience, the disease is underdiagnosed as many hips reach the state of secondary arthritis before the diagnosis of AVN. Especially in chemotherapy for leukemia associated with ON, the average patient age was as young as 14 years at the time of diagnosis [5].

As nontraumatic AVN of the hip affects both hips nonsimultaneously in up to 90% of the cases, it is mandatory also to examine the contralateral "silent hip" [6].

W. R. Drescher et al. (eds.), *Advances in Specialist Hip Surgery*,
https://doi.org/10.1007/978-3-030-61830-8_9

Based on epidemiologic studies in Japan, the crude incidence rate has been reported to be 2.51 cases per 100,000 person-years, and the number of new nontraumatic AVN patients in Japan (population: ~120 million) was estimated to be around 3200 cases per year [7].

9.3 Etiology

In a prospective study, 20% of the patients were diagnosed with AVN of the hip 1 year after solid organ transplantation and associated glucocorticoid therapy [8], with renal transplantations having the highest risk. Cigarette smokers had an odds ratio of 10.3 for being affected by AVN of the hip over nonsmokers [9]. Further etiologies of ON are systemic lupus erythematosus [10], chronic inflammatory bowel disease [11], and multiple sclerosis [12].

In a retrospective study in 105 pediatric patients with chemotherapy because of acute lymphoblastic or myeloid leukemia and non-Hodgkin lymphoma, the average age was 8 years at leukemia diagnosis [5]. After 17 months, 4 boys und 4 girls each (7.6%) between 10 and 17 years had 18 osteonecrotic lesions, 12 of which affected the hip joint.

Further etiologies of AVN are sickle cell anemia [13], Caisson's disease of the divers [1], and Gaucher's disease [14]. Bone marrow edema syndrome and ON has also been reported in association with pregnancy and postpartum [15, 16].

9.4 Pathogenesis

Impaired femoral head blood flow and a procoagulatory state of plasma could be experimentally shown after high-dose steroid treatment [17]. Systemic fat embolism has been described after renal transplantation and associated glucocorticoid therapy [18]. Thrombophilia and hypofibrinolysis were described in 12 cases of steroid-induced ON [19].

Hypertrophy of bone marrow fat cells could be shown after steroid and alcohol application in vitro [20]. Fat-cell hypertrophy was postulated to increase intraosseous pressure, compress capillaries and sinus, and thereby decrease local bone blood flow in this study.

The necrotic area is typically located at the end of the lateral epiphyseal arteries within the femoral head. In these vessels, pathologic changes have been shown [21]. Later on, gene expression of factors of bone formation and remodeling as well as bone morphogenetic proteins 2 and 7 has been shown to rise [22].

As to the animal model for ON, corticosteroid-induced ON was firstly developed in rabbits, in which high-dose methylprednisolone (MPSL) (20 mg/kg) can induce multifocal ON in conjunction with thrombocytopenia, hypofibrinogenemia, and hyperlipidemia [23]. Based on this animal model for ON, several investigations for the prevention of AVN have been reported, including combined effects of warfarin and lipid-lowering agent [24], antiplatelet drug [25], statin [26], and anti-vasospasm agent [27, 28].

Recently, a genome-wide association study (GWAS) has been performed using 1602 ON cases and 60,000 controls. Stratified GWASs based on the three subgroups of ON of the femoral head (ONFH) (corticosteroids, alcohol, idiopathic) were also performed. A novel ON locus was identified at chromosome 20q12, and *LINC01370* was the best candidate gene in this locus [29].

9.5 Pathology

One of the most characteristic pathologic findings in ON is a zone formation, comprising necrotic, reparative, and viable tissue [30]. A wedge-shaped necrotic area is seen in a subchondral area, which is surrounded by reparative tissue. This reparative tissue continues to the normal viable bone and bone marrow tissue (Fig. 9.1).

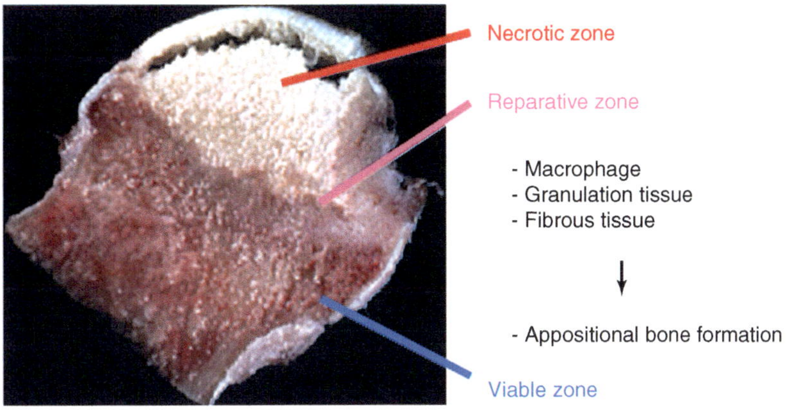

Fig. 9.1 Zone formation in ON. A wedge-shaped necrotic area is seen in a subchondral area, which is surrounded by the reparative tissue. This reparative tissue continues to the normal viable bone and bone marrow tissue. In the early phase of ON, the reparative tissue generally consists of infiltration macrophage, granulation tissue, and fibrous tissue, which can only be recognized on magnetic resonance imaging (MRI). Thereafter, bony repair such as appositional bone formation and creeping substitution occur, when radiograph can detect these bony changes as a sclerotic change

9.6 Diagnostic Criteria

First symptoms often are spontaneous groin pain eventually radiating to the knee [31]. According to the experience of the authors, the pain is extremely strong, unrelated to mechanic stress/weight bearing, and often occurs spontaneously in the night. At clinical examination of the range of motion (ROM), the hip often is extremely painful in many directions.

9.7 The ARCO and JIC Classification Systems

Very much established today is the ARCO classification consented by the Association Research Circulation Osseous (Table 9.1) [4]. The JIC classification for clinical differential therapy has been worked out by the Japanese Investigation Committee. Both systems are presented here as they very much supplement each other.

Stage ARCO 0 can only be detected histologically [32]. It is defined as a reversible stage without clinical symptoms. It should be thought of, when the contralateral hip has a later stage AVN as both hips are affected in up to 90% in an unsynchronized fashion. In this case, MRI of both hips is warranted.

In the reversible early stage ARCO 1, X-rays are without pathological findings. Gold standard is the MRI, preferably T1-weighted spin-echo and T2-weighted fat-suppressed spin-echo (FSE) or short T1 inversion recovery (STIR) sequences [33]. On MRI, stage 1 is characterized by unspecific signal changes.

An important differential diagnosis in this early stage is bone marrow edema syndrome [34, 35]. By peculiar history taking, especially searching for etiologic factors of ON, a detailed clinical examination, and simply thinking of AVN as a differential diagnosis, the early stage ARCO 1 can be secured by MRI examination.

Early diagnosis is very important; as for stage ARCO 1, a high rate of healing has been reported after the simple surgical therapy of core drilling [36].

ARCO stage 2 is the irreversible early stage (ARCO 2) In this stage, AVN of the hip can be diagnosed by X-ray examination. Enhanced bone

Table 9.1 The ARCO classification of AVN of the hip [4]

Stage		Characteristics
0		Bone biopsy results consistent with AVN (Ficat 1985) without radiographic pathology
I		Positive scintiscan or MRI, or both; lesions subdivided into medial, central, or lateral depending on the location of involvement of femoral head; no radiographic pathology
	I-A	<15% involvement of the femoral head
	I-B	15–30% involvement of the femoral head
	I-C	>30% involvement of the femoral head
II		Radiographic abnormalities (mottled appearance of the femoral head, osteosclerosis, cyst formation, and osteopenia); no signs of collapse of the femoral head on radiographs or computed tomography (CT) scan; positive scintiscan and MRI; no changes in acetabulum; lesions subdivided into medial, central, or lateral depending on the location of involvement of femoral head
	II-A	<15% involvement of the femoral head
	II-B	15–30% involvement of the femoral head
	II-C	>30% involvement of the femoral head
III		Crescent sign; lesions subdivided into medial, central, or lateral depending on the location of involvement of femoral head
	III-A	<15% crescent sign or <2 mm depression of femoral head
	III-B	15–30% crescent sign or 2–4 mm depression of femoral head
	III-C	>30% crescent sign or 4 mm depression of femoral head
IV		Articular surface flattened radiographically and joint space shows narrowing; changes in acetabulum with evidence of osteosclerosis, cyst formation, and marginal osteophytes

apposition on necrotic trabeculae makes the necrotic area less radiolucent. On MRI, the necrotic area is now delineated, and the "double-line sign" in T2-weighted sequences is pathognomonic [37]. The outer line of low signal intensity represents reactive bone while the inner line of higher signal intensity represents the vascularized zone of reparation.

Stage ARCO 3 is characterized by advancing resorption of dead bone trabeculae with mechanic weakening, subchondral fracture, and depression of the femoral head. The narrow radiolucent subchondral line on X-ray is pathognomonic for stage 3, and is termed "crescent sign" [37]. In case of uncertainty about the subchondral fracture, CT is recommended [38]. An important differential diagnosis in stage ARCO 3 is subchondral insufficiency fracture (SIF) in elderly osteoporotic and renal transplant patients [39]. The low-signal-intensity band in the T1-weighted coronary MR sequence is distinctive here [40].

The late stage ARCO 4 denominates secondary arthritis of the hip.

The stages ARCO 1–3 are subclassified by medial, central, or lateral localization of the necrotic lesion also addressing its size (Table 9.1).

The Japanese Investigation Committee (JIC) of ON proposed criteria for the diagnosis, classification, and staging of ON in 2001, by the working group of the Specific Disease Investigation Committee under the auspices of the Japanese Ministry of Health, Labor and Welfare [41].

9.8 Diagnosis: JIC criteria

The following five criteria were selected for the diagnosis of ON, since they all showed high specificity:

1. Collapse of the femoral head (including crescent sign) without joint space narrowing or acetabular abnormality on X-ray images
2. Demarcating sclerosis in the femoral head without joint space narrowing or acetabular abnormality
3. "Cold in hot" on bone scans
4. Low-intensity band on T1-weighted MRI (bandlike pattern)
5. Trabecular and bone marrow necrosis on histology

ON can be diagnosed if the patient fulfills two of these five criteria and does not have bone tumors, SIF, or dysplasia.

9.9 Differential Diagnosis

9.9.1 Subchondral Insufficiency Fracture

The entity of SIF has been described in both the osteoporotic elderly and renal transplant recipients [39, 42]. At the onset of pain, plain radiographs show no obvious findings but MRI reveals a bone marrow edema pattern with an associated irregular serpiginous low-signal-intensity line on the T1-weighted images. This irregular low-intensity line is one of the characteristic appearances in SIF [43]. Based on histological re-examination, the prevalence of SIF in cases with a preoperative diagnosis of osteoarthritis was 6.3% (460 out of 7349), and with ON was 11.1% (41 out of 369) [44].

9.10 The JIC 2001 Classification

The classification scheme consists of four types, based on their location on T1-weighted images or X-ray images.

1. Type A lesions occupy the medial one-third or less of the weight-bearing portion.
2. Type B lesions occupy the medial two-thirds or less of the weight-bearing portion.
3. Type C1 lesions occupy more than the medial two-thirds of the weight-bearing portion but do not extend laterally to the acetabular edge.
4. Type C2 lesions occupy more than the medial two-thirds of the weight-bearing portion and extend laterally to the acetabular edge. Staging is based on anteroposterior and lateral views of the femoral head on X-ray images.

Based on this classification, the collapse rate on each type has been reported (Fig. 9.2) [45].

9.11 Therapy

Core drilling (core decompression) is indicated for AVN patients with the reversible stage ARCO 1. This procedure leads to relief of intraosseous pressure and improvement of microcirculation. Neovascularization occurs in the necrotic lesion by penetrating the boundary of necrotic lesion. Wirtz et al. reported that a restitutio ad integrum can be achieved by core decompression of the femoral head in cases with transient bone marrow edema [36]. In stages ARCO 1 and 2, cases with less than 30% of necrotic lesion within the femoral head have the best prognosis.

Stem cell therapy is discussed in Chaps. 11 and 12 of this book.

Iloprost A long-term follow-up study showed that intravenous iloprost could relieve pain and reduce the necrotic lesion or bone marrow edema. However, there was no convincing evidence of prognostic improvement for AVN [46].

Bisphosphonates A prospective randomized multicenter study demonstrated that zoledronate had no protective effect on the onset of ON or the decrease of cases with surgical indication [47].

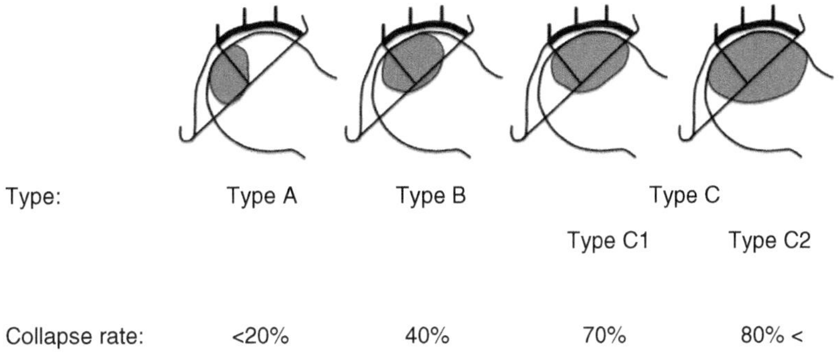

Fig. 9.2 Necrotic area location [45]

Intertrochanteric Osteotomy Previous reports have described various survival rates of intertrochanteric osteotomy. Flexion osteotomy is the most commonly used intertrochanteric osteotomy technique. We previously evaluated 70 hips treated with intertrochanteric flexion osteotomy, reporting that a 5-year survival rate was 90%, and after 10 years it was 81% [48]. A better survival rate was obtained in cases in stage ARCO 2 and with a necrotic angle of less than 200°. Reck et al. examined lower benefit of flexion osteotomy because of its poor prognosis [49]. They reported a 10-year survival rate of only 42.5%. It should be taken into account that the subsequent hip replacement is considerably difficult after osteotomy. Another report showed superior results at 10-year follow-up of cementless short-stem arthroplasty as an alternative treatment of intertrochanteric osteotomy [50].

In Japan, two operative procedures to preserve the original hip joint have been performed. One is intertrochanteric curved varus osteotomy of the femur, and the other is rotational osteotomy of the femoral head [51]. Both operations are performed in patients with a postoperative intact area of 34% or higher (Fig. 9.3) [52] according to the position and size of the intact area (Fig. 9.4).

Transtrochanteric Rotational Osteotomy The areas of necrosis can be accurately identified by using anteroposterior radiographs of the hip joint and Lauenstein radiographs (flexion, 90°; abduction, 45°). Osteotomy is performed in patients with a postoperative intact area ratio to the acetabular weight-bearing area of 34% or higher (Fig. 9.4). If the necrotic area is anteriorly located or is located in the middle or back of the head, an anterior rotational osteotomy, wherein the intact area remaining in the posterior portion is moved to the weight-bearing area, and a posterior rotational osteotomy, wherein the intact area remaining in the anterior portion is moved to the weight-bearing area, are performed, respectively. The femoral head can be rotated up to 90° anteriorly and up to 140° posteriorly. Several good clinical results have been reported [51–54].

Transtrochanteric Curved Varus Osteotomy This procedure is indicated in cases with a residual intact area in the lateral part of the femoral head with an intact area ratio to the acetabular weight-bearing area of 34% or more in a maximum abduction position. Good clinical results [55, 56] as well as leg-length discrepancies after this procedure have been reported [57].

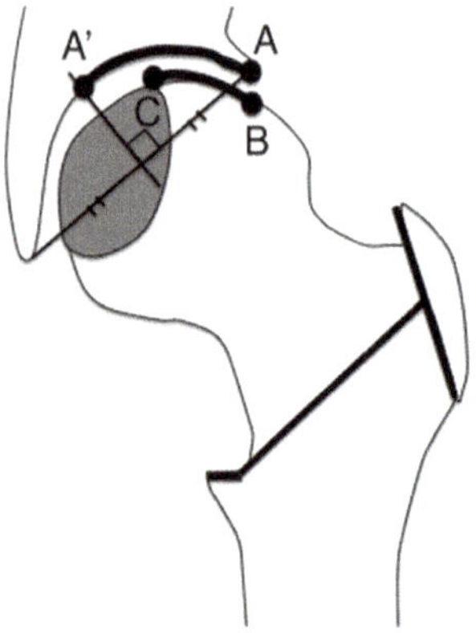

$$\text{Postoperative intact ratio (\%)} = \frac{B - C}{A - A'} \times 100$$

Fig. 9.3 Postoperative intact ratio. This is a calculation of the postoperative intact ratio. It is essential that the postoperative intact ratio be 34% or higher [52]

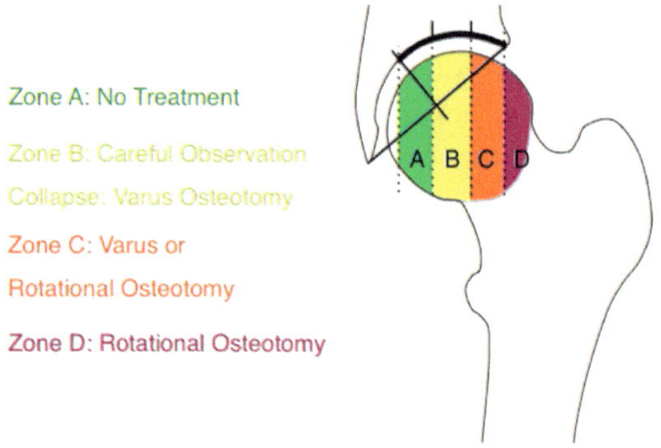

Fig. 9.4 Indication for femoral osteotomy. In principle, a curved varus osteotomy is performed in patients with an intact area ratio to the weight-bearing area of around 34% in a maximum abduction position, and an anterior rotation osteotomy or posterior rotation osteotomy is performed in patients other than those mentioned

Nonvascularized Bone Transplantation Rijnen et al. have suggested that this straightforward procedure does not impair subsequent total hip replacement [58]. A bone cylinder is obtained by a hollow drill from the lateral side of proximal femoral cortex to the necrotic lesion within the femoral neck. First, the necrotic lesion is completely removed, and is finally filled with impacted autograft bone chips. Rijnen et al. prospectively evaluated 28 hips in 27 patients in stages ARCO 2–4 at a mean follow-up of 42 months, reporting that subsequent hip replacement was performed in 8 hips. Of the remaining 20 hips, 90% of cases were clinically successful and 70% were radiologically successful. Patients aged less than 30 years had a better radiological outcome, while patients with subchondral collapse and a history of corticosteroid use had a poor prognosis. Seyler et al. reported that 18 of 22 hips in stage ARCO 2 survived at a mean follow-up of 36 months [59]. Mont et al. reported the contribution of bone substitute material (a combination of demineralized bone matrix, processed allograft bone chips, and a thermoplastic carrier) with bone morphogenetic protein through a window at the femoral head-neck junction [60]. Eighteen of 21 hips with a mean follow-up of 48 months were clinically successful at latest follow-up.

Vascularized Fibula Transplantation Previous studies showed good results of the vascularized grafting of fibular or iliac crest bone in the stage ARCO 2 or 3. A minimum 10-year follow-up study reported that the Harris hip score improved after vascularized fibular grafting, whereas only 10.5% of cases failed treatment and underwent conversion to total hip replacement [61]. In this study, postoperative subtrochanteric fracture was reported in two hips. Advanced surgical skill is required to insert grafting at the central position. In practice, revision surgery after vascularized fibular grafting is more difficult. The risk of fracture and the difficulty of revision surgery are similar to those of trabecular metal from the tantalum implant (Trabecular metal ON intervention implant, Zimmer Biomet, Warsaw/In, USA) [62]. Flörkemeier et al. reported that the survival rate with tantalum implant insertion was not superior to that of core decompression alone [63].

Short-Stem Hip Arthroplasty Short-stem hip arthroplasty is suitable for a sustainable long-term treatment strategy in young AVN patients, because it preserves the femoral neck. Short-stem hip arthroplasty is recommended to AVN patients due to encouraging midterm results [50]. In these cases, it seems to be important to evaluate the involvement of femoral head and neck on MRI. The increase of osteoblast formation and the alteration of trabecular bone properties in histopathology need to be taken into account even though these findings do not directly indicate ON [64].

Total Hip Arthroplasty In previous reports, complications and loosening after total hip replacement in AVN were variously described [65]. AVN associated with steroid, renal osteopathy, or sickle cell anemia has been reported to cause a higher rate of stem loosening after total hip replacement. Patients with immunosuppression have a higher rate of infection after total hip replacement. Regardless of etiology, 158 hips in 141 AVN patients had a mean Harris hip score of 84 at a mean follow-up of 103 months, and revision surgery was needed in 8.9% of these cases [66]. Recently, Kim et al. investigated 64 hips in 55 patients with a minimum 15 years of follow-up, reporting that the survivorship with an end point of revision of cementless modular stem was 93.8% at 16.8 years [67]. The good midterm results for ceramic-on-ceramic bearings were also prospectively reported in advanced AVN [68]. In addition, a previous study reported favorable midterm results of cementless short stems with ceramic-on-ceramic bearings [69].

Final Considerations of the Different Methods In our opinion, collateral damage of the selected technique has to be taken into account as the common end point will be total hip arthroplasty. The technique of free vascularized fibular grafting described by Urbaniak et al. requires drilling of a 2 cm wide channel from the lateral proximal femur through the femoral neck [70]. This involves the risk of subtrochanteric fracture [61].

Additionally, this makes a subsequent short-stem implantation impossible. Standard total hip arthroplasty can be even more difficult.

Flexion osteotomy can complicate or make subsequent hip arthroplasty very difficult.

References

1. Jones JP Jr, et al. The pathophysiologic role of fat in dysbaric osteonecrosis. Clin Orthop Relat Res. 1993;296:256–64.
2. Mankin HJ. Nontraumatic necrosis of bone (osteonecrosis). N Engl J Med. 1992;326(22):1473–9. https://doi.org/10.1056/NEJM199205283262206.
3. Kim YH, et al. Contemporary total hip arthroplasty with and without cement in patients with osteonecrosis of the femoral head. J Bone Joint Surg Am. 2003;85-A(4):675–81.
4. Mont MA, Hungerford DS. Non-traumatic avascular necrosis of the femoral head. J Bone Joint Surg Am. 1995;77(3):459–74.
5. Salem KH, et al. Avascular necrosis after chemotherapy for haematological malignancy in childhood. Bone Joint J. 2013;95-B(12):1708–13. https://doi.org/10.1302/0301-620X.95B12.30688.
6. Bradway JK, Morrey BF. The natural history of the silent hip in bilateral atraumatic osteonecrosis. J Arthroplast. 1993;8(4):383–7.
7. Yamaguchi R, et al. Incidence of nontraumatic osteonecrosis of the femoral head in the Japanese population. Arthritis Rheum. 2011;63(10):3169–73. https://doi.org/10.1002/art.30484.
8. Marston SB, et al. Osteonecrosis of the femoral head after solid organ transplantation: a prospective study. J Bone Joint Surg Am. 2002;84-A(12):2145–51.
9. Takahashi S, et al. Pronounced risk of nontraumatic osteonecrosis of the femoral head among cigarette smokers who have never used oral corticosteroids: a multicenter case-control study in Japan. J Orthop Sci. 2012;17(6):730–6. https://doi.org/10.1007/s00776-012-0293-x.
10. Nakamura J, et al. Development of new osteonecrosis in systemic lupus erythematosus patients in association with long-term corticosteroid therapy after disease recurrence. Clin Exp Rheumatol. 2010;28(1):13–8.
11. Hauzeur JP, et al. Osteonecrosis in inflammatory bowel diseases: a review of the literature. Acta Gastroenterol Belg. 2009;72(3):327–34.
12. Ce P, et al. Avascular necrosis of the bones: an overlooked complication of pulse steroid treatment of multiple sclerosis. Eur J Neurol. 2006;13(8):857–61. https://doi.org/10.1111/j.1468-1331.2006.01375.x.
13. Hernigou P, et al. The natural history of asymptomatic osteonecrosis of the femoral head in adults with sickle cell disease. J Bone Joint Surg Am. 2006;88(12):2565–72. https://doi.org/10.2106/JBJS.E.01455.
14. Katz K, et al. The natural history of osteonecrosis of the femoral head in children and adolescents who have Gaucher disease. J Bone Joint Surg Am. 1996;78(1):14–9.
15. Ugwonali OF, et al. Bilateral osteonecrosis of the femoral head associated with pregnancy: four new cases and a review of the literature. Orthopedics. 2008;31(2):183.
16. Aigner N, et al. Bone marrow edema syndrome in postpartal women: treatment with iloprost. Orthop Clin North Am. 2009;40(2):241–7. https://doi.org/10.1016/j.ocl.2008.10.007.
17. Drescher W, et al. Femoral head blood flow reduction and hypercoagulability under 24-h megadose steroid treatment in pigs. J Orthop Res. 2004;22(3):501–8. https://doi.org/10.1016/j.orthres.2003.10.002.
18. Jones JP Jr. Intravascular coagulation and osteonecrosis. Clin Orthop Relat Res. 1992;(277):41–53.
19. Glueck CJ, et al. Thrombophilia and hypofibrinolysis: pathophysiologies of osteonecrosis. Clin Orthop Relat Res. 1997;334:43–56.
20. Cui Q, et al. Steroid-induced adipogenesis in a pluripotential cell line from bone marrow. J Bone Joint Surg Am. 1997;79(7):1054–63.
21. Saito S, et al. Early arteriopathy and postulated pathogenesis of osteonecrosis of the femoral head. The intracapital arterioles. Clin Orthop Relat Res. 1992;(277):98–110.
22. Tingart M, et al. Influence of factors regulating bone formation and remodeling on bone quality in osteonecrosis of the femoral head. Calcif Tissue Int. 2008;82(4):300–8. https://doi.org/10.1007/s00223-008-9111-z.
23. Yamamoto T, et al. Effects of pulse methylprednisolone on bone and marrow tissues: corticosteroid-induced osteonecrosis in rabbits. Arthritis Rheum. 1997;40(11):2055–64. https://doi.org/10.1002/art.1780401119.
24. Motomura G, et al. Combined effects of an anticoagulant and a lipid-lowering agent on the prevention of steroid-induced osteonecrosis in rabbits. Arthritis Rheum. 2004;50(10):3387–91. https://doi.org/10.1002/art.20517.
25. Yamaguchi R, et al. Effects of an anti-platelet drug on the prevention of steroid-induced osteonecrosis in rabbits. Rheumatology (Oxford). 2012;51(5):789–93. https://doi.org/10.1093/rheumatology/ker197.
26. Nishida K, et al. Pitavastatin may reduce risk of steroid-induced osteonecrosis in rabbits: a preliminary histological study. Clin Orthop Relat Res. 2008;466(5):1054–8. https://doi.org/10.1007/s11999-008-0189-4.
27. Ikemura S, et al. Preventive effects of the anti-vasospasm agent via the regulation of the Rho-kinase pathway on the development of steroid-induced osteonecrosis in rabbits. Bone. 2013;53(2):329–35. https://doi.org/10.1016/j.bone.2012.12.050.

28. Drescher W, et al. Methylprednisolone enhances contraction of porcine femoral head epiphyseal arteries. Clin Orthop Relat Res. 2004;423:112–7.
29. Sakamoto Y, et al. Genome-wide association study of idiopathic osteonecrosis of the femoral head. Sci Rep. 2017;7(1):15035. https://doi.org/10.1038/s41598-017-14778-y.
30. Yamamoto T, et al. The prevalence and clinicopathological appearance of extension of osteonecrosis in the femoral head. J Bone Joint Surg Br. 1999;81(2):328–32.
31. Ficat RP. Idiopathic bone necrosis of the femoral head. Early diagnosis and treatment. J Bone Joint Surg Br. 1985;67(1):3–9.
32. Delling G. [Pathohistology of femoral head necrosis]. Orthopade. 2007;36(5):404, 406–8, 410–13. https://doi.org/10.1007/s00132-007-1080-9.
33. Saini A, Saifuddin A. MRI of osteonecrosis. Clin Radiol. 2004;59(12):1079–93. https://doi.org/10.1016/j.crad.2004.04.014.
34. Hofmann S, et al. Bone-marrow oedema syndrome and transient osteoporosis of the hip. An MRI-controlled study of treatment by core decompression. J Bone Joint Surg Br. 1993;75(2):210–6.
35. Kramer J, et al. [Femoral head necrosis]. Radiologe. 2009;49(5):410–8. https://doi.org/10.1007/s00117-009-1831-1.
36. Wirtz C, et al. [MRI-controlled outcome after core decompression of the femur head in aseptic osteonecrosis and transient bone marrow edema]. Z Orthop Ihre Grenzgeb. 1998;136(2):138–46. https://doi.org/10.1055/s-2008-1051296.
37. Mitchell DG, et al. Femoral head avascular necrosis: correlation of MR imaging, radiographic staging, radionuclide imaging, and clinical findings. Radiology. 1987;162(3):709–15. https://doi.org/10.1148/radiology.162.3.3809484.
38. Yeh LR, et al. Diagnostic performance of MR imaging in the assessment of subchondral fractures in avascular necrosis of the femoral head. Skelet Radiol. 2009;38(6):559–64. https://doi.org/10.1007/s00256-009-0659-0.
39. Yamamoto T, Bullough PG. Subchondral insufficiency fracture of the femoral head: a differential diagnosis in acute onset of coxarthrosis in the elderly. Arthritis Rheum. 1999;42(12):2719–23. https://doi.org/10.1002/1529-0131(199912)42:12<2719::AID-ANR31>3.0.CO;2-X.
40. Ikemura S, et al. MRI evaluation of collapsed femoral heads in patients 60 years old or older: differentiation of subchondral insufficiency fracture from osteonecrosis of the femoral head. AJR Am J Roentgenol. 2010;195(1):W63–8. https://doi.org/10.2214/AJR.09.3271.
41. Sugano N, et al. The 2001 revised criteria for diagnosis, classification, and staging of idiopathic osteonecrosis of the femoral head. J Orthop Sci. 2002;7(5):601–5. https://doi.org/10.1007/s007760200108.
42. Vande Berg BC, et al. Transient epiphyseal lesions in renal transplant recipients: presumed insufficiency stress fractures. Radiology. 1994;191(2):403–7. https://doi.org/10.1148/radiology.191.2.8153313.
43. Yamamoto T, et al. Subchondral insufficiency fracture of the femoral head: histopathologic correlation with MRI. Skelet Radiol. 2001;30(5):247–54.
44. Yamamoto T, et al. Histopathological prevalence of subchondral insufficiency fracture of the femoral head. Ann Rheum Dis. 2008;67(2):150–3. https://doi.org/10.1136/ard.2006.066878.
45. Ohzono K, et al. Natural history of nontraumatic avascular necrosis of the femoral head. J Bone Joint Surg Br. 1991;73(1):68–72.
46. Classen T, et al. Long-term clinical results after iloprost treatment for bone marrow edema and avascular necrosis. Orthop Rev (Pavia). 2016;8(1):6150. https://doi.org/10.4081/or.2016.6150.
47. Lee YK, et al. Does zoledronate prevent femoral head collapse from osteonecrosis? A prospective, randomized, open-label, multicenter study. J Bone Joint Surg Am. 2015;97(14):1142–8. https://doi.org/10.2106/JBJS.N.01157.
48. Drescher W, et al. Survival analysis of hips treated with flexion osteotomy for femoral head necrosis. J Bone Joint Surg Br. 2003;85(7):969–74.
49. Reck F, et al. [Analysis of 10-year survival after flexion osteotomy for femoral head necrosis]. Z Orthop Unfall. 2007;145(4):448–51. https://doi.org/10.1055/s-2007-965268.
50. Floerkemeier T, et al. Cementless short stem hip arthroplasty METHA(R) as an encouraging option in adults with osteonecrosis of the femoral head. Arch Orthop Trauma Surg. 2012;132(8):1125–31. https://doi.org/10.1007/s00402-012-1524-5.
51. Sugioka Y. Transtrochanteric anterior rotational osteotomy of the femoral head in the treatment of osteonecrosis affecting the hip: a new osteotomy operation. Clin Orthop Relat Res. 1978;(130):191–201.
52. Miyanishi K, et al. Prediction of the outcome of transtrochanteric rotational osteotomy for osteonecrosis of the femoral head. J Bone Joint Surg Br. 2000;82(4):512–6.
53. Sugioka Y, Yamamoto T. Transtrochanteric posterior rotational osteotomy for osteonecrosis. Clin Orthop Relat Res. 2008;466(5):1104–9. https://doi.org/10.1007/s11999-008-0192-9.
54. Zhao G, et al. Radiological outcome analyses of transtrochanteric posterior rotational osteotomy for osteonecrosis of the femoral head at a mean follow-up of 11 years. J Orthop Sci. 2013;18(2):277–83. https://doi.org/10.1007/s00776-012-0347-0.
55. Ito H, et al. Long-term results of conventional varus half-wedge proximal femoral osteotomy for the treatment of osteonecrosis of the femoral head. J Bone Joint Surg Br. 2012;94(3):308–14. https://doi.org/10.1302/0301-620X.94B3.27814.
56. Zhao G, et al. Radiological outcome analysis of transtrochanteric curved varus osteotomy for osteonecrosis of the femoral head at a mean follow-up of 12.4 years. J Bone Joint Surg Br. 2010;92(6):781–6. https://doi.org/10.1302/0301-620X.92B6.23621.

57. Ikemura S, et al. Leg-length discrepancy after trans-trochanteric curved varus osteotomy for osteonecrosis of the femoral head. J Bone Joint Surg Br. 2007;89(6):725–9. https://doi.org/10.1302/0301-620X.89B6.18499.
58. Rijnen WH, et al. Treatment of femoral head osteonecrosis using bone impaction grafting. Clin Orthop Relat Res. 2003;(417):74–83. https://doi.org/10.1097/01.blo.0000096823.67494.64.
59. Seyler TM, et al. Nonvascularized bone grafting defers joint arthroplasty in hip osteonecrosis. Clin Orthop Relat Res. 2008;466(5):1125–32. https://doi.org/10.1007/s11999-008-0211-x.
60. Mont MA, et al. Outcome of nonvascularized bone grafting for osteonecrosis of the femoral head. Clin Orthop Relat Res. 2003;(417):84–92. https://doi.org/10.1097/01.blo.0000096826.67494.38.
61. Yoo MC, et al. Long-term follow-up of vascularized fibular grafting for femoral head necrosis. Clin Orthop Relat Res. 2008;466(5):1133–40. https://doi.org/10.1007/s11999-008-0204-9.
62. Stronach BM, et al. Subtrochanteric femur fracture after core decompression and placement of a tantalum strut for osteonecrosis of the femoral head. J Arthroplast. 2010;25(7):1168.e5–7. https://doi.org/10.1016/j.arth.2009.08.008.
63. Floerkemeier T, et al. Clinical and radiological outcome of the treatment of osteonecrosis of the femoral head using the osteonecrosis intervention implant. Int Orthop. 2011;35(4):489–95. https://doi.org/10.1007/s00264-009-0940-9.
64. Tingart M, et al. Analysis of bone matrix composition and trabecular microarchitecture of the femoral metaphysis in patients with osteonecrosis of the femoral head. J Orthop Res. 2009;27(9):1175–81. https://doi.org/10.1002/jor.20873.
65. Fink B, Ruther W. [Partial and total joint replacement in femur head necrosis]. Orthopade. 2000;29(5):449–56.
66. Hungerford MW, et al. Outcome of uncemented primary femoral stems for treatment of femoral head osteonecrosis. Orthop Clin North Am. 2009;40(2):283–9. https://doi.org/10.1016/j.ocl.2008.10.006.
67. Kim SM, et al. Cementless modular total hip arthroplasty in patients younger than fifty with femoral head osteonecrosis: minimum fifteen-year follow-up. J Arthroplast. 2013;28(3):504–9. https://doi.org/10.1016/j.arth.2012.08.005.
68. Lee YK, et al. Mid-term results of the BIOLOX delta ceramic-on-ceramic total hip arthroplasty. Bone Joint J. 2017;99-B(6):741–8. https://doi.org/10.1302/0301-620X.99B6.BJJ-2016-0486.R3.
69. Kim YH, et al. Cementless metaphyseal fitting anatomic total hip arthroplasty with a ceramic-on-ceramic bearing in patients thirty years of age or younger. J Bone Joint Surg Am. 2012;94(17):1570–5. https://doi.org/10.2106/JBJS.K.00697.
70. Aldridge JM 3rd, et al. Free vascularized fibular grafting for the treatment of postcollapse osteonecrosis of the femoral head. Surgical technique. J Bone Joint Surg Am. 2004;86-A(Suppl 1):87–101.

Femoral Osteotomies for Osteonecrosis of the Femoral Head

10

Jae-Young Lim, Yong-Chan Ha, and Kyung-Hoi Koo

10.1 Introduction

Osteonecrosis of the femoral head usually affects young adults and frequently leads to degenerative arthritis of the hip [1, 2]. This disease is becoming more prevalent after the increasing use of steroids for organ transplantation or as an adjuvant therapy for leukemia and other myelogenous diseases [3–5]. The advanced state of the disease frequently necessitates total hip arthroplasty (THA) [6–8]. However, THA might not be durable at long term in young active patients. As its alternatives, several methods of proximal femoral osteotomies have been introduced to preserve the hip joint [9–11]. The principle of these techniques is to move the necrotic portion from the weight-bearing region to a nonweight-bearing region. Among them, transtrochanteric curved varus osteotomy (TCVO) [11] and transtrochanteric rotational osteotomy (TRO) [9] are well known and most commonly used.

Nishio and Sugioka introduced TCVO in 1971 [11]. A curved osteotomy is made between the greater and lesser trochanters, and the femoral head is rotated into a varus position. The reported success rates of this technique ranged from 90 to 97.3% [12–14].

Sugioka introduced another osteotomy, TRO, in 1978 [9]. In this procedure, a transtrochanteric osteotomy is made, and the femoral head fragment is rotated anteriorly. Reportedly, the success rate varied widely ranging from 17 to 100% [15–18].

In this chapter, surgical techniques of the two osteotomies are described, and indication and reported results are reviewed.

10.2 Surgical Technique of Transtrochanteric Rotational Osteotomy

According to the traditional surgical technique of TRO, a U-shaped incision and cancellous screws were used. We describe a modified surgical technique by Ha et al. [1], which uses a Y-shaped skin incision and a 120° compression hip screw. This modified technique has two advantages. First, the Y-shaped incision provides a better exposure of the anterior capsule. Second, the use of a 120° compression hip screw can minimize the risk of fixation failure and nonunion. It also reduces the hospital length of stay and allows an early ambulation. After the greater trochanter is osteotomized, the joint capsule is circumferentially incised to expose the femoral neck and head. Second, the osteotomy is made in the transtrochanteric area while preserving the posterior

J.-Y. Lim · Y.-C. Ha (✉)
Department of Orthopaedic Surgery, Chung-Ang University College of Medicine, Seoul, South Korea

K.-H. Koo
Department of Orthopaedic Surgery, Seoul National University Bundang Hospital, Seongnam, South Korea

Department of Orthopedic Surgery, Seoul National University College of Medicine, Seoul, South Korea
e-mail: khkoo@snu.ac.kr

W. R. Drescher et al. (eds.), *Advances in Specialist Hip Surgery*,
https://doi.org/10.1007/978-3-030-61830-8_10

branch of the medial circumflex artery. Then the femoral head is rotated anteriorly by 60° to 90°, as well as varisation.

10.2.1 Patient Positioning

The patient is placed in the lateral decubitus position on a standard operating room table with the pelvis stabilized in neutral position. Intraoperative fluoroscopy is used to confirm the appropriate osteotomy line and the position of the compression hip screw.

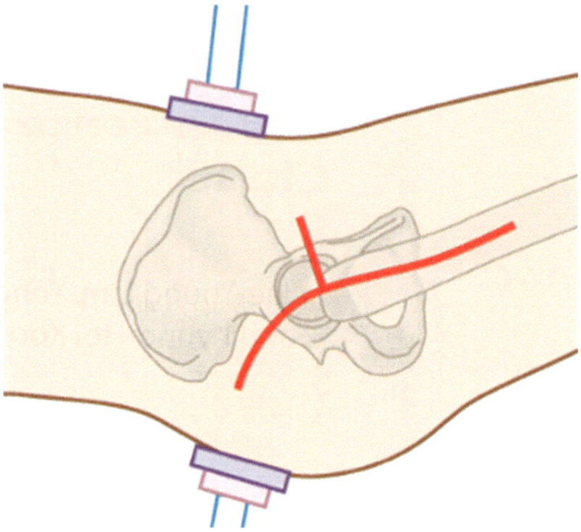

Fig. 10.1 The patient is placed in the lateral decubitus position and the pelvis is secured with holding devices and pads. The Y-shaped skin incision is centered at the greater trochanter. The posterior portion of the incision is started at a point that is level with the posterior superior iliac spine and along a line parallel to the posterior edge of the greater trochanter. The incision is extended distally to the center of the greater trochanter and then to a point 10–15 cm distal to the greater trochanter, in line with the femoral shaft. The anterior portion of the incision is made from the greater trochanter to the anterior superior iliac spine (reproduced with permission and copyright of Springer)

10.2.2 Skin Incision

A Y-shaped skin incision is made. The posterior limb of the incision starts at the posterior superior iliac spine, proceeds to the greater trochanter, and then extends 10–15 cm distally in line with the axis of the femur. The anterior limb of the incision starts from the center of the greater trochanter to the anterior iliac spine by a length of 5–8 cm (Fig. 10.1). The length of the incision is adjusted according to the size and obesity of the patient.

10.2.3 Fascia Incision

The fascia lata and the gluteus maximus fascia are incised in line with the skin incision. Then gluteus maximus muscle fibers are bluntly divided, giving access to the gluteus medius and the external rotators of the hip.

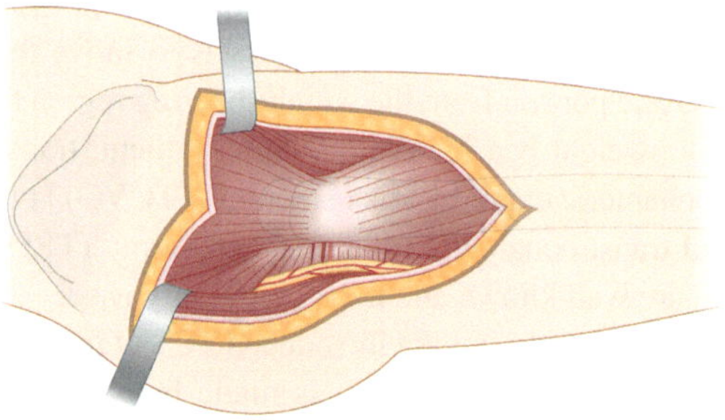

Fig. 10.2 The gluteus maximus fascia is incised in line with the posterior portion of the skin incision, and the muscle fibers of the gluteus maximus are bluntly divided. Fibers of the fascia lata are divided in line with the anterior portion of the skin incision. The fat tissues covering the external rotators and the trochanteric bursa are removed to expose the sciatic nerve along its course beneath the piriformis muscle and over the short external rotators distally (reproduced with permission and copyright of Springer)

10.2.4 Exposure of the External Rotators and Sciatic Nerve

Remove the fat tissue covering the external rotators, divide the trochanteric bursa, and bluntly sweep it posteriorly to expose the sciatic nerve along its course beneath the piriformis muscle and over the short external rotators distally. The nerve is protected during the operation (Fig. 10.2).

10.2.5 Osteotomy of the Greater Trochanter

The greater trochanter is osteotomized between the gluteus medius and piriformis posteriorly and between the gluteus medius and vastus lateralis anteriorly with an oscillating saw.

10.2.6 Exposure of the Hip Joint Capsule and Capsulotomy

Expose the superior portion of the hip joint capsule by dissecting the gluteus minimus from the capsule. Expose the posterior capsule by cutting the tendons of the piriformis and obturator internus at the trochanteric insertion. Expose the inferior capsule by cutting the quadratus femoris, superior gemellus, and inferior gemellus muscles. To avoid damage to the medial femoral circumflex artery, cut the quadratus femoris, superior gemellus, and inferior gemellus at their muscle fibers 2 cm apart from their femoral insertions. Expose the anterior capsule by developing the interval between the gluteus medius and vastus lateralis muscles. Once the complete exposure of the hip joint capsule is obtained, a circumferential capsulotomy is performed. The capsulotomy line should be about 1 cm apart from the acetabular rim to avoid injury of the acetabular labrum. During the capsulotomy hold the capsule using a forceps and separate it from the underlying femoral head to avoid injury of the femoral head cartilage (Fig. 10.3).

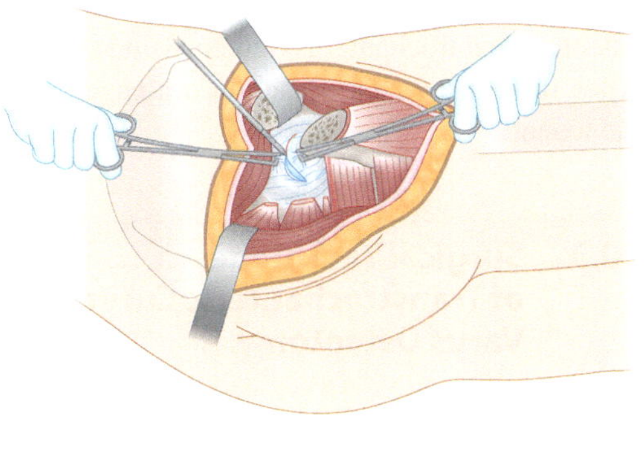

Fig. 10.3 After complete exposure of the hip joint capsule, the joint capsule is incised circumferentially. The capsulotomy line is 1 cm away from the acetabular rim to protect the acetabular labrum and to obtain adequate rotation of the femoral head (reproduced with permission and copyright of Springer)

10.2.7 Transtrochanteric Osteotomies

Make two transtrochanteric osteotomies. The first osteotomy is made about 10 mm distal to the intertrochanteric crest. The osteotomy line should be inclined at 20° from the line perpendicular to the femoral neck to place the femoral head in a varus angulation. The second osteotomy is made near the upper one-third of the lesser trochanter at 90° to the first osteotomy line (Fig. 10.4a).

10.2.8 Rotation of the Proximal Segment

The proximal fragment is rotated anteriorly by 90° with care to avoid excessive stretching or

a

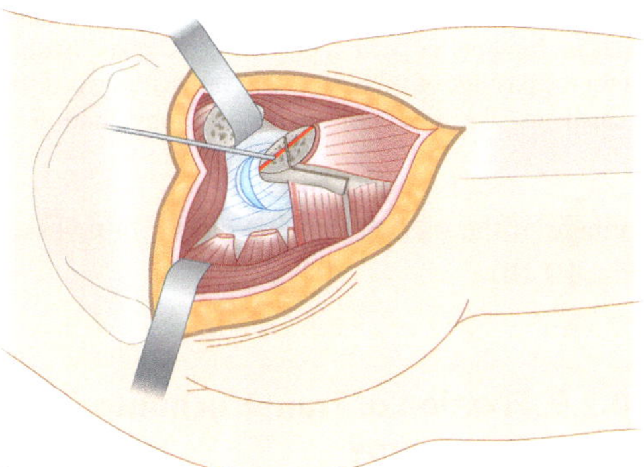

b

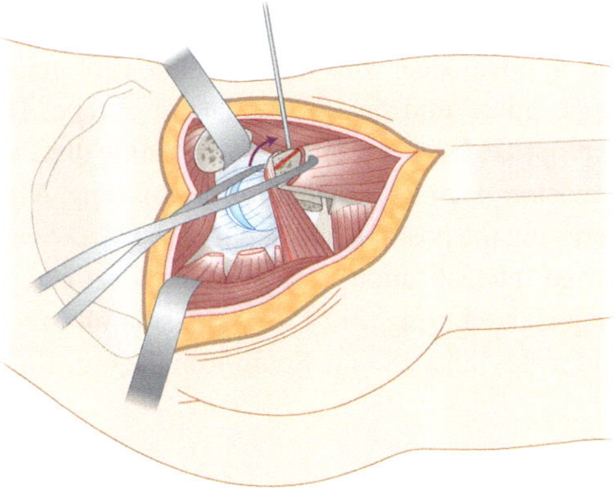

Fig. 10.4 A Kirschner wire is placed in the proximal segment (**a**). The proximal fragment is rotated anteriorly 90° (arrow in **b**), with care taken to avoid excessive stretching of or damage to the medial femoral circumflex vessels. The rotated proximal segment is temporarily fixed with the use of clamps or Kirschner wires (**b**) (reproduced with permission and copyright of Springer)

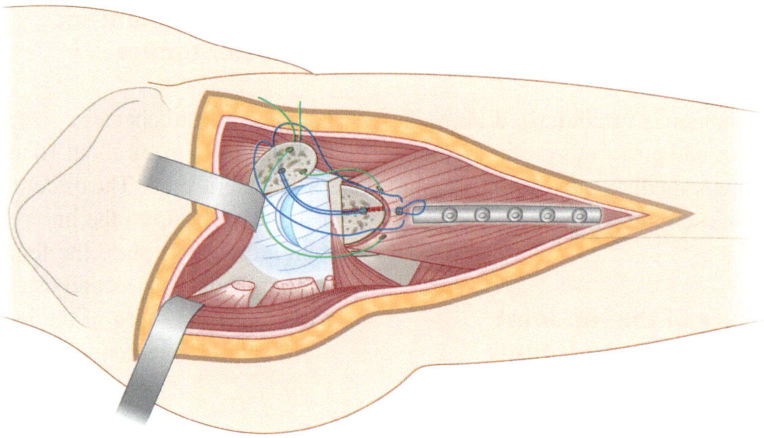

Fig. 10.5 After rotating the proximal fragment, the guide pin is positioned with the use of a 120° fixed-angle guide that is anchored on the midportion of the lateral femoral cortex. After verifying the position and depth of the lag screw in both the anteroposterior and mediolateral planes, the osteotomy is fixed with the use of a 120° compression hip screw and plate. The trochanteric fragment is reattached with the use of a number 16 stainless steel wire. A hole is drilled in the lateral femoral cortex and a hole is made in the superior portion of the osteotomized trochanter for the passage of vertical wires. Another hole is drilled 1 cm below the first trochanteric osteotomy line in the proximal part of the femur, and two holes are drilled in the anterior and posterior portions of the osteotomized trochanter for the passage of transverse wires. The two ends of the U-shaped vertical wire are passed through the hole in the lateral femoral cortex and the hole in the superior portion of the osteotomized trochanter. The two free ends are then passed in opposite directions through the loop in the lateral cortex. The two transverse wires are passed through the hole below the trochanteric osteotomy and then through the two holes in the anterior and posterior portions of the osteotomized trochanter (reproduced with permission and copyright of Springer)

damage of the medial femoral circumflex vessels (Fig. 10.4b).

10.2.9 Fixation of Transtrochanteric Osteotomy

After rotating the proximal fragment, the guide pin is positioned with the use of a 120° fixed-angle guide midway on the lateral cortex. The appropriate lag screw length and reaming distance are determined with the aid of fluoroscopy. After verifying the position and depth of the screw with image intensification in both planes, the osteotomy is fixed using a 120° compression hip screw and plate (Solco, Seoul, South Korea) (Fig. 10.5).

10.2.10 Reattachment of the Greater Trochanter

For reattachment of the trochanteric fragment, a folding vertical number 16 stainless steel wire is used. One side of the folding vertical wire is inserted in the hole drilled in the lateral cortex below the abductor tubercle and the hole in the osteotomized trochanter, and the other side of folding end makes a loop at the lateral cortex. Each of the two ends is crossed loop in different directions, tightening the wires and tying the knots with Kirschner wire bow. Then the transverse wire that is inserted in the hole drilled in the anteroposterior cortex and the two holes in the osteotomized trochanter is tightened and twisted. After inserting a closed suction drainage, close the wound.

10.3 Surgical Technique of Transtrochanteric Curved Varus Osteotomy

Transtrochanteric curved varus osteotomy is performed by making a curved osteotomy between the greater and the lesser trochanters, which has a merit to prevent elevation of the greater trochanter and lateral displacement of the femoral shaft which may cause decreased tension of the gluteus medius muscle. The head segment is rotated into a varus position by about 30° in the coronal plane.

10.3.1 Operative Position

The patient is placed in the lateral decubitus position. An image intensifier is used during the fixation of the osteotomy.

10.3.2 Skin Incision

A Kocher-Langenbeck incision is made. The length of incision ranges from 15 to 20 cm according to the constitution and obesity of the patient.

10.3.3 Fascia Incision and Exposure of Trochanteric Crest

The fascia lata and the gluteus maximus fascia are incised in line with the skin incision. Then, gluteus maximus muscle fibers are bluntly divided, giving access to the gluteus medius muscle and the external rotators of the hip. The trochanteric bursa and underlying fat tissue are removed to expose the intertrochanteric crest. Then, the lesser trochanter is exposed subperiosteally. During this process, care should be taken not to damage the medial femoral circumflex artery.

10.3.4 Osteotomy and Varization of the Proximal Segment

Draw a downward convex curved line using Bovie cautery between the tip of the greater trochanter and the center of the lesser trochanter. The rotational distance should be determined before operation. The distance is marked on the distal and the proximal bone fragments using Bovie cautery. Then, the osteotomy is performed

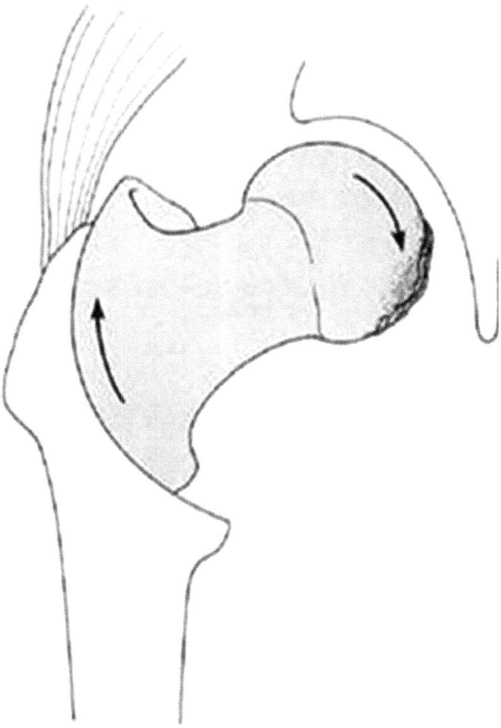

Fig. 10.6 The transtrochanteric curved osteotomy is made between the greater and the lesser trochanters and the proximal fragment is rotated into a varus position (reproduced with permission and copyright of Springer)

with a reciprocating saw along the planned osteotomy line. The proximal bone fragment is rotated until the two points marked on the proximal and distal bone fragments meet so that the femoral head is rotated into a varus position (Fig. 10.6). The varus position is maintained using clamps.

10.3.5 Fixation of Bone Fragments

A longitudinal incision is made on the vastus lateralis muscle. Insert a guide pin and confirm the varus angle, the position of pins, and the direction and length of the pins using an image intensifier. A lag screw with appropriate length is selected and reamed along the guide pin. Then, the osteotomy is fixed using a 120° compression hip screw and plate (Solco, Seoul, South Korea) (Fig. 10.7).

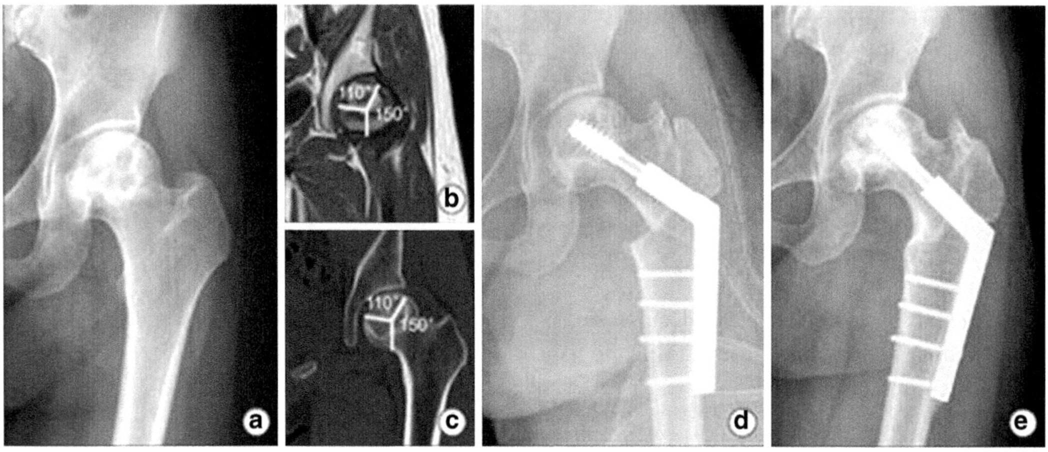

Fig. 10.7 A 28-year-old woman had osteonecrosis in the left femoral head. (**a**) Preoperative anteroposterior hip radiograph. (**b**, **c**) The angle of the necrotic area in the mid-coronal images of computed tomography and magnetic resonance imaging was 110°. The angle between the central vertical line of the femoral head and the lateral margin of the necrotic portion was 150°. (**d**) Immediate postoperative anteroposterior hip radiograph after curved intertrochanteric varus osteotomy. (**e**) Follow-up radiograph taken 6 years after the operation showing no progressing collapse or osteophyte formation around the femoral head

10.3.6 Comparison Between TCVO and TRO

There is no randomized clinical trial comparing TCVO and TRO. To date, only one study retrospectively compared the results of these two osteotomy techniques. Lee et al. compared 85 patients (91 hips) treated with TRO and 58 patients (65 hips) that were treated with TCVO [19]. The TCVO group had shorter operation time, and less blood loss. Postoperative collapse was observed in 26 TRO hips (28.6%) and in 7 TCVO hips (10.8%). Osteophyte formation was found in 34 TRO hips (37.4%) and in 13 TCVO hips (20%). Fifteen TRO hips (16.5%) and 7 TCVO hips (10.8%) underwent conversion to THA. The survival rate at 9 years with an endpoint of radiographic collapse was 68.7% in the TRO group, and 84.7% in the TCVO group. With conversion to THA as the endpoint, the survival rate was 82.2% in the TRO group and 89.2% in the TCVO group.

Their comparison showed that TCVO was better than TRO in most aspects.

There are several principal differences between these two osteotomies. In TRO, the greater trochanter should be osteotomized and the joint capsule should be circumferentially incised. Accordingly, it requires longer operation time and causes more bleeding.

10.3.7 Indication

The reported outcomes after the osteotomies were inconsistent [12–18]. Inappropriate patient selection is the major reason for poor outcomes after the osteotomy [15, 17]. In order to improve its success rate, more efficient patient selection is mandatory.

Patient's age, body mass index (BMI), stage of disease, size of the necrotic portion, and remaining viable portion of the femoral head are known factors affecting the result after osteotomy.

10.3.7.1 Patient's Age and Body Mass Index

Patient's age and BMI are the affecting factors of the outcomes after the osteotomy. In a previous study, secondary collapse was more frequent in older (>40 years) patients and overweight (BMI >24 kg/m^2) patients [20].

After the osteotomy, an intact and viable portion of the femoral head is established in the weight-bearing region. Secondary collapse occurs due to the stress fracture in this portion, which is usually thin and beak shaped. Age-related osteopenia begins around the age of 40 years and progressively worsens [21]. In patients with high BMI, an excessive load is applied on the femoral head, which leads to a stress fracture and secondary collapse of the newly formed weight-bearing portion.

10.3.7.2 Stage of the Disease

Osteotomies should be performed in the early stages of the disease before marked collapse of the femoral head: Ficat stage IIB (a crescentic subchondral fracture or slight flattening of the femoral head) or stage III (a definite head collapse without joint space narrowing) [22, 23].

10.3.7.3 Size of Necrotic Portion

Small lesions usually do not progress even without any medical or surgical intervention [24]. However, hips with a large lesion preoperatively have a higher risk of subsequent femoral head collapse after the osteotomy [25]. Thus, the osteotomies should be performed in medium-size lesions with a combined necrotic angle between 190° and 240° (Fig. 10.8) [26], or type B lesions involving the medial two-thirds or less of the weight-bearing portion according to the Japanese Investigation Committee (JIC) classification [27]. The extent of necrotic portion should be measured on MRI for accurate measurement of necrotic portion.

10.3.7.4 Viable Portion of the Femoral Head

The femoral head should have a sufficient viable portion to restore adequate weight-bearing area after the osteotomy [28, 29]. Adequate size of viable bone for TRO is an arc of >120° between the central vertical line of the femoral head and the posterior margin of the necrotic portion on a midsagittal MRI scan (Fig. 10.7). Meanwhile, the size for TCVO is an arc of >150° between the central vertical line of the femoral head and the lateral margin of the necrotic portion on the mid-coronal MRI scan.

Previous studies have demonstrated variable rates of failure after transtrochanteric rotational osteotomy. While studies from Japan and Korea have reported satisfactory results, the results from Western countries have not been favorable.

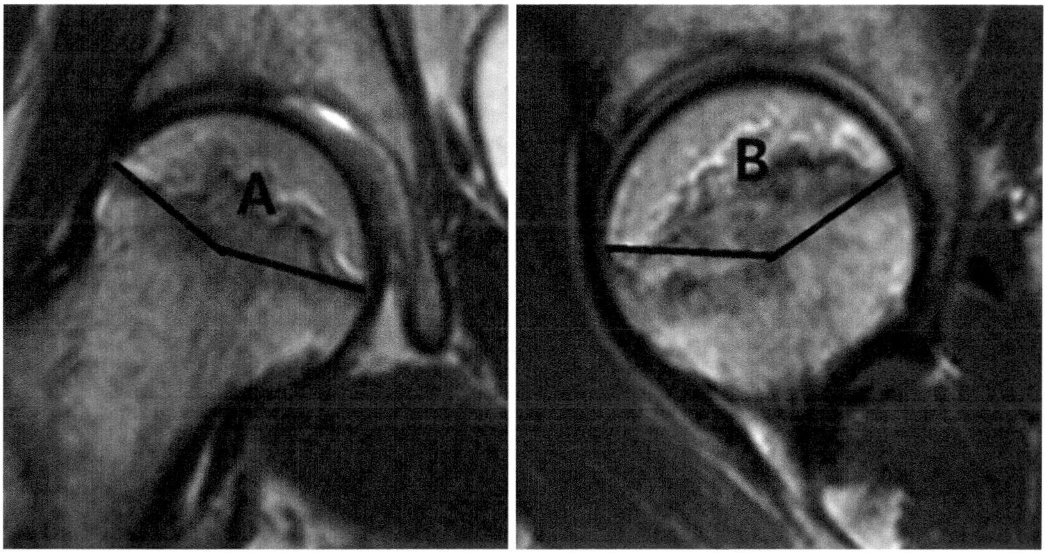

Fig. 10.8 Calculation of the combined necrotic angle from magnetic resonance imaging scans. *A* The angle of necrotic area in the mid-coronal image. *B* The angle of necrotic area in the midsagittal image. The combined necrotic angle = *A* + *B*

10.4 Conclusion

We recommend the use of TCVO for the treatment of femoral head osteonecrosis in patients who have (1) hip pain, (2) an age less than 40 years, (3) a body mass index less than 24 kg/m^2, (4) Ficat stage IIA or III disease, (5) medium-sized lesion (combined necrotic angle between 190° and 240° or JIC type B lesion), and (6) adequate viable bone (>150° between the central vertical line and the lateral margin of the necrotic portion on the mid-coronal MRI).

References

1. Gutierrez F, Padilla S, Masia M, Flores J, Boix V, Merino E, et al. Osteonecrosis in patients infected with HIV: clinical epidemiology and natural history in a large case series from Spain. J Acquir Immune Defic Syndr. 2006;42(3):286–92. https://doi.org/10.1097/01.qai.0000225012.53568.20. PubMed PMID: 16763523.
2. Shimizu K, Moriya H, Akita T, Sakamoto M, Suguro T. Prediction of collapse with magnetic resonance imaging of avascular necrosis of the femoral head. J Bone Joint Surg Am. 1994;76(2):215–23. PubMed PMID: 8113255.
3. Shibatani M, Fujioka M, Arai Y, Takahashi K, Ueshima K, Okamoto M, et al. Degree of corticosteroid treatment within the first 2 months of renal transplantation has a strong influence on the incidence of osteonecrosis of the femoral head. Acta Orthop. 2008;79(5):631–6. https://doi.org/10.1080/17453670810016641. PubMed PMID: 18839369.
4. Shigemura T, Nakamura J, Kishida S, Harada Y, Ohtori S, Kamikawa K, et al. Incidence of osteonecrosis associated with corticosteroid therapy among different underlying diseases: prospective MRI study. Rheumatology. 2011;50(11):2023–8. https://doi.org/10.1093/rheumatology/ker277. PubMed PMID: 21865285.
5. Arlet J. Nontraumatic avascular necrosis of the femoral head. Past, present, and future. Clin Orthop Relat Res. 1992;277:12–21. PubMed PMID: 1555331.
6. Baek SH, Kim SY. Cementless total hip arthroplasty with alumina bearings in patients younger than fifty with femoral head osteonecrosis. J Bone Joint Surg Am. 2008;90(6):1314–20. https://doi.org/10.2106/JBJS.G.00755. PubMed PMID: 18519326.
7. Kim YH, Choi Y, Kim JS. Cementless total hip arthroplasty with ceramic-on-ceramic bearing in patients younger than 45 years with femoral-head osteonecrosis. Int Orthop. 2010;34(8):1123–7. https://doi.org/10.1007/s00264-009-0878-y. PubMed PMID: 19784647; PubMed Central PMCID: PMC2989073.
8. Fye MA, Huo MH, Zatorski LE, Keggi KJ. Total hip arthroplasty performed without cement in patients with femoral head osteonecrosis who are less than 50 years old. J Arthroplast. 1998;13(8):876–81. PubMed PMID: 9880179.
9. Sugioka Y. Transtrochanteric anterior rotational osteotomy of the femoral head in the treatment of osteonecrosis affecting the hip: a new osteotomy operation. Clin Orthop Relat Res. 1978;(130):191–201. PubMed PMID: 639389.
10. Atsumi T, Muraki M, Yoshihara S, Kajihara T. Posterior rotational osteotomy for the treatment of femoral head osteonecrosis. Arch Orthop Trauma Surg. 1999;119(7–8):388–93. https://doi.org/10.1007/s004020050007. PubMed PMID: WOS:000083877700007.
11. Nishio A, Sugioka Y. A new technique of the varus osteotomy at the upper end of the femur. Orthop Traumatol. 1971;20:381–6.
12. Sakano S, Hasegawa Y, Torii Y, Kawasaki M, Ishiguro N. Curved intertrochanteric varus osteotomy for osteonecrosis of the femoral head. J Bone Joint Surg Br. 2004;86(3):359–65. PubMed PMID: 15125122.
13. Ikemura S, Yamamoto T, Jingushi S, Nakashima Y, Mawatari T, Iwamoto Y. Leg-length discrepancy after transtrochanteric curved varus osteotomy for osteonecrosis of the femoral head. J Bone Joint Surg Br. 2007;89(6):725–9. https://doi.org/10.1302/0301-620X.89B6.18499. PubMed PMID: 17613494.
14. Zhao G, Yamamoto T, Ikemura S, Motomura G, Mawatari T, Nakashima Y, et al. Radiological outcome analysis of transtrochanteric curved varus osteotomy for osteonecrosis of the femoral head at a mean follow-up of 12.4 years. J Bone Joint Surg Br. 2010;92(6):781–6. https://doi.org/10.1302/0301-620X.92B6.23621. PubMed PMID: 20513873.
15. Inao S, Ando M, Gotoh E, Matsuno T. Minimum 10-year results of Sugioka's osteotomy for femoral head osteonecrosis. Clin Orthop Relat Res. 1999;368:141–8. PubMed PMID: 10613162.
16. Koo KH, Song HR, Yang JW, Yang P, Kim JR, Kim YM. Trochanteric rotational osteotomy for osteonecrosis of the femoral head. J Bone Joint Surg Br. 2001;83(1):83–9. PubMed PMID: 11245544.
17. Dean MT, Cabanela ME. Transtrochanteric anterior rotational osteotomy for avascular necrosis of the femoral head. Long-term results. J Bone Joint Surg Br. 1993;75(4):597–601. PubMed PMID: 8331115.
18. Tooke SM, Amstutz HC, Hedley AK. Results of transtrochanteric rotational osteotomy for femoral head osteonecrosis. Clin Orthop Relat Res. 1987;(224):150–7. PubMed PMID: 3665235.
19. Lee YK, Park CH, Ha YC, Kim DY, Lyu SH, Koo KH. Comparison of surgical parameters and results between curved varus osteotomy and rotational osteotomy for osteonecrosis of the femoral head. Clin Orthop Surg. 2017;9(2):160–8. https://doi.org/10.4055/cios.2017.9.2.160. PubMed PMID: 28567217; PubMed Central PMCID: PMC5435653.

20. Ha YC, Kim HJ, Kim SY, Kim KC, Lee YK, Koo KH. Effects of age and body mass index on the results of transtrochanteric rotational osteotomy for femoral head osteonecrosis: surgical technique. J Bone Joint Surg Am. 2011;93(Suppl 1):75–84. https://doi.org/10.2106/JBJS.J.01215. PubMed PMID: 21411688.
21. Parfitt AM. Age-related structural changes in trabecular and cortical bone: cellular mechanisms and biomechanical consequences. Calcif Tissue Int. 1984;36(Suppl 1):S123–8. PubMed PMID: 6430512.
22. Sugano N, Takaoka K, Ohzono K, Matsui M, Saito M, Saito S. Rotational osteotomy for non-traumatic avascular necrosis of the femoral head. J Bone Joint Surg Br. 1992;74(5):734–9. PubMed PMID: 1527125.
23. Hisatome T, Yasunaga Y, Takahashi K, Ochi M. Progressive collapse of transposed necrotic area after transtrochanteric rotational osteotomy for osteonecrosis of the femoral head induces osteoarthritic change. Mid-term results of transtrochanteric rotational osteotomy for osteonecrosis of the femoral head. Arch Orthop Trauma Surg. 2004;124(2):77–81. https://doi.org/10.1007/s00402-003-0610-0. PubMed PMID: 14658077.
24. Mont MA, Zywiel MG, Marker DR, McGrath MS, Delanois RE. The natural history of untreated asymptomatic osteonecrosis of the femoral head: a systematic literature review. J Bone Joint Surg Am. 2010;92(12):2165–70. https://doi.org/10.2106/JBJS.I.00575. PubMed PMID: 20844158.
25. Mont MA, Fairbank AC, Krackow KA, Hungerford DS. Corrective osteotomy for osteonecrosis of the femoral head. J Bone Joint Surg Am. 1996;78(7):1032–8. PubMed PMID: 8698720.
26. Ha YC, Jung WH, Kim JR, Seong NH, Kim SY, Koo KH. Prediction of collapse in femoral head osteonecrosis: a modified Kerboul method with use of magnetic resonance images. J Bone Joint Surg Am. 2006;88(Suppl 3):35–40. https://doi.org/10.2106/JBJS.F.00535. PubMed PMID: 17079365.
27. Sugano N, Atsumi T, Ohzono K, Kubo T, Hotokebuchi T, Takaoka K. The 2001 revised criteria for diagnosis, classification, and staging of idiopathic osteonecrosis of the femoral head. J Orthop Sci. 2002;7(5):601–5. https://doi.org/10.1007/s007760200108. PubMed PMID: 12355139.
28. Atsumi T, Kuroki Y. Modified Sugioka's osteotomy: more than 130 degrees posterior rotation for osteonecrosis of the femoral head with large lesion. Clin Orthop Relat Res. 1997;(334):98–107. PubMed PMID: 9005901.
29. Hiranuma Y, Atsumi T, Kajiwara T, Tamaoki S, Asakura Y. Evaluation of instability after transtrochanteric anterior rotational osteotomy for nontraumatic osteonecrosis of the femoral head. J Orthop Sci. 2009;14(5):535–42. https://doi.org/10.1007/s00776-009-1363-6. PubMed PMID: 19802664.

Stem Cell Therapy for the Treatment of Hip Osteonecrosis

11

Philippe Hernigou and Wolf R. Drescher

11.1 Introduction

Osteonecrosis of the femoral head (ONFH) is a progressive pathologic process affecting young patients (from 30 to 50 years old). It is a painful disease based on traumatic or nontraumatic etiology [1]. It is caused by death of all cells within bone in relation with multifactorial factors associated with genetic predisposition and exposure to risk factors including corticosteroid [2, 3], alcohol abuse [4], hemoglobinopathy, previous trauma, chemotherapy [5], Gaucher's disease, coagulopathies [6], and other diseases. It is estimated that 10% of total hip replacements (THR) are performed every year to treat this disease [7], but their outcome has been demonstrated to be less satisfactory than in other etiologies and their durability limited in such young patients. Consequently, it is increasingly focused on early interventions to avoid or at least delay THR. Core decompression (CD) was the most frequent surgical treatment but the use of new regenerative techniques has recently been proposed for early osteonecrosis stages. The strategy was proposed 30 years ago [8] and is driven by the hypothesis that stem cells can repopulate the trabecular dead bone, and "revitalize" and remodel necrotic bone [9, 10].

The aim of this chapter is to explain the rationale of autologous bone marrow concentrate grafting injected through the channel of core decompression; the possibility to expand ex vivo autologous bone marrow-derived stem cells; the results and mechanism of healing of hip osteonecrosis; and the safety of cell therapy.

P. Hernigou (✉)
Hôpital Henri Mondor, University Paris East (UPEC), Creteil, France

W. R. Drescher
Department of Orthopedics, RWTH Aachen University Hospital, Aachen, Germany

Orthopedic Surgery of the Lower Limb and Arthroplasty, Rummelsberg Hospital, Schwarzenbruck, Germany
e-mail: Wolf.Drescher@sana.de

11.2 Technique of Hip Osteonecrosis Treatment by Mesenchymal Stem Cells

The patient is supine on a radiolucent operating table with general anesthesia. Fluoroscopic imaging is used to ensure adequate anterior-posterior views and frog-leg lateral views. The operative hip and iliac crest are draped in a sterile manner into the surgical field.

11.2.1 Bone Marrow Aspiration

Bone marrow can be aspirated from the anterior or posterior iliac wing. The anatomy of the iliac wings was evaluated to perform bone marrow

W. R. Drescher et al. (eds.), *Advances in Specialist Hip Surgery*,
https://doi.org/10.1007/978-3-030-61830-8_11

aspiration. The spongious bone's thickness of the iliac wing is an important factor for the placement of a trocar between the tables of the iliac bone. Sectors can be obtained by demarcating lines traced from the iliac crest through the center of the hip trochanter. The thickness of the spongious bone has been reported in a map. Sector 2, sector 3, and sector 6 are more favorable for a 3 mm diameter trocar. Sector 1, sector 4, and sector 5 are the areas presenting the thinnest parts. This system of sector predicts unsafe and safe areas for trocar placement [11, 12].

Collection of bone marrow is accomplished by a 10 cm^3 syringe. Preparation of the syringe and needle involves rinsing with heparin solution. Aspiration in small fractions [13] reduces dilution by peripheral blood. All aspirates are pooled in bags containing anticoagulant solution. Once collected, the marrow is placed in a centrifuge to concentrate the mononuclear fraction that contains the mesenchymal progenitor cells.

11.2.2 Intraosseous Injection of Mesenchymal Stem Cells

Patients are placed on an operating table with image intensifier and C-arm [14]. With a percutaneous approach, the decompression is performed with a 4 mm diameter trocar. A 5 mm incision is made on the lateral trochanter. The position is confirmed by fluoroscopy. When the starting point has been chosen to reach the osteonecrosis, the trocar is pushed forward under biplanar fluoroscopy while checking the position of the tip to reach the necrotic lesion. Since, at early stages, the radiographs show little or any evidence of necrosis, the preoperative MRI is used together with the intensifier views, to determine the site of the lesion. The trocar is advanced into the necrotic lesions with mallet taps. The necrosis can be entered with the trocar but it should not be advanced too close to the subchondral bone to avoid collapse (less than 5 mm). Then, after removing the inner core of the trocar, the 4 mm trocar position is checked in the necrotic portion of the femoral head. The bone marrow is injected into the femoral head using the trocar. Although the diameter of the trocar is small compared with the trephines normally used for core decompression, femoral head pressure measurements have shown that even a small hole relieved the intraosseous pressure. Due to the sclerotic lesions of osteonecrosis, it may require some pressure to inject the concentrate bone marrow from the syringe. If excessive resistance is met, then the trocar can be retracted while confirming that the end of the trocar remains within the necrotic area. This increases the volume of the space to inject the mesenchymal stems cells in the correct area. Bone marrow injection itself should be slow to avoid increased pressure in the femoral head. In patients, no complications were observed: no reduction in oxygen saturation, and no change in pulse rate or in blood pressure. After injecting the contents of the syringe, to avoid the bone marrow solution from flowing retrogradely due to pressure gradients, the hip is put in internal rotation. Then, to prevent the retrograde backflow, the trocar is reinserted into the previous channel at a different angle in order to push some cancellous bone into the tract.

11.2.3 Postoperative Care

Patients are discharged home after the day of surgery. They are allowed to weight bear with the use of crutches for approximately 1 week or 2 weeks in patients who undergo bilateral procedures. Some patients may have an increase in pain 1 month after the injection. This pain is unlikely to last more than 2 months and the majority of patients have significant pain relief within a few weeks.

11.3 The Results of Femoral Head Necrosis Repair with Progenitor Cells

Original Description The introduction of stem cells for avascular necrosis treatment was proposed in 1987 [8] and first results were reported in the English literature in 2002 [15]. A retrospective review of 189 hips described the technique using a trephine approach to enter the necrosis under fluoroscopy and inject concentrated bone marrow into the necrotic area. Excellent results were found in patients who were stage I or II (pre-collapse). Nine out of 145 hips required hip arthroplasty at a minimum of 5-year follow-up [15]. However, in hips that had already collapsed (stage III or IV), 25 of 44 hips required THA.

11.4 Randomized Trials in Different Patients

Since this study, some studies have prospectively compared the results of standard core decompression and core decompression with autologous bone marrow introduction. In 2004, Gangji et al. in a prospective randomized controlled trial compared the results of core decompression with core decompression with bone marrow (CDBM) [16]. The study specifically looked at patients with stage I–II AVN, and excluded all patients with post-collapse AVN. Eight hips underwent core decompression and ten hips underwent CDBM. The patients' age and underlying cause of AVN were similar. During the 24-month period, the CDBM group had a statistically significant decrease in pain. The Lequesne and WOMAC indices were also significantly improved. At follow-up, five of eight hips in the core decompression group collapsed compared to only one of ten in the CDBM group. The author also found that the volume of involvement of AVN of the femoral head in the CDBM group had significantly decreased from 15.6% pre-op to 10.1% at 24 months. In the core decompression group, it significantly increased from 16.7% pre-op to 20.6% ($P = 0.036$). Finally, both methods were found to have no major complications. This paper was followed up in 2011 with 5 years of clinical follow-up [17]. At 5-year follow-up, 8 of the 11 hips in the CD group had progressed to collapse, while in the bone marrow group only 3 of the 13 progressed to collapse.

In a prospective trial of Sen et al., 25 hips had core decompression and 26 hips CDBM [18]. Patient follow-up was a minimum of 2 years. At the final follow-up, the BM group had higher Harris Hip Score. The authors noted that etiologies significantly affected outcome and that patients with poor pre-op scores, edema, and effusion on MRI had better results in the bone marrow group.

Zhao et al. looked at a similar group of patients [19]. Fifty-one hips had core decompression and 53 hips CDBM. Ten patients in the core decompression group progressed. Only two hips in the bone marrow group required further surgery. Patients who had CDBM also had a higher Harris Hip Score at final follow-up. No significant complications appeared in either group.

However, these studies as many others [20] suffer from bias (different causes of ON, procedures performed in different patients), short follow-up, and different outcome measures. There was also a lack of standardization for cell harvest and cell processing, as well as for cell count.

11.5 Randomized Trials in the Same Patients

There is only one series [21] with very-long-term follow-up comparing both treatments (CD and BM) in the same patients on each side, respectively; surgery was performed at the same time on the same stages of ON in the same disease, and with the same team counting the cells with the same technique. This was possible due to the high number of osteonecrosis treated in this center (more than 10,000 during the past three decades). The efficiency of cell therapy was gauged on several parameters: on repairing the disease (MRI and/or histology), on delaying collapse and total hip replacement, and on the risk of arthroplasty revision and low hip function after multiple revisions or complications. 125 patients (78 males and 47 women) with bilateral symptomatic osteonecrosis (ON) at the same pre-collapse stage on each side (stage I or II) were included from 1988 to 1998 in this study. Osteonecrosis was related to corticosteroids. The osteonecrosis volume was measured with MRI; the smaller ON was treated with decompression and the contralateral larger ON with percutaneous mesenchymal cell (MSC) obtained from bone marrow concentration. The average number of MSCs (counted as colony-forming units—fibroblast) that was injected in each hip was 90,000 ± 25,000 cells (ranging as 45,000–180,000 cells). At the most recent follow-up (average 25 years ranging from 20 to 30 years), bone marrow implantation had decreased number of primary total hip replacements: 95 hips (76%) in the CD group had total hip replacement whereas it was necessary only for 30 hips (24%) in the bone marrow group ($p < 0.0001$). For the 90 hips treated with success with bone marrow, the mean volume of repair on MRI at follow-up was 16.4 cm^3 (ranging from 12 to 21 cm^3) corresponding to a decrease in average volume from 22.4 cm^3 (range 35–15 cm^3) preoperatively to 6 cm^3 (range 12–0 cm^3) at most recent follow-up; as percentage, the volume decreased from 45 to 12%. Bone marrow implantation decreased the need for revision and subsequent revision of hip replacement: At the most recent follow-up (25 years after the first surgery, ranging from 20 to 30 years), among the 125 hips operated with bone marrow, 2 of 30 THA had revision (second THA). For the 125 hips operated with decompression without cells, 45 of 95 THA required revision (second THA) at a mean follow-up of 18 years (ranging from 10 to 28 years), and 5 of these 45 needed a re-revision.

11.6 Cytotherapy of Hip Osteonecrosis: Challenges and Prospects

Important variations of the number of MSCs are observed in patients [22] and may be a limit of the technique: Decreased MSCs have been described in patients with corticosteroid-associated hip osteonecrosis. MSCs were shown to be high in some hematological disorders as sickle cell disease. It varied also depending on patient age.

- *Tissue engineering* is probably one of the solutions [23] to bring a regular number of cells to the patient. In a classical approach, tissue engineering consists of harvesting bone marrow, isolating MSCs by their adherence to tissue culture plastic, and expanding and differentiating those cells in culture to a sufficient number. But the ex vivo amplification and further administration of MSCs, in contrast to bone marrow cell concentrates, are controlled by regulatory authorities, namely the US Food and Drug Administration (FDA) and the European Medicines Agency (EMA). This autologous approach for isolation and osteogenic differentiation of MSCs is however highly demanding in terms of logistics, production, and safety of culture conditions leading to a costly therapeutic procedure. However, usually the number of MSCs expanded after 3 weeks of tissue culture is about five million MSCs per mL. So according to the reported culturing time, ranging from 10 days to 3 weeks, the number of cultured MSCs could range from 100,000 to 20 million cells. Such treatment has been started by the authors in France. This work is supported by the 7th Framework Program of the European Commission through the REBORNE (Regenerating Bone defects using New biomedical Engineering approaches) project (Health-2009-1.4.2-241879).
- *Allogenic bone marrow-derived stem cell therapy:* A unique advantage of MSCs is their potential for allogenic cell delivery in immunocompetent patients. Their immune-privileged characteristic is partially due to the lack of expression of major histocompatibility complex (MHC) II antigens that are responsible for immune rejection, although MHC II expression could be induced by IFN-γ stimulation. In addition, MSCs lack the expression of co-stimulatory molecules that activate T cells, including CD40, CD80, and CD86. MSCs have immunomodulatory effects of inhibiting the proliferation of T cells and B cells. The use of allogenic instead of autologous MSCs for the treatment of AVN appears attractive because of logistic and economic advantages given that these cells might be available as “off-the-shelf” product. However, allogenic MSCs have the danger of disease

transmission or immunological rejection, as present in organ transplantation. Therefore, a risk-benefit analysis of allogenic MSC-based strategies in populations of patients has to be addressed. Hernigou and colleagues [24] previously reported on the use of allogenic stem cells in osteonecrosis treatment. They reported on a patient who had osteonecrosis of the humeral head secondary to sickle cell disease. Treatment with a bone marrow allograft led to a favorable outcome and total repair of osteonecrosis after a follow-up of 4 years. The transplantation was performed in February 1992 after administration of a conditioning regimen of busulfan (16 mg per kilogram of body weight), cyclophosphamide (200 mg per kilogram of body weight), and lymphoid irradiation to suppress immune response and to eliminate the hematopoietic precursors. The bone marrow donor was an HLA-identical sibling for whom a mixed-leukocyte culture was nonreactive; the donor was heterozygous for sickle cell anemia. Such a treatment with expanded allogenic stem cells could decrease the price of the procedure.

- *Can technical devices help?* Can point-of-care devices in the future simplify the procedure of concentrating the bone marrow aspirate and of achieving a standardized and sufficient number of MSCs for implantation. Preliminary research has shown promising data [25].

11.7 Discussion

Autologous bone marrow transplantation was proposed for the treatment of osteonecrosis. Bone marrow mononuclear cell efficiency may be related to the number of stem cells with osteogenic properties. Another explanation for efficiency of bone marrow implantation is that injected stromal cells secrete cytokines, resulting in angiogenesis and improvement in osteogenesis. Finally, bone marrow-derived mononuclear cells are able to elicit formation of new blood vessels by the presence of endothelial cell progenitors or hemangioblasts in this cell fraction. This may be due to both supply of progenitor cells and angiogenic cytokines produced by bone marrow cells. Endothelial progenitors can actively engage in vasculogenesis in tissue devoid of vessels, and in neoangiogenesis from the preexisting capillaries. Besides the generation of new capillaries, the growing endothelia enhance mobilization and growth of mesenchymal progenitors through the angiopoietin 1-Tie2 pathway, which generates pericytes and vascular mural cells required for new vessel growth and stabilization. A broad capacity of differentiation of perivascular mesenchymal cells has been shown, and participation of perivascular mesenchymal progenitors in the repair of adjacent tissues has been described in both experimental models and humans. On its turn, local ischemia that activates the HIF1a signaling and mobilization of circulating progenitors through the SDF1-dependent pathway may supply permanent stimuli for blood vessel repair and supply new cells for bone regeneration.

Adult MSCs usually represent a heterogeneous population of cells, with a positive immunophenotype for STRO-1, CD73, CD146, and CD106 and a negative one for CD11b, CD45, CD34, CD31, and CD117. MSCs act via multifaceted pathways that are not completely understood to date to augment regeneration, including mechanisms that mediate homing of administered MSCs to sites of injury. Two main functions of MSCs can be distinguished. The first is the secretory or "trophic" function of MSCs, which includes the secretion of a wide spectrum of factors with immunomodulatory, anti-inflammatory, antiapoptotic, proangiogenic, proliferative, or chemoattractive capacities, among others. Second, administered MSCs can orchestrate a differentiation process with differentiated or undifferentiated cells for functional tissue restoration.

11.8 Conclusion

In future research, some questions should be addressed. For example, is the differentiation potential of MSCs from different sources (bone marrow, fat, periosteum) the same? Are their functional abilities after repeated culture the same? How different are bones formed by implanted MSCs from normal bones in terms of histology and biomechanics? In addition, the risk of forming cancer at the implanted site should be evaluated. Hernigou and co-workers [26, 27] found that patients treated with cell therapy do not have a greater incidence of cancer than the rest of the population. They analyzed the occurrence of cancer by follow-up, cell number, sites of cancer, age, gender, and pathology that was treated. They found that the risk of cancer was not increased in patients with longer follow-ups or in patients who had received higher number of MSCs. However, this study was performed with autologous MSCs from bone marrow; no report has been done when allogenic MSCs or expanded MSCs are implanted with long-term follow-up.

References

1. Mont MA, Hungerford DS. Non-traumatic avascular necrosis of the femoral head. J Bone Joint Surg Am. 1995;77(3):459–74.
2. Hernigou P, Beaujean F. Abnormalities in the bone marrow of the iliac crest in patients who have osteonecrosis secondary to corticosteroid therapy or alcohol abuse. J Bone Joint Surg Am. 1997;79(7):1047–53.
3. Hernigou P, Beaujean F, Lambotte JC. Decrease in the mesenchymal stem-cell pool in the proximal femur in corticosteroid-induced osteonecrosis. J Bone Joint Surg Br. 1999;81(2):349–55.
4. Yoon BH, Jones LC, Chen CH, Cheng EY, Cui Q, Drescher W, Fukushima W, Gangji V, Goodman SB, Ha YC, Hernigou P, Hungerford M, Iorio R, Jo WL, Khanduja V, Kim H, Kim SY, Kim TY, Lee HY, Lee MS, Lee YK, Lee YJ, Mont MA, Sakai T, Sugano N, Takao M, Yamamoto T, Koo KH. Etiologic classification criteria of ARCO on femoral head osteonecrosis part 2: alcohol-associated osteonecrosis. J Arthroplast. 2019;34(1):169–174.e161. https://doi.org/10.1016/j.arth.2018.09.006.
5. Salem KH, Brockert AK, Mertens R, Drescher W. Avascular necrosis after chemotherapy for haematological malignancy in childhood. Bone Joint J. 2013;95-B(12):1708–13. https://doi.org/10.1302/0301-620X.95B12.30688.
6. Yamamoto T, Hirano K, Tsutsui H, Sugioka Y, Sueishi K. Corticosteroid enhances the experimental induction of osteonecrosis in rabbits with Shwartzman reaction. Clin Orthop Relat Res. 1995;(316):235–43.
7. Merschin D, Hane R, Tohidnezhad M, Pufe T, Drescher W. Bone-preserving total hip arthroplasty in avascular necrosis of the hip—a matched-pairs analysis. Int Orthop. 2018;42(7):1509–16. https://doi.org/10.1007/s00264-018-3896-9.
8. Hernigou P, Trousselier M, Roubineau F, Bouthors C, Chevallier N, Rouard H, Flouzat-Lachaniette CH. Stem cell therapy for the treatment of hip osteonecrosis: a 30-year review of progress. Clin Orthop Surg. 2016;8(1):1–8. https://doi.org/10.4055/cios.2016.8.1.1.
9. Hernigou P. Bone transplantation and tissue engineering, part IV. Mesenchymal stem cells: history in orthopedic surgery from Cohnheim and Goujon to the Nobel Prize of Yamanaka. Int Orthop. 2015;39(4):807–17. https://doi.org/10.1007/s00264-015-2716-8.
10. Hernigou P, Daltro G, Hernigou J. Hip osteonecrosis: stem cells for life or behead and arthroplasty? Int Orthop. 2018;42(7):1425–8. https://doi.org/10.1007/s00264-018-4026-4.
11. Hernigou J, Alves A, Homma Y, Guissou I, Hernigou P. Anatomy of the ilium for bone marrow aspiration: map of sectors and implication for safe trocar placement. Int Orthop. 2014;38(12):2585–90. https://doi.org/10.1007/s00264-014-2353-7.
12. Hernigou J, Picard L, Alves A, Silvera J, Homma Y, Hernigou P. Understanding bone safety zones during bone marrow aspiration from the iliac crest: the sector rule. Int Orthop. 2014;38(11):2377–84. https://doi.org/10.1007/s00264-014-2343-9.
13. Hernigou P, Homma Y, Flouzat Lachaniette CH, Poignard A, Allain J, Chevallier N, Rouard H. Benefits of small volume and small syringe for bone marrow aspirations of mesenchymal stem cells. Int Orthop. 2013;37(11):2279–87. https://doi.org/10.1007/s00264-013-2017-z.
14. Hernigou P, Thiebaut B, Housset V, Bastard C, Homma Y, Chaib Y, Flouzat Lachaniette CH. Stem cell therapy in bilateral osteonecrosis: computer-assisted surgery versus conventional fluoroscopic technique on the contralateral side. Int Orthop. 2018;42(7):1593–8. https://doi.org/10.1007/s00264-018-3953-4.
15. Hernigou P, Beaujean F. Treatment of osteonecrosis with autologous bone marrow grafting. Clin Orthop Relat Res. 2002;(405):14–23.
16. Gangji V, Hauzeur JP, Matos C, De Maertelaer V, Toungouz M, Lambermont M. Treatment of osteonecrosis of the femoral head with implantation of autologous bone-marrow cells. A pilot study. J Bone Joint Surg Am. 2004;86-A(6):1153–60.
17. Gangji V, De Maertelaer V, Hauzeur JP. Autologous bone marrow cell implantation in the treatment of non-traumatic osteonecrosis of the femoral head: five year follow-up of a prospective controlled study. Bone. 2011;49(5):1005–9. https://doi.org/10.1016/j.bone.2011.07.032.
18. Sen RK, Tripathy SK, Aggarwal S, Marwaha N, Sharma RR, Khandelwal N. Early results of core decompression and autologous bone marrow mononuclear cells instillation in femoral head osteonecrosis: a randomized control study. J Arthroplast.

2012;27(5):679–86. https://doi.org/10.1016/j.arth.2011.08.008.
19. Zhao D, Cui D, Wang B, Tian F, Guo L, Yang L, Liu B, Yu X. Treatment of early stage osteonecrosis of the femoral head with autologous implantation of bone marrow-derived and cultured mesenchymal stem cells. Bone. 2012;50(1):325–30. https://doi.org/10.1016/j.bone.2011.11.002.
20. Piuzzi NS, Chahla J, Jiandong H, Chughtai M, LaPrade RF, Mont MA, Muschler GF, Pascual-Garrido C. Analysis of cell therapies used in clinical trials for the treatment of osteonecrosis of the femoral head: a systematic review of the literature. J Arthroplast. 2017;32(8):2612–8. https://doi.org/10.1016/j.arth.2017.02.075.
21. Hernigou P, Dubory A, Homma Y, Guissou I, Flouzat Lachaniette CH, Chevallier N, Rouard H. Cell therapy versus simultaneous contralateral decompression in symptomatic corticosteroid osteonecrosis: a thirty year follow-up prospective randomized study of one hundred and twenty five adult patients. Int Orthop. 2018;42(7):1639–49. https://doi.org/10.1007/s00264-018-3941-8.
22. Hernigou P, Guerin G, Homma Y, Dubory A, Chevallier N, Rouard H, Flouzat Lachaniette CH. History of concentrated or expanded mesenchymal stem cells for hip osteonecrosis: is there a target number for osteonecrosis repair? Int Orthop. 2018;42(7):1739–45. https://doi.org/10.1007/s00264-018-4000-1.
23. Gomez-Barrena E, Rosset P, Gebhard F, Hernigou P, Baldini N, Rouard H, Sensebe L, Gonzalo-Daganzo RM, Giordano R, Padilla-Eguiluz N, Garcia-Rey E, Cordero-Ampuero J, Rubio-Suarez JC, Stanovici J, Ehrnthaller C, Huber-Lang M, Flouzat-Lachaniette CH, Chevallier N, Donati DM, Ciapetti G, Fleury S, Fernandez MN, Cabrera JR, Avendano-Sola C, Montemurro T, Panaitescu C, Veronesi E, Rojewski MT, Lotfi R, Dominici M, Schrezenmeier H, Layrolle P. Feasibility and safety of treating non-unions in tibia, femur and humerus with autologous, expanded, bone marrow-derived mesenchymal stromal cells associated with biphasic calcium phosphate biomaterials in a multicentric, non-comparative trial. Biomaterials. 2018;196:100. https://doi.org/10.1016/j.biomaterials.2018.03.033.
24. Hernigou P, Bernaudin F, Reinert P, Kuentz M, Vernant JP. Bone-marrow transplantation in sickle-cell disease. Effect on osteonecrosis: a case report with a four-year follow-up. J Bone Joint Surg Am. 1997;79(11):1726–30.
25. Woodell-May JE, Tan ML, King WJ, Swift MJ, Welch ZR, Murphy MP, McKale JM. Characterization of the cellular output of a point-of-care device and the implications for addressing critical limb ischemia. Biores Open Access. 2015;4(1):417–24. https://doi.org/10.1089/biores.2015.0006.
26. Hernigou P, Homma Y, Flouzat-Lachaniette CH, Poignard A, Chevallier N, Rouard H. Cancer risk is not increased in patients treated for orthopaedic diseases with autologous bone marrow cell concentrate. J Bone Joint Surg Am. 2013;95(24):2215–21. https://doi.org/10.2106/JBJS.M.00261.
27. Hernigou P, Flouzat Lachaniette CH, Delambre J, Chevallier N, Rouard H. Regenerative therapy with mesenchymal stem cells at the site of malignant primary bone tumour resection: what are the risks of early or late local recurrence? Int Orthop. 2014;38(9):1825–35. https://doi.org/10.1007/s00264-014-2384-0.

12 Alternative Head-Preserving Procedure for Osteonecrosis of the Femoral Head: Tissue Engineering, Future Perspective

Shin-Yoon Kim

12.1 Etiology, Pathophysiology, and Pathogenesis of Osteonecrosis of the Femoral Head

Osteonecrosis of the femoral head (ONFH) is the death of the cellular portion of the bone, with subsequent structural changes, leading to progressive collapse of the femoral head followed by degenerative arthritis of the hip joint. Diverse conditions have been associated with the development of secondary ON, including corticosteroids, alcohol abuse, trauma (femoral neck fracture), gout, diabetes, sickle cell anemia, dysbarism, hyperlipidemia, pancreatic, radiation, systemic lupus erythematosus, and Caisson's disease [1, 2]. ONFH affects primarily young adults and bilateral involvement is more than 50%. The disease typically affects epiphyseal bone on the convex side of a joint, likely due to lack of collateral circulation, and most commonly affects the femoral head, although it can affect the femoral condyles, humeral head, proximal tibia, vertebra, and small bones of the hand and foot.

The precise pathogenesis of ONFH is not clear, but it has been suggested that a common pathogenesis of ONFH involves an interruption of the circulation of blood to the femoral head, thus leading to ischemic insult and bone collapse. Ischemia can be produced by vascular interruption (fractures or dislocations), thrombotic occlusion (intravascular coagulation), or extravascular compression (marrow fat enlargement). Current evidence suggests that intravascular coagulation and microcirculatory thrombotic occlusion likely provide a final common pathway for nontraumatic osteonecrosis. Many authors believe that it is the result of the combined effects of metabolic factors and local factors affecting blood supply such as vascular damage, increased intraosseous pressure, and mechanical stresses [3–5]. Until now, studies about osteonecrosis have suggested that alcohol and steroid use may cause osteonecrosis by increasing adipogenesis and decreasing osteogenesis of bone marrow stromal cells [6, 7]. Corticosteroids and alcohol are able to induce a pluripotent bone marrow cell line to differentiate into adipocytes in vitro preferentially. Increased adipogenesis causes venous sinusoidal compression, which leads to venous congestion, intraosseous hypertension, impaired arterial inflow, and ultimately infarction [8] (Fig. 12.1). The pathophysiology includes decreased blood flow and ischemia by the above pathogenesis. Ischemia leads to death of osteocytes followed by a repairing process. Biochemical sequences of necrosis are as follows: there is low nutrition; low oxygen tension; decreased osteoblast and alkaline phosphatase activity; imbalance between osteo-

S.-Y. Kim (✉)
Department of Orthopedic Surgery, School of Medicine, Kyungpook National University Hospital, Daegu, South Korea
e-mail: syukim@knu.ac.kr

W. R. Drescher et al. (eds.), *Advances in Specialist Hip Surgery*,
https://doi.org/10.1007/978-3-030-61830-8_12

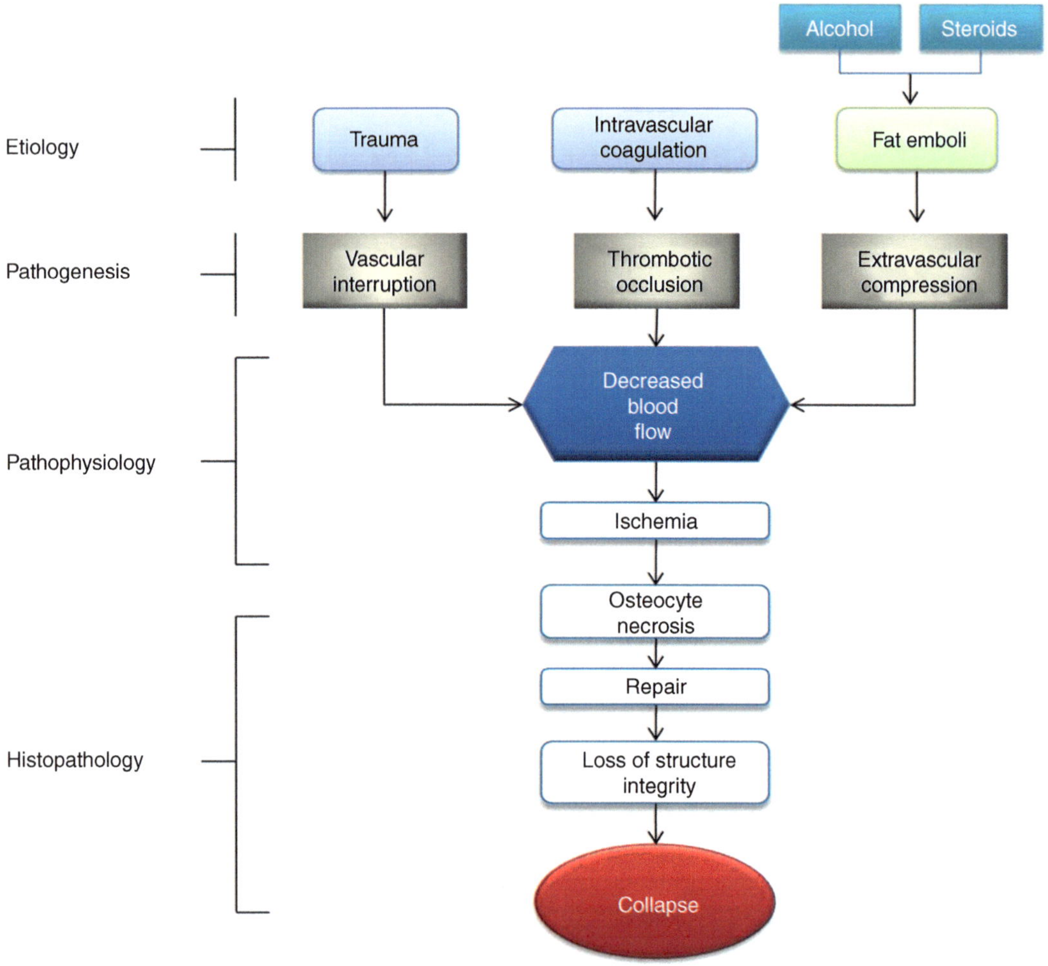

Fig. 12.1 Etiology, pathogenesis, pathophysiology, and histopathology of osteonecrosis that result in joint collapse. Aaron RK. Osteonecrosis: etiology, pathophysiology, and diagnosis. In: Callaghan J, Rosenberg A, Rubash H, eds The Adult Hip New York, NY: Raven Press. 1998; 451–66 [3]

blast and osteoclast coupling; increased activity of osteoclast, fibroblast, adipocyte, and chondrocyte; and failure of the repair process. Biomechanical sequences to collapse are as follows. Decreased rate of deformation to load in necrosis results in decreased compliance of the cartilage and adjacent bone due to uneven mechanical transmission from joint surface to trabecular bone. These factors increase hip joint stress abnormally and stress will concentrate along the interface of necrotic bone and normal bone leading to sclerotic band formation, microfracture of the bone, and collapse of the femoral head eventually. The schematic drawing shows the etiology, pathogenesis, pathophysiology, and histopathology of osteonecrosis that result in collapse of femoral head.

12.2 Prognosis and Intervention

The prognosis of ONFH with or without various femoral head-preserving procedures is usually influenced by the stage, size, and location of the lesion.

Natural history without any intervention has been encouraging in hips with early stage, small size, and medial-located lesion [9].

However, ONFH with advanced, extensive, lateral-located (weight-bearing portion) lesions showed early collapse and subsequent osteoarthritic change, eventually leading to hip arthroplasty. Advanced lesions are defined as lesions Ficat III and IV [10]; extensive lesions are Steinberg [11] and ARCO [12] class C (>50% involvement), Kerboul [13] combined necrotic angle >200°, Koo [14] combined necrotic angle of >240°, and revised Japanese Investigation Committee classification [15] of C1 or C2. Until present, unmet needs include a simple, easy, reproducible option to prevent collapse and to preserve the own femoral head in these advanced or extensive lesions of ONFH.

There are numerous options to prevent the collapse of ONFH (Fig. 12.2): observation, core decompression, multiple drilling, cancellous impaction graft, vascularized or non-vascularized bone graft, transtrochanteric osteotomy (TRO), and cell-based therapy. Hip arthroplasty is the last choice in post-collapsed and progressed lesions with advanced osteoarthritis. Each has the theoretical rationale to relieve pain, to halt the progression to collapse, and to enhance the repair process to normal trabecular bone.

Core decompression is performed as a gold standard head-preserving surgical procedure [16]. Theoretically, it can lower the elevated bone marrow pressure and new bone can grow through the tract encouraging revascularization and repair. The efficacy of core decompression remains controversial. Recently, it is only used for small-sized, medial (non-weight-bearing portion) located, and pre-collapsed lesions. Multiple drilling, especially a percutaneous technique, was performed instead of core decompression with a similar rationale to core decompression with simple and less invasive technique [17]. Non-vascularized fibula or tibia bone grafting was performed to heal the necrotic lesion and to prevent collapse by strutting effect. Non-vascularized bone grafting was effective only in small- to medium-size and pre-collapsed lesion in non-weight-bearing portion [18]. Vascularized fibular [19] or vascularized iliac [20] bone grafting aiming the strutting effect and a more rapid induction of primary callus formation in the subchondral bone as result of more robust revascularization and increased the osteoinductive potential. They showed better clinical and radiographic results than non-vascularized bone grafting. Transtrochanteric rotational osteotomy

1. Observation
2. Core decompression
3. Multiple drilling
4. Nonvascularized Bone graft
5. Vascularized Bone [fibula. iliac] graft
6. Transtrochanteric Osteotomy
7. Cell Therapy-BM, adipose MSCs
8. Tissue Engineering9.
9. PEMF, ESW, Hyperbaric Oxygen
10. Phamaceuticals
11. Arthroplasty

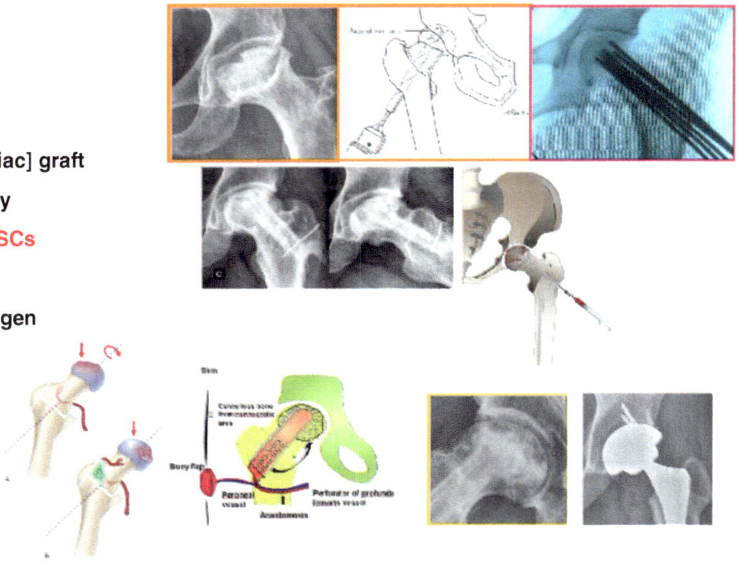

Fig. 12.2 Various treatment options for osteonecrosis of the femoral head

(TRO) involves transposing an intact area to a weight-bearing portion of the joint, thus resulting in transfer of the necrotic area to a non-weight-bearing area [21]. Vascularized bone grafting and TRO had favorable results after long-term follow-up in lesions of medium to large size, weight-bearing portion located, and pre-collapsed necrosis. However, these procedures require very-high-demanding techniques, long operation time, and long-term rehabilitation period associated with unpredictable results and high rates of complications [22–24].

Core decompression showed better clinical results than nonoperative management [16]. Vascularized bone grafting had significantly better results than core decompression [25]. Vascularized bone grafting had significantly better results than non-vascularized bone grafting especially in large lesions of ONFH [26, 27]. However, there are no clear answers yet: Which option is best? Which case is the ideal indication of each option?

Can the outcomes of each option be reproducible?

Multiple drilling tried based on percutaneous technique had showed better or similar outcomes compared with core decompression [17]. Growth factor like BMP was injected into the necrotic area after core decompression [28]. Electrical stimulation, electric shock wave, hyperbaric oxygen, thrombolytic agents, and bisphosphonates have tried to relieve pain due to their possible advantages as adjuvant therapy.

12.3 Cell-Based Therapy

More recently, cell-based therapy with or without additional surgery, scaffold, and growth factors has been helping to relieve pain, increase function, repair the necrotic lesion, improve the survivorship of femoral heads, and reduce the need for hip arthroplasty.

Multipotent mesenchymal stem cells (MSCs) have the ability to maintain mitotic multiplication while being capable of differentiating into various cellular types, such as osteoblasts, osteocytes, chondrocytes, and adipocytes [29]. There are abnormalities in number or in function of bone progenitor cells in bone marrow [30] and decreased numbers of circulating endothelial precursor cells and colony-forming units in patients with osteonecrosis [31]. On the other hand, the capillaries within the necrotic femoral head serving as conduits for stem cell and osseous cell delivery in the bone remodeling unit are believed to be occluded by emboli or thrombosis [32].

There can be an imbalance between osteoblast formation and osteoclast resorption in patients with osteonecrosis [33]. The theoretical background of cell therapy in ON is that implanted MSCs can repopulate trabecular bone and subsequently revitalize and remodel the necrotic bone. Experimentally, MSCs transplanted have shown to enhance tissue regeneration areas of necrotic bone [34].

Cell therapy is usually performed in conjunction with the classical core decompression procedure and involves harvesting of autologous bone marrow aspirate, isolation of its mononuclear cell fraction, and injection of it into the necrotic zone of the femoral head through the canal of the preceding core decompression. The hypothesis of this strategy is based on multipotent MSCs in the bone marrow aspirate that could repopulate the trabeculae of the necrotic zone within the femoral head, enhancing regeneration and remodeling of the necrotic bone [35].

These findings prompted researchers to develop a new approach for the treatment of ONFH, based on implantation into the necrotic zone of the femoral head of a concentrated bone marrow preparation, containing endothelial progenitor cells promoting angiogenesis and MSCs promoting osteogenesis [36].

With a greater number of MSCs in the autologous bone marrow concentrate injected into the necrotic lesion, a more favorable outcome will be possible. Usually bone marrow aspirate contains various cell types with very low percentage (0.01%) of MSCs [37]. In contrast, a highly concentrated autologous bone marrow aspirate may contain a large number of MSCs (ranging from 1160 per mL to 4900 per mL) [38]. However, the exact number of MSCs that is required to induce remodeling and repair of the osteonecrotic zone is unknown yet [39].

12.4 Clinical Trial Cell-Based Therapy for ONFH

There were several clinical trials of BMAC or culture-expanded BMSC implantation directly into the lesion, intra-arterial or intravenous delivery. Cells were implanted alone or in combination with autologous bone graft, porous tantalum rod, platelet-rich plasma, fibrin glue, free fibular graft, or vascularized iliac graft with b-TCP granules. Clinical trials were case series, cohort study, and prospective randomized trial with or without control.

There are three categories in cell-based therapy for ONFH. First, there is local injection of BMAC containing osteoprogenitor cells/MSCs with variable-size core decompression. Hernigou was a pioneer of cell therapy for ONFH. They added BMAC to core decompression [31]. Similar series reported positive results of BMAC implantation for treatment of ONFH in the form of case series, [38] cohort study [39], and prospective randomized studies [40, 41]. However, BMAC is a mixture of various mononuclear cells, of which a very small fraction (0.01%) comprises MSCs [37]. Combination of BMACs with autologous bone graft [42, 43], fibrin glue [44], and PRP [45] was used in other clinical trials. Second category is to implant the ex vivo culture-expanded BMSCs instead of BMSCs. Culture-expanded BMSCs can be implanted directly into the lesion [46, 47]. This strategy has advantages such as controlling the number of cells, if it is not sufficient, and use of committed state of pre-osteoblast instead of fully differentiated osteoblast. However, transformation of implanted cells is a potential serious complication in the implantation of culture-expanded MSCs. Other studies combined implantation of ex vivo-expanded BMSCs cultured with b-TCP granules and free fibular vascularized graft [48] or vascularized iliac bone graft [49]. Third category is intra-arterial injection of peripheral blood stem cells mobilized by granulocyte colony-stimulating factor with [50] or without [51] mechanical support (porous tantalum rod).

The number of BMSCs and methods of application are heterogeneous in each individual trial. The number of implanted cells is also different without regarding the necrotic area or volume. Most studies did not show how many cells were implanted. Only two studies reported the number of culture BMSCs as 2×106 or $0.5–1 \times 10^8$. Scaffolds in the form of hydrogel (fibrin glue) or solid forms (β-TCP granules) may help to retain the cells at the lesion site and promote osteoconduction or osteoinduction.

A recent meta-analysis and systemic review of human clinical trials using cell-based therapy seems to show reasonable, if not remarkable, effects on early-stage (Ficat I or II) ONFH in terms of symptomatic relief, less radiographic progression of femoral head collapse, improved Harris Hip Score, low rate of complications, and lower conversion to THA compared with core decompression alone [52].

The classification of ONFH in almost all clinical trials is by Ficat staging; therefore, the most important prognostic factors for progression of ONFH such as location and extent of necrosis are not reflected. Concerns should be focused on cell-based therapy that can preserve the head in large advanced necrotic lesion located in lateral weight portion which is known to have poor prognosis, especially in young patients.

12.5 Author's Tissue Engineering Technology

Orthopedic hip surgeons should decide to intervene with appropriate procedures to prevent collapse and preserve own femoral head or to leave without any unnecessary procedures. The recent Japanese group guideline indicates to leave without any intervention JIC A (medial) and B (central) lesion of Ficat stages I and II, and try TRO in JIC C1 (lateral) or C2 (far lateral) lesion in Ficat stages I, IIa, and IIb, and hip arthroplasty in advanced Ficat stages III and IV. However, if the patients are of young active age, even though the necrotic lesion is large, located in lateral weight portion and even in advanced stage (unmet needs condition), every effort should be made to prevent collapse and preserve own femoral head.

We introduce a new tissue engineering technique using ex vivo culture-expanded BM MSC seeding in calcium metaphosphate beads as an alternative minimal invasive procedure instead of technically challenging technique such as VFG or VIG and TRO in present unmet needs condition.

Our techniques involve the following:

1. Two weeks before scheduled cell implantation, we performed aspiration of 10 mL of bone marrow from iliac crest at an interval of 2 cm and collection of mononuclear cells. These cells expanded and differentiated to preosteoblast ex vivo using the osteogenic media for 10–14 days. Usually, passage 3 cells were implanted (Fig. 12.3).
2. Porous bead-form scaffolds were made of calcium metaphosphate (CMP) with a diameter of 4–6 mm and BMSCs were seeded in an average density of 1.2 million (range 1–2 million)/mL into 10–15 beads for 7 days in heat-inactivated autologous serum at clean bench room (Fig. 12.4).
3. Drill the core tract with a diameter of 12–16 mm instead of standard 10 mm or 2–4 mm usually done in cell therapy (Fig. 12.5). This wide core tract can reduce an elevated bone marrow pressure and congestion in ON and can support a space for removal of the necrotic lesion as possible. A 3–4 cm longitudinal incision over the greater trochanteric ridge is sufficient. Entry point of core tract should be proximal to lesser trochanter to avoid stress-riser-induced fracture due to core tract. Avoid penetrating into hip joint when inserting the guide pin or when making core tract using a biplanar image intensifier.

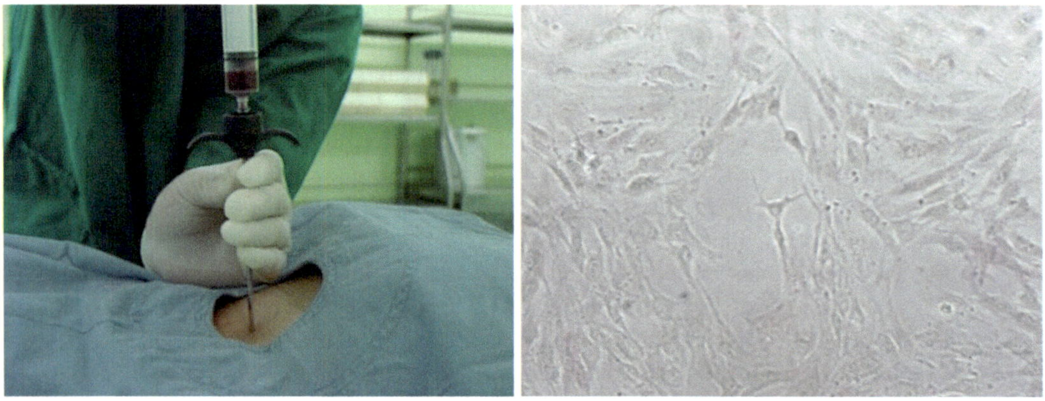

Fig. 12.3 Bone marrow aspiration along the iliac crest and showing preosteoblast after passage 3 in culture plate

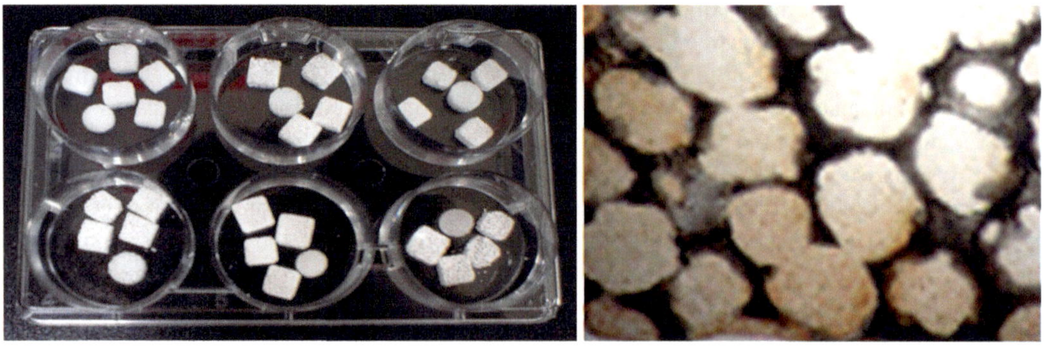

Fig. 12.4 Left: Porous bead-form (round) scaffolds were made of calcium metaphosphate (CMP). Right: Cells (yellow) seeded in scaffold (black)

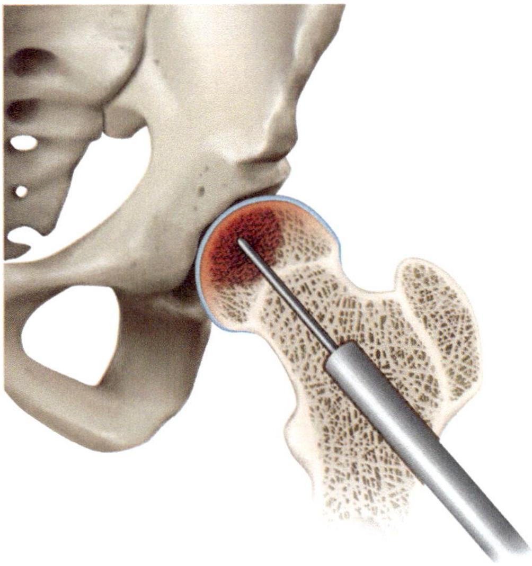

Fig. 12.5 Insertion of guide pin to the center of necrosis; 12–16 mm diameter core tract is made using the reamer. Near the entry point, cancellous bone graft is done using curved curette

4. Remove the necrotic lesion thoroughly using a low-speed burr or curved curettage into the circumferential direction. Make empty space like a mushroom. The sclerotic border should be removed thoroughly also (Fig. 12.6).
5. Cancellous bone can be achieved from proximal metaphysis of femur near the entry of the core tract. This cancellous bone is packed using an impactor in subchondral area underneath the joint (Fig. 12.7).
6. The entrance of core tract is occluded with a same-diameter CMP rod for prevention of invasion of epithelial cells into core tract and as a bone graft substitute (Fig. 12.8).
7. Postoperatively, there was no prophylaxis for deep vein thrombosis in all patients.

The surgical time was within 30 min. Non-weight-bearing ambulation was possible from day 1 after surgery. Partial weight bearing with a walker or two crutches was allowed after 3 weeks

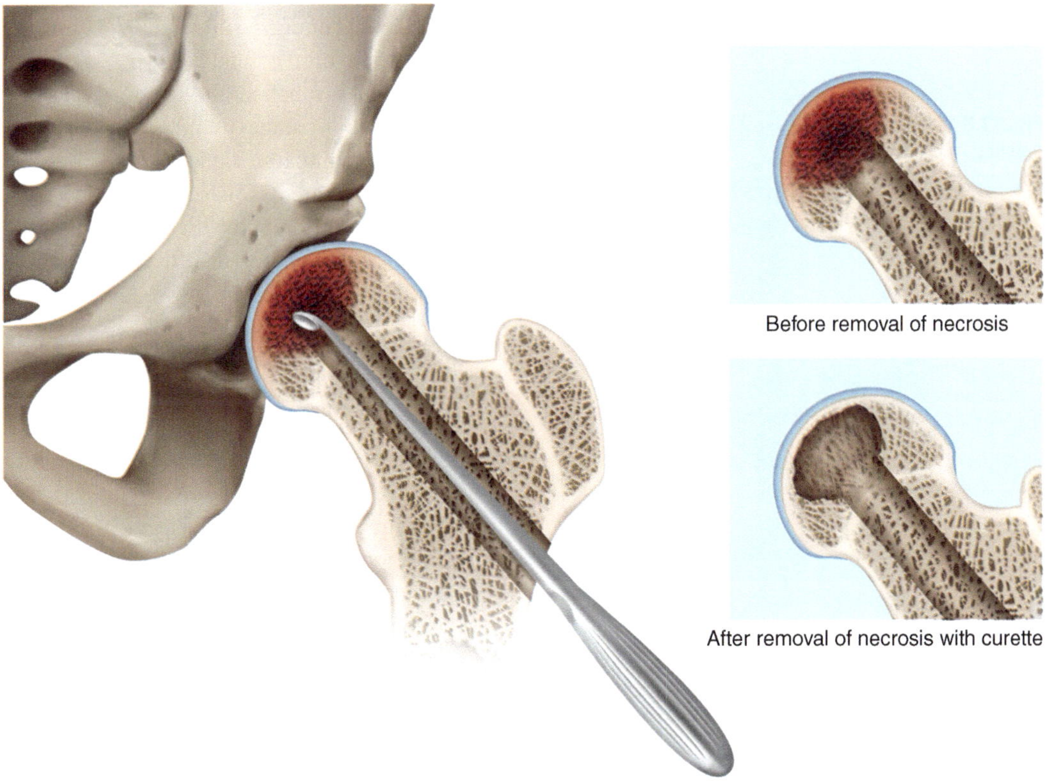

Fig. 12.6 Mushroomlike defect is made through removing of necrosis using the reamer or curved curette

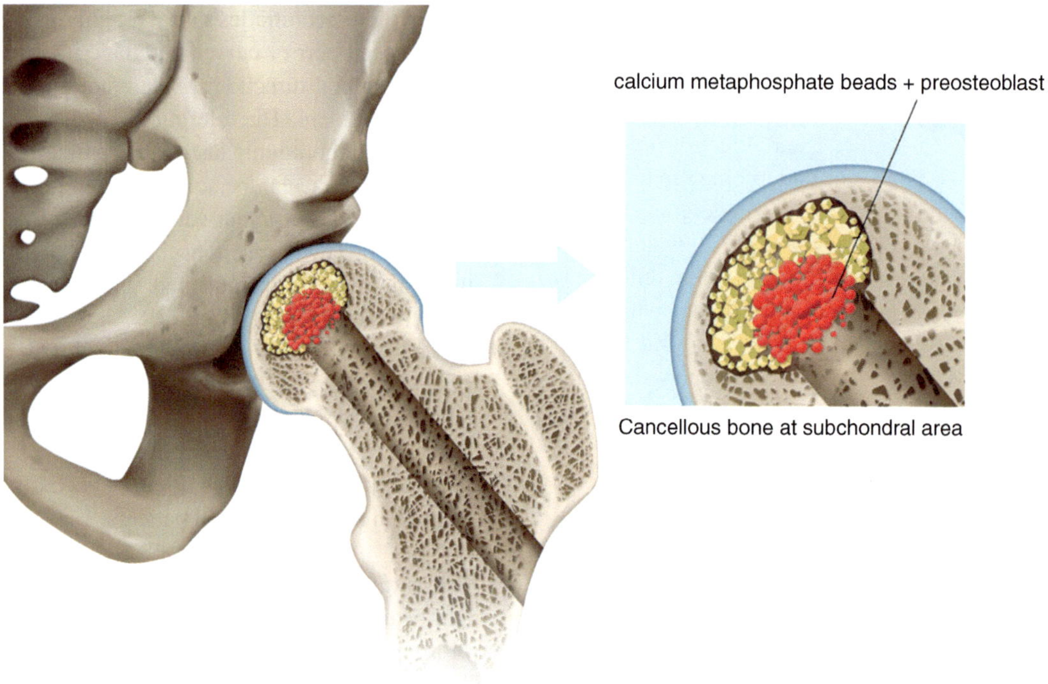

Fig. 12.7 Cancellous bone graft is packed underneath the subchondral area using impactor and the CMP beads with adhering preosteoblasts (ex vivo expanded bone marrow stromal cells) were implanted loosely in mushroom-shaped empty space through core tract

Fig. 12.8 Schematic drawing of tissue engineering technique

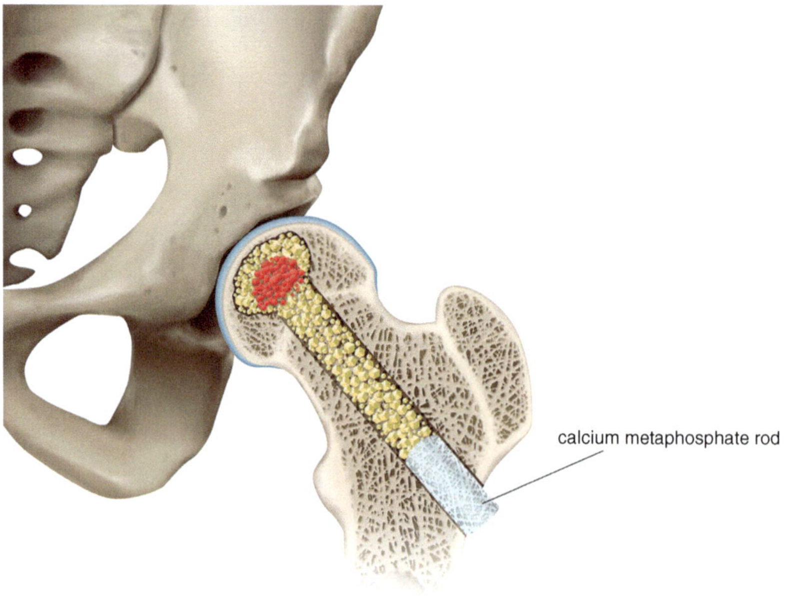

and full weight bearing was permitted after 6 weeks postoperatively.

We had tried bench-to-bedside translation case series in nine hips of seven patients who had a large lesion (ARCO: IIc in five hips and IVc in four hips) in weight-bearing area (JIC: C1 in four hips, and C2 in five hips) (unpublished data). The age of the patients ranged from 16 to 37. Associated factors were steroid in four hips, idiopathic in three hips, alcoholic in one hip, and traumatic in one hip. Koo combined necrotic angle on MRI was more than 200° in all hips (range 200°–380°). Minimum follow-up period was 10 years (range 14–16 years). Two hips with IIc lesion progressed to IVc with dome depression >2 mm and were converted to THR. The other seven hips did not progress to advanced osteoarthritis radiographically. Follow-up radiographs 14 years after operation showed disappearance of necrotic portion and sclerotic band with reappearance of trabecular pattern. Degenerative changes progressed slowly with parallel congruity. MRI showed evidence of regeneration of necrotic bone and signal change to normal marrow image (Fig. 12.9a–c).

The schematic summary is as follows (Fig. 12.10).

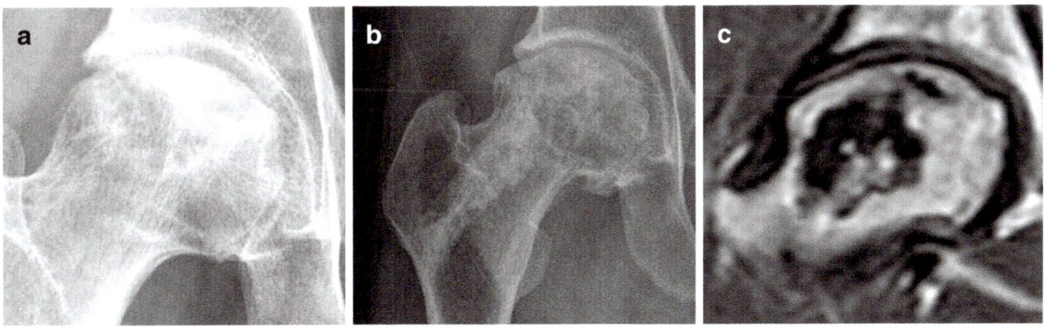

Fig. 12.9 Changes of femoral head. (**a**) Preoperative radiograph, (**b**) radiograph of 14 years after operation, (**c**) MRI: of 14 years after operation

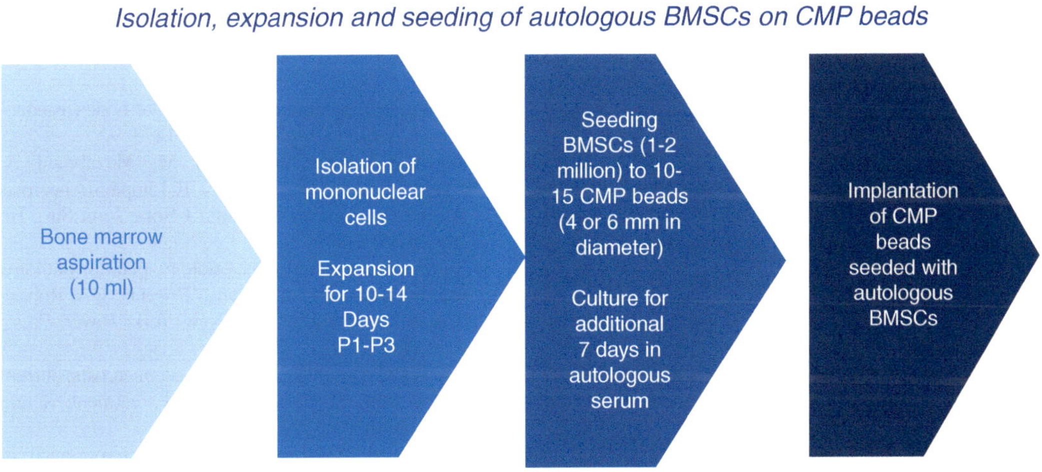

Fig. 12.10 Schematics for preparing the implants with cells and scaffold

12.6 Discussion and Future Perspective

Ideal treatment of osteonecrosis is to preserve the own femoral head without collapse. More ideal point is to convert the dead bone to viable bone. Every intervention is better if it is without invasiveness, and with less donor-site morbidity, small incision, short operation time, and short period rehabilitation. There is no ideal intervention fulfilling all the above advantages. Recently, cell-based therapy has become an attractive option with the mentioned advantages.

Thirty to fifty percent of implanted MSCs or BMAC can remain at the site of implantation after 24 h and cells can survive 12 weeks even in avascular environment [34]. Implanted MSCs are expected to differentiate to osteoblasts; however, most of the cells implanted undergo death within a short period. Before cell death, they exert a paracrine effect [53]. The MSCs secrete bioactive cytokines and chemokines that act on immunomodulation, angiogenesis/arteriogenesis, anti-apoptosis, antioxidation, and cell migration/stimulation [54]. Hypoxia can stimulate MSCs to secrete angiogenetic factors, attract or recruit MSCs to the ischemic site, and mediate trophic activities [55]. The action modes of MSCs are transdifferentiation, cell fusion, mitochondrial transfer, and microvesicle (exosome) formation [56]. The theoretically possible advantages of our technique are wide decompression, use of culture-expanded MSCs at committed stage to fully differentiated osteoblast (preosteoblast), adding autologous cancellous bone graft, use of autologous serum at final cell seeding to scaffold, osteoconduction of calcium metaphosphate used as scaffold, and guided bone regeneration by prevention of epithelial cell invasion by filling the entry. Further issues of cell-based therapy are to mobilize stem cells from niche to lesion site using G-CSF or GFDFgM-CSF before, during, and after the procedure; to deliver appropriate number of appropriate (sources) cells; to add combined procedures; and to use carrier or growth factors. Also study design such as level of evidence, appropriate number of patients and control group involved, and standardization of classification of ON should be clear. MSC-based products are complex and heterogeneous. The variability in donor and tissue sources, manufacturing processes, phenotypic cell markers, and bioactivity has the potential to significantly impact the product and prevents a direct comparison of therapeutic protocols. Bone marrow is not the sole source of MSC-based products; research on the use of adipose-derived MSCs and allogenic use of umbilical cord or placental tissue-derived MSCs is ongoing [57]. Tissue or cell-derived ECM, deeper understanding of the role of niche (interaction of MSCs and microenvironment), and adding ideal growth factors such as BMP or VEGF [58] will be more attractive alternatives to the regeneration of bone in necrotic area.

There are Clinical Trials.gov: XCEL-MTOSTEO-ALPHA, PREOB, CD133+ cells, and BioCUE on the internet. Recently, MSC-based products have increased significantly. The product should be sufficient to demonstrate acceptable levels of safety and efficacy for ensuring public health. CTPs and TEPs are going through the equal regulatory process.

Even with all of these considerations, and in spite of only limited clinical success, the future of the field of tissue engineering for ONFH will be a promising option.

References

1. Mankin HJ. Nontraumatic necrosis of bone (osteonecrosis). N Engl J Med. 1992;326:1473–9.
2. Merle d'Aubigne R, Postel M, Mazabraud A, Massias P, Gueguen J, France P. Idiopathic necrosis of the femoral head in adults. J Bone Joint Surg Br. 1965;47:612–33.
3. Aaron RK. Osteonecrosis: etiology, pathophysiology, and diagnosis. In: Callaghan J, Rosenberg A, Rubash H, editors. The adult hip. New York: Raven Press; 1998. p. 451–66.
4. Chang CC, Greenspan A, et al. Osteonecrosis: current perspectives on pathogenesis and treatment. Semin Arthritis Rheum. 1993;23(1):47–69.
5. Hungerford DS, Lennox DW. The importance of increased intraosseous pressure in the development of osteonecrosis of the femoral head: implications for treatment. Orthop Clin North Am. 1985;16(4):635–54.
6. Wang Y, Li Y, et al. Alcohol-induced adipogenesis in bone and marrow: a possible mechanism for osteonecrosis. Clin Orthop Relat Res. 2003;(410):213–24.

7. Wang GJ, Cui Q, et al. The Nicolas Andry award. The pathogenesis and prevention of steroid-induced osteonecrosis. Clin Orthop Relat Res. 2000;370:295–310.
8. Laroche M. Intraosseous circulation from physiology to disease. Joint Bone Spine. 2002;69(3):262–9.
9. Jergesen HE, Kahn AS. The natural history of untreated asymptomatic hips in patients who have non-traumatic osteonecrosis. J Bone Joint Surg Am. 1997;79:359–63.
10. Ficat RP, Arlet J, Hungerford DS, editors. Necrosis of the femoral head. In: Ischemia and necroses of bone. Baltimore: Williams & Wilkins; 1980. p. 53–74.
11. Steinberg ME, Hayken GD, Steinberg DR. A quantitative system for staging avascular necrosis. J Bone Joint Surg. 1995;77B:34–41.
12. Gardniers JWM. ARCO committee on terminology and staging. ARCO Newsl. 1993;5:79–82.
13. Kerboul M, Thomone J, Postel M, et al. The conservative surgical treatment of idiopathic aseptic necrosis of the femoral head. J Bone Joint Surg. 1974;56-B:291–6.
14. Koo KH, Kim R. Quantifying the extent of osteonecrosis of the femoral head: a new method using MRI. J Bone Joint Surg. 1995;77-B:875–80.
15. Sugano N, Atsumi T, Ohzono K, Kubo T, Hotokebuchi T, Takaoka K. The 2001 revised criteria for diagnosis, classification, and staging of idiopathic osteonecrosis of the femoral head. J Orthop Sci. 2002;7:601–5.
16. Mont MA, Carbone JJ, Fairbank AC. Core decompression versus nonoperative management for osteonecrosis of the hip. Clin Orthop. 1996;324: 169–78.
17. Mont MA, Ragland PS, Etienne G. Core decompression of the femoral head for osteonecrosis using percutaneous multiple small-diameter drilling. Clin Orthop Relat Res. 2004;429:131–8.
18. Buckley PD, Gearen PF, Petty RW. Structural bone grafting for early atraumatic avascular necrosis of the femoral head. J Bone Joint Surg Am. 1991;73:1357–64.
19. Urbaniak JR, Coogan PG, Gunneson EB, Nunley JA. Treatment of osteonecrosis of the femoral head with free vascularized fibular grafting. A long-term follow-up study of one hundred and three hips. J Bone Joint Surg Am. 1995;77:681–94.
20. Chen CC, Lin CL, Chen WC, Shih HN, Ueng SW, Lee MS. Vascularized iliac bone grafting for osteonecrosis with segmental collapse of the femoral head. J Bone Joint Surg Am. 2009;91(10):2390–4.
21. Sugioka Y. Transtrochanteric anterior rotational osteotomy of the femoral head in the treatment of osteonecrosis affecting the hip: a new osteotomy operation. Clin Orthop Relat Res. 1978;130:191–201.
22. Urbaniak JR. Donor-site morbidity with use of vascularized autogenous fibular grafts. J Bone Joint Surg Am. 1996;78:204–11.
23. Aluisio FV, Urbaniak JR. Proximal femur fractures after free vascularized fibular grafting to the hip. Clin Orthop. 1998;356:192–201.
24. Dailiana ZH, Gunneson EE, Urbaniak JR. Heterotopic ossification after treatment of femoral head osteonecrosis with free vascularized fibular graft. J Arthroplast. 2003;18:83–8.
25. Scully SP, Aaron RK, Urbaniak JR. Survival analysis of hips treated with core decompression or vascularized fibular grafting because of avascular necrosis. J Bone Joint Surg Am. 1998;80:1270–5.
26. Plakseychuk AY, Kim SY, Park BC, Varitimidis SE, Rubash HE, Sotereanos DG. Vascularized compared with nonvascularized fibular grafting for the treatment of osteonecrosis of the femoral head. J Bone Joint Surg Am. 2003;85:589–96.
27. Kim SY, Kim YG, Kim PT, Ihn JC, Cho BC, Koo KH. Vascularized compared with nonvascularized fibular grafts for large osteonecrotic lesions of the femoral head. J Bone Joint Surg Am. 2005;87:2012–59.
28. Lieberman JR, Conduah A, Urist MR. Treatment of osteonecrosis of the femoral head with core decompression and human bone morphogenetic protein. Clin Orthop Relat Res. 2004;429:139–452.
29. Baksh D, Song L, Tuan RS. Adult mesenchymal stem cells: characterization, differentiation, and application in cell and gene therapy. J Cell Mol Med. 2004;8(3):301–10.
30. Gangji V, Hauzeur JP, Schoutens A, Hinsenkamp M, Appelboom T, Egrise D. Abnormalities in the replicative capacity of osteoblastic cells in the proximal femur of patients with osteonecrosis of the femoral head. J Rheumatol. 2003;30(2):348–51.
31. Hernigou P, Beaujean F. Treatment of osteonecrosis with autologous bone marrow grafting. Clin Orthop Relat Res. 2002;405:14–23.
32. Jones JP Jr. Fat embolism and osteonecrosis. Orthop Clin North Am. 1985;16(4):595–633.
33. Tian L, Baek S-H, Jang JA, Kim S-Y. Imbalanced bone turnover markers and low bone mineral density in patients with osteonecrosis of the femoral head. Int Orthop. 2018;42:1545–9.
34. Yan Z, Hang D, Guo C, Chen Z. Fate of mesenchymal stem cells transplanted to osteonecrosis of femoral head. J Orthop Res. 2009;27(4):442–6.
35. Hernigou P, Manicom O, Poignard A, Nogier A, Filippini P, De Abreu L. Core decompression with marrow stem cells. Oper Tech Orthop. 2004;14(2):68–74.
36. Gangji V, Hauzeur JP, Matos C, De Maertelaer V, Toungouz M, Lambermont M. Treatment of osteonecrosis of the femoral head with implantation of autologous bone-marrow cells. A pilot study. J Bone Joint Surg Am. 2004;86-A(6):1153–60.
37. Jones EA, English A, Kinsey SE, Straszynski L, Emery P, Ponchel F, McGonagle D. Optimization of a flow cytometry-based protocol for detection and phenotypic characterization of multipotent mesenchymal stromal cells from human bone marrow. Cytometry B Clin Cytom. 2006;70:391–9.
38. Hernigou P, Poignard A, Zilber S, Rouard H. Cell therapy of hip osteonecrosis with autologous bone marrow grafting. Indian J Orthop. 2009;43(1):40–5.

39. Daltro GC, Fortuna V, de Souza ES, Salles MM, Carreira AC, Meyer R, Freire SM, Borojevic R. Efficacy of autologous stem cell-based therapy for osteonecrosis of the femoral head in sickle cell disease: a five-year follow-up study. Stem Cell Res Ther. 2015;6:110.
40. Gangji V, De Maertelaer V, Hauzeur JP. Autologous bone marrow cell implantation in the treatment of non-traumatic osteonecrosis of the femoral head: five-year follow-up of a prospective controlled study. Bone. 2011;49(5):1005–9.
41. Sen RK, Tripathy SK, Aggarwal S, Marwaha N, Sharma RR, Khandelwal N. Early results of core decompression and autologous bone marrow mononuclear cells instillation in femoral head osteonecrosis: a randomized control study. J Arthroplast. 2012;27:679–86.
42. Kang JS, Moon KH, Kim BS, Kwon DG, Shin SH, Shin BK, Ryu DJ. Clinical results of auto-iliac cancellous bone grafts combined with implantation of autologous bone marrow cells for osteonecrosis of the femoral head: a minimum 5-year follow-up. Yonsei Med J. 2013;54:510–5.
43. Ma Y, Wang T, Liao J, Gu H, Lin X, Jiang Q, Bulsara MK, Zheng M, Zheng Q. Efficacy of autologous bone marrow buffy coat grafting combined with core decompression in patients with avascular necrosis of femoral head: a prospective, double-blinded, randomized, controlled study. Stem Cell Res Ther. 2014;5:115.
44. Lim YW, Kim YS, Lee JW, Kwon SY. Stem cell implantation for osteonecrosis of the femoral head. Exp Mol Med. 2013;45(11):e61.
45. Martin JR, Houdek MT, Sierra RJ. Use of concentrated bone marrow aspirate and platelet rich plasma during minimally invasive decompression of the femoral head in the treatment of osteonecrosis. Croat Med J. 2013;54:219–24.
46. Zhao D, Cui D, Wang B, Tian F, Guo L, Yang L, Liu B, Yu X. Treatment of early stage osteonecrosis of the femoral head with autologous implantation of bone marrow-derived and cultured mesenchymal stem cells. Bone. 2012;50:325–30.
47. Persiani P, de Cristo C, Graci J, Noia G, Gurzì M, Villani C. Stage-related results in treatment of hip osteonecrosis with core-decompression and autologous mesenchymal stem cells. Acta Orthop Belg. 2015;81:406–12.
48. Kawate K, Yajima H, Ohgushi H, Kotobuki N, Sugimoto K, Ohmura T, Kobata Y, Shigematsu K, Kawamura K, Tamai K, Takakura Y. Tissue-engineered approach for the treatment of steroid-induced osteonecrosis of the femoral head: transplantation of autologous mesenchymal stem cells cultured with beta-tricalcium phosphate ceramics and free vascularized fibula. Artif Organs. 2006;30:960–2.
49. Aoyama T, Goto K, Kakinoki R, Ikeguchi R, Ueda M, Kasai Y, Maekawa T, Tada H, Teramukai S, Nakamura T, Toguchida J. An exploratory clinical trial for idiopathic osteonecrosis of femoral head by cultured autologous multipotent mesenchymal stromal cells augmented with vascularized bone grafts. Tissue Eng Part B Rev. 2014;20:233–42.
50. Mao Q, Wang W, Xu T, Zhang S, Xiao L, Chen D, Jin H, Tong P. Combination treatment of biomechanical support and targeted intra-arterial infusion of peripheral blood stem cells mobilized by granulocyte-colony stimulating factor for the osteonecrosis of the femoral head: a randomized controlled clinical trial. J Bone Miner Res. 2015;30:647–56.
51. Mao Q, Jin H, Liao F, Xiao L, Chen D, Tong P. The efficacy of targeted intraarterial delivery of concentrated autologous bone marrow containing mononuclear cells in the treatment of osteonecrosis of the femoral head: a five-year follow-up study. Bone. 2013;57:509–16.
52. Papakostidis C, Tosounidis TH, Jones E, Giannoudis PV. The role of "cell therapy" in osteonecrosis of the femoral head. A systematic review of the literature and meta-analysis of 7 studies. Acta Orthop. 2016;87(1):72–8.
53. Gnecchi M, Zhang Z, Ni A, Dzau VJ. Paracrine mechanisms in adult stem cell signaling and therapy. Circ Res. 2008;103:1204.
54. Rehman J, Traktuev D, Li J, Merfeld-Clauss S, Temm-Grove CJ, Bovenkerk JE, et al. Secretion of angiogenic and antiapoptotic factors by human adipose stromal cells. Circulation. 2004;109:1292.
55. Fan L, Liu R, Li J, Shi Z, Dang X, Wang K. Low oxygen tension enhances osteogenic potential of bone marrow-derived mesenchymal stem cells with osteonecrosis-related functional impairment. Stem Cells Int. 2015;2015:950312.
56. Phinney DG, Pittenger MF. Concise review: MSC-derived exosomes for cell-free therapy. Stem Cells. 2017;35(4):851–8.
57. Murphy MB, Moncivais K, Caplan AI. Mesenchymal stem cells: environmentally responsive therapeutics for regenerative medicine. Exp Mol Med. 2013;45:e54.
58. Kang ML, Kim JE, Im GI. Vascular endothelial growth factor-transfected adipose-derived stromal cells enhance bone regeneration and neovascularization from bone marrow stromal cells. J Tissue Eng Regen Med. 2017;11:337–48.

Part V

Arthritis of the Hip: Primary Hip Arthroplasty

13 Ceramic-on-Ceramic Total Hip Arthroplasty

Byung-Ho Yoon, Yong-Han Cha, Soong Joon Lee, Javad Parvizi, and Kyung-Hoi Koo

13.1 Introduction

Total hip arthroplasty (THA) is the most successful procedure to treat end-stage osteoarthritis of the hip. The use of contemporary bearings, highly cross-linked polyethylene, metal-on-metal (MoM), and ceramic-on-ceramic (CoC) bearings, which were expected to minimize wear and subsequent osteolysis, enabled surgeons to perform THA in young and active patients [1–4]. Among the contemporary bearings, MoM bearings were almost abandoned due to serious adverse local or systemic reactions [5, 6]. The CoC articulations offer superior wear properties and biocompatibility [7].

13.2 Evolution of Ceramic-on-Ceramic Bearings

In the 1970s, the first-generation CoC bearing was developed in France and Germany. The results of THA using the early-generation ceramic bearings were not satisfactory due to insufficient fixation of the acetabular cup and excessive wear [8]. The lack of bone-ingrown stability of the mono-block cup design and large grain size of the ceramic were thought to be the causes of failure [9–11].

To overcome these problems, third-generation alumina ceramic was developed, and a taper fixation of the ceramic liner in a metal-backed component was adopted in 1995. The mechanical properties of ceramic materials have been improved by hot isostatic pressing, laser marking, and nondestructive proof-testing, which translated to reduced grain size and increased strength of the ceramic composite [12]. Since then, alumina CoC bearings (Biolox Forte; CeramTec, Plochingen, Germany) were popularly used for THA of young patients [13]. This design has generated excellent survival and patient satisfaction compared to conventional metal-on-polyethylene bearing. However,

B.-H. Yoon
Department of Orthopedic Surgery, Inje University College of Medicine, Seoul Paik Hospital, Seoul, South Korea

Y.-H. Cha
Department of Orthopedic Surgery, Eulji University Hospital, Daejeon, South Korea

S. J. Lee
Department of Orthopedic Surgery, Seoul National University College of Medicine, SMG-SNU Borame Medical Center, Seoul, South Korea

J. Parvizi
Department of Orthopedic Surgery, Rothman Orthopaedic Institute, Philadelphia, PA, USA

K.-H. Koo (✉)
Department of Orthopaedic Surgery, Seoul National University Bundang Hospital, Seongnam, South Korea

Department of Orthopedic Surgery, Seoul National University College of Medicine, Seoul, South Korea
e-mail: khkoo@snu.ac.kr

W. R. Drescher et al. (eds.), *Advances in Specialist Hip Surgery*,
https://doi.org/10.1007/978-3-030-61830-8_13

ceramic fracture and squeaking appeared as major concerns of the third-generation alumina ceramic bearings [14].

13.3 Ceramic Head Fracture

A 28 mm short-neck head of pure alumina ceramic has a high risk for fracture. In 2008, Koo et al. reported five head fractures (1.4%) among 367 cementless THAs with the use of 28 mm alumina CoC bearing [15]. All fractures occurred in short-neck heads and involved the circumferential portion along the inner edge of the head bore (Fig. 13.1). The same finding was reported by registry studies. In a UK registry data involving 222,852 THAs with the use of contemporary CoC bearings, the use of 28 mm head was the highest risk factor for ceramic fracture (0.382%) [2]. In the Danish Hip Arthroplasty Registry data, ceramic component fracture occurred in 0.35% and all of them occurred in 28 mm femoral heads [4].

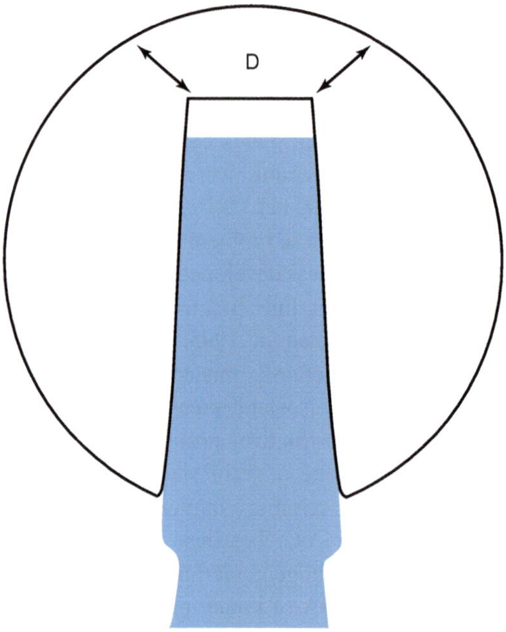

Fig. 13.1 Head bore is a tapered hole in the ceramic modular femoral head. When using a short-neck taper, the contact area between the bore of the ceramic head and the trunnion of the femoral stem is located high, nearest to the dome

In 2004, Delta ceramic (Biolox Delta; CeramTec), a composite of 82% alumina, 17% zirconia, and 1% mixed oxides, was developed to reduce the rate of ceramic fracture [16]. This newest ceramic composite has a smaller grain size (less than 0.8 μm), higher bending strength, and increased toughness than previous alumina ceramic [17]. The strong toughness of Delta ceramic allowed the use of larger femoral heads and thinner liners, which increased the range of motion and reduced the rate of dislocation.

Recently, midterm results of THA with the use of Delta ceramic bearings have been reported [1, 3, 18–22]. The risk of head fracture has been reduced with the use of Delta ceramic (Table 13.1).

No fracture was seen in the Delta ceramic heads in the UK Registry data, and only one fracture was noted in 28 mm Delta heads in the Danish Registry data [2, 4].

13.4 Ceramic Liner Fracture

Although the use of Delta ceramic markedly reduced the incidence of ceramic head fracture, it did not significantly reduce the incidence of liner fracture. The overall survivorship of ceramic liners was similar between alumina and Delta ceramics. In the registry data from the UK, the fracture incidence was 0.112% (35/31258) in alumina liners and 0.126% (101/80170) in Delta liners [2]. The incidence of ceramic liner fracture from single-cohort studies ranged from 0 to 1.2% in alumina liners and from 0 to 0.8% in Delta liners (Table 13.1).

Incomplete/asymmetric seating of the ceramic liner into the metal shell and dent of metal shell is a possible cause for liner fracture [23, 24]. Surgeons should be cautious to achieve firm symmetric seating of the liner along the Morse taper inside the metal cup [14, 22, 25, 26]. Heavy body weight has been reported as a risk for the liner fracture. The risk may be attributable to the difficulty of liner insertion during the operation of patients with high body mass index [22, 27, 28].

Table 13.1 Incidence of third- and fourth-generation ceramic fracture from single-cohort studies which had used cementless total hip arthroplasty

Study name	Ceramic bearing information	N of hips	N of head fracture	N of liner fracture	Mean follow-up (years)
Lee 2017	Delta: 36 mm (39 hips), 32 mm (247 hips)	286	0 (0%)	1 (0.3%)	5.6
Lim 2017	Delta: 36 mm (472 hips), 32 mm (277 hips)	749	0 (0%)	2 (0.3%)	6.5
Salo 2017	Delta: 40 mm (102 hips), 36 mm (222 hips), 32 mm (12 hips)	336	0 (0%)	0 (0%)	2.1
Hamilton 2015	Delta: 36 mm (168 hips), 28 mm (177 hips)	345	0 (0%)	3 (0.8%)	5.3
Aoude 2015	Delta: 36 mm (98 hips), 28 mm (35 hips)	133	0 (0%)	0 (0%)	6
Park 2015	Forte: 36 mm (366 hips), 28 mm (211 hips)	577	14 (2.4%)	7 (1.2%)	5.9
Lee 2014	Forte: 32 mm (55 hips), 28 mm (52 hips)	107	0 (0%)	0 (0%)	6.3
Kiyama 2013	Forte: 36 mm (23 hips), 32 mm (149 hips), 28 mm (11 hips)	183	0 (0%)	1 (0.6%)	5.6
Amanatullah 2011	Forte: 32 mm (135 hips), 28 mm (61 hips)	196	1 (0.5%)	2 (1%)	5
Mesko 2011	Forte: 36 mm (152 hips), 32 mm (699 hips), 28 mm (79 hips)	930	0 (0%)	3 (0.3%)	5.9
Garcia-Rey 2009	Forte: 32 mm (300 hips), 28 mm (37 hips)	337	0 (0%)	1 (0.3%)	5.6
Lusty 2007	Forte: 32 mm (278 hips), 28 mm (23 hips)	301	0 (0%)	1 (0.3%)	6.5

The use of a multi-bearing metal shell, which can be coupled with hard liners as well as polyethylene liner, appeared as a risk factor for malseating of the ceramic liner. This type of metal shell has an inner taper angle of 10° [1, 21]. In 2017, Lee et al. compared malseating rate of ceramic liners between two metal shell designs: one with an inner taper angle of 18° and the other with an inner taper angle of 10°. The malseating rate in the 10° metal shell was higher than that in the 18° metal shell (23.3% vs. 0%) (Fig. 13.2) [29]. Currently, most manufacturers have adopted 18° as the inner taper angle of metal shells for ceramic liner.

Thin metal shell is a risk factor of liner malseating. During firm impaction of a thin metal shell into sclerotic and inelastic acetabulum, a permanent deformation of the metal shell can occur. This deformation induces an uneven contact between the metal shell and the ceramic liners, which can lead to malseating and subsequent fracture of the ceramic liner [30]. This deformation of the thin acetabular component may not make a problem when coupled with a polyethylene liner, which is soft and elastic and easily slides into the deformed metal shell. However, the ceramic liner is plastic and would not be completely seated into the deformed metal shell [31].

13.5 Squeak

The squeaking has been reported as a complication of modern CoC bearings. Although the methods of measuring squeaking are not standardized, the incidence of squeaking after CoC THA ranged from 0.5 to 17% in the literature [23, 32, 33]. The exact mechanism of squeaking is unrevealed, but it seems to be multifactorial. To date, three contributing factors, (a) metal shell design, (b) metal shell position, and (c) patient's constitution, have been known for the development of squeaking. A squeak occurs when the fluid film, which separates the ceramic head from the ceramic liner, is disrupted to allow a friction at the joint and to excite an audible vibration. The lubrication by synovial film is broken in specific conditions such as joint separation due to impingement, stripe wear, edge loading, and metal transfer [33–35].

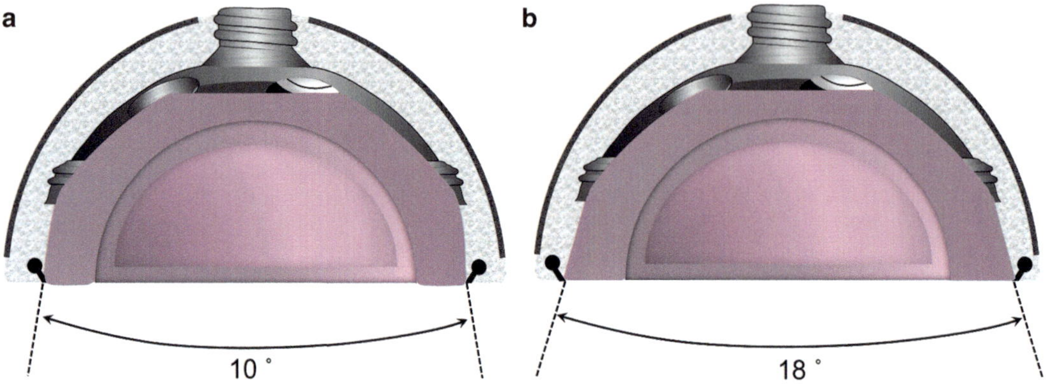

Fig. 13.2 (**a**) The acetabular metal shell had a 10° inner taper angle. (**b**) The acetabular metal shell had a 18° inner taper angle

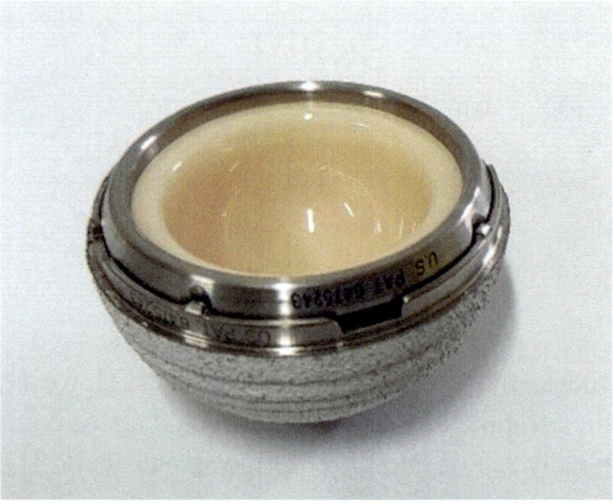

Fig. 13.3 Titanium-backed ceramic liner to prevent impingement between the stem neck and the ceramic liner rim

The acetabular cup with an elevated metal rim (Trident® system; Stryker Orthopaedics, Mahwah, NJ, USA) has been known as a risk for squeaking (Fig. 13.3) [36]. This metal shell was designed to prevent an impingement between stem neck and brittle ceramic liner. However, it was associated with a reduced range of motion, leading to metal-to-metal contact between the stem neck and rim of metal shell. The metal-to-metal contact generates metal debris, which disrupts the fluid-film lubrication in the ceramic bearing surface and leads to squeaking. The neck-rim impingement increases the chance of lever out of the ceramic head, which leads to edge loading, stripe wear, and squeaking. Furthermore, elevated metal rim increases the resonance, which amplifies squeaking [35, 36].

Walter et al. showed that excessive or insufficient anteversion or inclination of the acetabular cup was associated with squeaking [37]. In their study, 94% of non-squeaking patients had 25° ± 10° of cup anteversion and 45° ± 10° of cup abduction, while 35% of squeaking patients had this range of cup position. Stem neck-metal shell impingement and edge loading in improperly positioned metal shells were the possible explanations for the squeaking.

Mai et al. reported that patients who had squeaking were taller than those who did not have [38]. Sexton et al. also reported that taller, heavier, and younger patients were more likely to squeak [39]. In the meta-analysis by Stanat and Capozzi, high body mass index was the only significant patient risk factor of squeaking [40].

13.6 Conclusions

Contemporary CoC bearings offer major advantages over other bearings. When surgeons use CoC bearings for THA, they should choose optimal implants, should be cautious about adequate positioning of implants, and should not make a scratch on the ceramic surface during the operation to minimize the risk of fracture and squeaking.

References

1. Lee YK, Ha YC, Yoo JI, Jo WL, Kim KC, Koo KH. Mid-term results of the BIOLOX delta ceramic-on-ceramic total hip arthroplasty. Bone Joint J. 2017;99-B(6):741–8.
2. Howard DP, Wall PDH, Fernandez MA, Parsons H, Howard PW. Ceramic-on-ceramic bearing fractures in total hip arthroplasty: an analysis of data from the National Joint Registry. Bone Joint J. 2017;99-B(8):1012–9.
3. Lim SJ, Ryu HG, Eun HJ, Park CW, Kwon KB, Park YS. Clinical outcomes and bearing-specific complications following fourth-generation alumina ceramic-on-ceramic total hip arthroplasty: a single-surgeon series of 749 hips at a minimum of 5-year follow-up. J Arthroplast. 2018;33(7):2182–6.e1.
4. Varnum C, Pedersen AB, Kjaersgaard-Andersen P, Overgaard S. Comparison of the risk of revision in cementless total hip arthroplasty with ceramic-on-ceramic and metal-on-polyethylene bearings. Acta Orthop. 2015;86(4):477–84.
5. White PB, Meftah M, Ranawat AS, Ranawat CS. A comparison of blood metal ions in total hip arthroplasty using metal and ceramic heads. J Arthroplast. 2016;31(10):2215–20.
6. Lee YK, Yoon BH, Choi YS, Jo WL, Ha YC, Koo KH. Metal on metal or ceramic on ceramic for cementless total hip arthroplasty: a meta-analysis. J Arthroplast. 2016;31(11):2637–45.e1.
7. Sentuerk U, von Roth P, Perka C. Ceramic on ceramic arthroplasty of the hip: new materials confirm appropriate use in young patients. Bone Joint J. 2016;98-B(1 Suppl A):14–7.
8. Mahoney OM, Dimon JH 3rd. Unsatisfactory results with a ceramic total hip prosthesis. J Bone Joint Surg Am. 1990;72(5):663–71.
9. Nich C, Sariali E-H, Hannouche D, Nizard R, Witvoet J, Sedel L, et al. Long-term results of alumina-on-alumina hip arthroplasty for osteonecrosis. Clin Orthop Relat Res. 2003;(417):102–11.
10. Callaway GH, Flynn W, Ranawat CS, Sculco TP. Fracture of the femoral head after ceramic-on-polyethylene total hip arthroplasty. J Arthroplast. 1995;10(6):855–9.
11. Morlock M, Nassutt R, Janssen R, Willmann G, Honl M. Mismatched wear couple zirconium oxide and aluminum oxide in total hip arthroplasty. J Arthroplast. 2001;16(8):1071–4.
12. Skinner HB. Ceramic bearing surfaces. Clin Orthop Relat Res. 1999;(369):83–91.
13. Boutin P. [Total arthroplasty of the hip by fritted aluminum prosthesis. Experimental study and 1st clinical applications]. Rev Chir Orthop Reparatrice Appar Mot. 1972;58(3):229–46.
14. Kang BJ, Ha YC, Hwang SC, Lee YK, Koo KH. Midterm results of large diameter Biolox forte ceramic head on delta ceramic liner articulation in total hip arthroplasty. J Arthroplast. 2014;29(12):2412–4.
15. Koo KH, Ha YC, Jung WH, Kim SR, Yoo JJ, Kim HJ. Isolated fracture of the ceramic head after third-generation alumina-on-alumina total hip arthroplasty. J Bone Joint Surg Am. 2008;90(2):329–36.
16. Pitto RP, Garland M, Sedel L. Are ceramic-on-ceramic bearings in total hip arthroplasty associated with reduced revision risk for late dislocation? Clin Orthop Relat Res. 2015;473(12):3790–5.
17. Stewart TD, Tipper JL, Insley G, Streicher RM, Ingham E, Fisher J. Long-term wear of ceramic matrix composite materials for hip prostheses under severe swing phase microseparation. J Biomed Mater Res B Appl Biomater. 2003;66(2):567–73.
18. Yoon BH, Park IK. Atraumatic fracture of the BIOLOX delta ceramic liner in well-fixed total hip implants. Orthopedics. 2018;41(6):e880–e3.
19. Abdel MP, Heyse TJ, Elpers ME, Mayman DJ, Su EP, Pellicci PM, et al. Ceramic liner fractures presenting as squeaking after primary total hip arthroplasty. J Bone Joint Surg Am. 2014;96(1):27–31.
20. Taheriazam A, Mohajer MA, Aboulghasemian M, Hajipour B. Fracture of the alumina-bearing couple delta ceramic liner. Orthopedics. 2012;35(1):e91–3.
21. Hamilton WG, McAuley JP, Dennis DA, Murphy JA, Blumenfeld TJ, Politi J. THA with Delta ceramic on ceramic: results of a multicenter investigational device exemption trial. Clin Orthop Relat Res. 2010;468(2):358–66.
22. Baek SH, Kim WK, Kim JY, Kim SY. Do alumina matrix composite bearings decrease hip noises and bearing fractures at a minimum of 5 years after THA? Clin Orthop Relat Res. 2015;473(12):3796–802.
23. Salo PP, Honkanen PB, Ivanova I, Reito A, Pajamaki J, Eskelinen A. High prevalence of noise following Delta ceramic-on-ceramic total hip arthroplasty. Bone Joint J. 2017;99-B(1):44–50.
24. Rambani R, Kepecs DM, Makinen TJ, Safir OA, Gross AE, Kuzyk PR. Revision total hip arthroplasty for fractured ceramic bearings: a review of best practices for revision cases. J Arthroplast. 2017;32(6):1959–64.
25. Langdown AJ, Pickard RJ, Hobbs CM, Clarke HJ, Dalton DJ, Grover ML. Incomplete seating of the liner with the Trident acetabular system: a cause for concern? J Bone Joint Surg Br. 2007;89(3):291–5.
26. Bascarevic Z, Vukasinovic Z, Slavkovic N, Dulic B, Trajkovic G, Bascarevic V, et al. Alumina-on-alumina ceramic versus metal-on-highly cross-linked polyethylene bearings in total hip arthroplasty: a comparative study. Int Orthop. 2010;34(8):1129–35.
27. Choy WS, Kim KJ, Lee SK, Bae KW, Hwang YS, Park CK. Ceramic-on-ceramic total hip arthroplasty: minimum of six-year follow-up study. Clin Orthop Surg. 2013;5(3):174–9.
28. Elkins JM, Pedersen DR, Callaghan JJ, Brown TD. Do obesity and/or stripe wear increase ceramic liner fracture risk? An XFEM analysis. Clin Orthop Relat Res. 2013;471(2):527–36.
29. Lee YK, Kim KC, Jo WL, Ha YC, Parvizi J, Koo KH. Effect of inner taper angle of acetabular metal

shell on the malseating and dissociation force of ceramic liner. J Arthroplast. 2017;32(4):1360–2.
30. Squire M, Griffin WL, Mason JB, Peindl RD, Odum S. Acetabular component deformation with press-fit fixation. J Arthroplast. 2006;21(6 Suppl 2):72–7.
31. Hothan A, Huber G, Weiss C, Hoffmann N, Morlock M. Deformation characteristics and eigen frequencies of press-fit acetabular cups. Clin Biomech. 2011;26(1):46–51.
32. D'Antonio JA, Capello WN, Naughton M. Ceramic bearings for total hip arthroplasty have high survivorship at 10 years. Clin Orthop Relat Res. 2012;470(2):373–81.
33. Park YS, Park SJ, Lim SJ. Ten-year results after cementless THA with a sandwich-type alumina ceramic bearing. Orthopedics. 2010;33(11):796.
34. Taylor S, Manley MT, Sutton K. The role of stripe wear in causing acoustic emissions from alumina ceramic-on-ceramic bearings. J Arthroplast. 2007;22(7 Suppl 3):47–51.
35. Walter WL, O'Toole GC, Walter WK, Ellis A, Zicat BA. Squeaking in ceramic-on-ceramic hips: the importance of acetabular component orientation. J Arthroplast. 2007;22(4):496–503.
36. Swanson TV, Peterson DJ, Seethala R, Bliss RL, Spellmon CA. Influence of prosthetic design on squeaking after ceramic-on-ceramic total hip arthroplasty. J Arthroplast. 2010;25(6 Suppl):36–42.
37. Walter WL, Insley GM, Walter WK, Tuke MA. Edge loading in third generation alumina ceramic-on-ceramic bearings: stripe wear. J Arthroplast. 2004;19(4):402–13.
38. Mai K, Verioti C, Ezzet KA, Copp SN, Walker RH, Colwell CW Jr. Incidence of 'squeaking' after ceramic-on-ceramic total hip arthroplasty. Clin Orthop Relat Res. 2010;468(2):413–7.
39. Sexton SA, Yeung E, Jackson MP, Rajaratnam S, Martell JM, Walter WL, et al. The role of patient factors and implant position in squeaking of ceramic-on-ceramic total hip replacements. J Bone Joint Surg Br. 2011;93(4):439–42.
40. Stanat SJ, Capozzi JD. Squeaking in third- and fourth-generation ceramic-on-ceramic total hip arthroplasty: meta-analysis and systematic review. J Arthroplast. 2012;27(3):445–53.

14 Highly Cross-Linked Polyethylene Bearing

Seung-Hoon Baek and Shin-Yoon Kim

Total hip arthroplasty (THA) is the most effective treatment for patients with advanced osteonecrosis of the femoral head (ONFH). There have been a number of studies reporting variable outcomes after THA in these patients. In the literature, the results of THA in ONFH patients were worse than those with osteoarthritis and several factors unique to ONFH were proposed to contribute to the poor results [1–4]. Young age of the patient, deficient number, and osteoblastic activity of bone marrow stem cells (BMSCs) in the proximal femur were suggested as risk factors for poor outcome in ONFH patients [5–8]. Moreover, a recent study showed that systemic bone metabolism is compromised in ONFH patients [9]. However, there is a controversy whether osteogenic potentials of BMSCs are defective in patients with idiopathic or alcohol-associated ONFH [10, 11]. Some authors proposed that ONFH patients have poor capacity of osteointegration at the implant-bone interface to obtain sufficient and durable implant fixation [12, 13].

In early studies, the results of THA were suboptimal in ONFH patients irrespective of the fixation method, cemented versus cementless [14–23]. In a study of cementless THA using Harris-Galante type I (HG-I) prosthesis (Zimmer, Warsaw, IN), 15-year survival was 70% for revision of any implant as the end point [22]. Another study on cementless THA with the use of porous coated anatomic (PCA) stem (Howmedica, Rutherford, NJ) showed a failure rate of 20.5% for revision of any component as the end point at a mean follow-up of 7.2 years [4]. At an average follow-up of 8 years after cemented THA, failure rate was 39% [16]. Use of undersized stem, poor stem design, inappropriate stem surface, poor cementing technique, and excessive wear of polyethylene liner were thought to be reasons for the high rate of failure in these studies.

Along with the introduction of contemporary cementless stem designs, which have proximal porous coating and tapered geometry, and third-generation cementing techniques, the long-term survivorship of THA in ONFH patients has been substantially improved [24–27]. Kim et al. [27] reported 98% survivorship at 18 years after THA using cementless profile stem (DePuy, Leeds, England) or cemented elite stem (DePuy) in ONFH patients. Polyethylene wear and periacetabular osteolysis appeared as the main causes of failure. Min et al. [28] reported 95.8% of survivorship for cementless HG Multilock stem (Zimmer) at 10-year follow-up. Even with the high survival of cementless stem, periacetabular osteolysis developed in 38 and 31% of cups was revised.

In addition to the potential risk for hampered implant fixation, ONFH usually affects young and

S.-H. Baek · S.-Y. Kim (✉)
Department of Orthopedic Surgery,
School of Medicine, Kyungpook National University,
Kyungpook National University Hospital, Daegu,
South Korea
e-mail: sbaek@knu.ac.kr; syukim@knu.ac.kr

W. R. Drescher et al. (eds.), *Advances in Specialist Hip Surgery*,
https://doi.org/10.1007/978-3-030-61830-8_14

middle-aged individuals, who have a high activity, risk of excessive wear, and consequent osteolysis. To address wear of conventional polyethylene and wear-related osteolysis, alternative bearing surfaces including ceramic-on-ceramic (COC), metal-on-metal, and highly cross-linked polyethylene (HXLPE) were developed (Fig. 14.1).

We have reported excellent midterm follow-up results after THA using COC bearing [29, 30] and MOM bearing surface [31] in ONFH patients. The MOM bearings were almost abandoned due to serious adverse reaction to metal debris [32, 33], while ceramic fracture and squeaking appeared as matters of concern after the use of COC bearing [34–38].

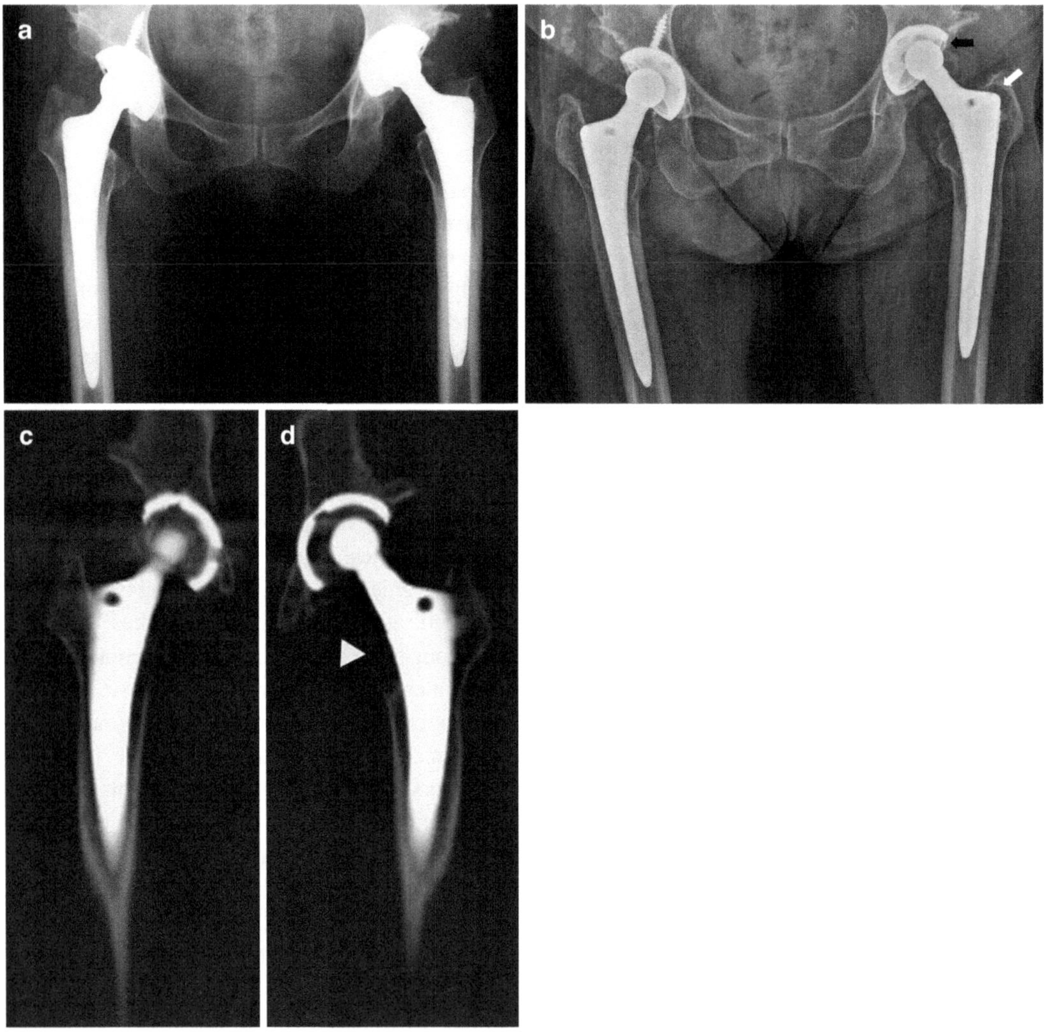

Fig. 14.1 (**a**) A 50-year-old woman underwent THA using conventional polyethylene on the left hip due to osteoarthritis. One year later, she underwent THA on the right hip with the use of HXLPE. (**b**) Radiograph at 19 years after left THA (18 years after right THA) shows eccentric wear of conventional polyethylene (black arrow) and osteolysis in the greater trochanter (white arrow) on the left side. (**c**) Three-dimensional CT scan shows no osteolysis in the right hip. (**d**) CT scan shows polyethylene wear and focal osteolysis in the left greater trochanter

14.1 Highly Cross-Linked Polyethylene (HXLPE)

Conventional polyethylene is irradiated with 2.5–4.0 Mrad during the manufacturing process. Free radicals are generated by the irradiation and are gradually oxidized. This oxidation weakens the mechanical strength and reduces wear resistance of the polyethylene [39]. HXLPE is irradiated at 5–10 Mrad to increase cross-linking between free radicals [40]. Thermal techniques enhance the cross-linking of free radicals [40]. Remelting breaks down crystallized molecules and induces more cross-linking of free radicals. However, excessive heating of remelting can weaken the mechanical strength of the polyethylene. Annealing heats polyethylene slightly below the melting temperature to preserve the mechanical properties of HXLPE [41, 42]. Even after the thermal treatments, residual free radicals may be oxidized later and the mechanical properties can be compromised [43]. Fracture of remelted HXLPE liner and later degradation of HXLPE still appeared as concerns [44, 45]. Second-generation HXLPE has been developed to minimize these problems of the first-generation HXLPE. In the second-generation HXLPE, gamma rays are used instead of electron beam. Sequential irradiation and annealing are repeated three times. Another option was the incorporation of vitamin E to reduce the oxidation of polyethylene. Vitamin E is blended before compression molding or diffused into consolidated HXLPE.

14.2 First-Generation HXLPE in Patients with ONFH

There have been only a few midterm outcome studies after THA using HXLPE bearing. Kim et al. [46] evaluated 71 ONFH patients (73 hips) who underwent THAs using 28 mm pure alumina head and HXLPE (Marathon®, DePuy) as bearing couples. Patients' mean age was 46 years at the time of arthroplasty and CT scans were performed at the mean follow-up of 8.5 years, because the best method to identify osteolysis is CT scan [47]. Radiological evaluation may underestimate the prevalence and extent of osteolysis [48]. In that study of Kim et al., the mean linear penetration was 0.05 ± 0.02 mm/year and no hip showed aseptic loosening or osteolysis. Lee et al. [49] assessed 109 patients (113 hips) who underwent THAs using bearing couple of 28 mm metal head on HXLPE liner (Longevity®, Zimmer). After a mean follow-up of 7.8 years, the annual wear was 0.031 ± 0.02 mm/year and acetabular osteolysis was seen in 10.6% (Fig. 14.2). Min et al. [50] evaluated 127 ONFH patients (162 hips; mean age 51.5 years) who underwent THAs using 28 mm metal head and HXLPE (Durasul®, Zimmer). After a mean follow-up of 7.2 years, the annual wear was 0.037 mm/year. Although most midterm studies performed in patients with ONFH provided promising results with reduced wear and low prevalence of osteolysis, further studies with longer term follow-up are warranted.

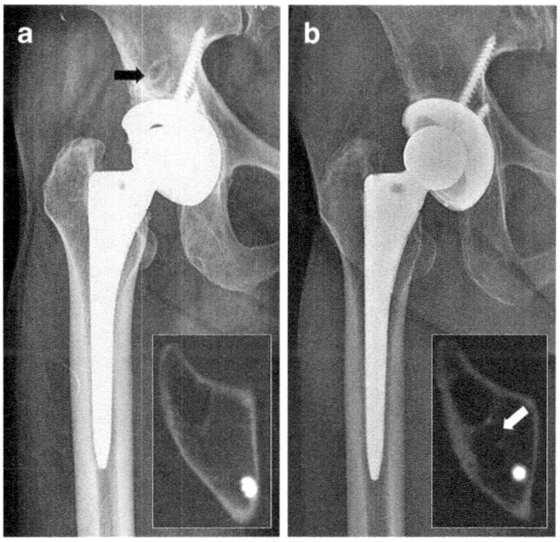

Fig. 14.2 (**a**) Radiograph and CT scan taken at 2 years after THA using HXLPE show subchondral cyst (black arrow) at the ilium. (**b**) Radiograph and CT scan taken at 14 postoperative years. Osteolysis is not definite on radiograph but is seen on CT scan (white arrow)

14.3 Long-Term Results of First-Generation HXLPE

Long-term (>10 years) follow-up studies of HXLPE showed excellent survivorship and radiological results (Table 14.1) [48, 51–58]. Babovic and Trousdale [51] reported 10-year follow-up results of 50 young (<50 years of age) patients (54 hips), who underwent THA with 28 mm femoral head and HXLPE bearings. The survival rate was 100%, there was no visible osteolysis on radiographs, and linear wear rate was 0.02 mm/year. Stambough et al. reviewed 72 patients (75 hips), who were younger than 50 years (mean, 41.2) and underwent THA using 28 mm femoral head-on-HXLPE bearing [59]. At 10-year follow-up, the linear and volumetric wear rates were 0.01 mm/year and 12.79 mm^3/year, respectively. No hip was revised due to osteolysis.

14.4 Results of Second-Generation HXLPE

To date, there is a lack of studies on the second-generation HXLPE and long-term follow-up studies are not available. Nebergall et al. [60] conducted a randomized controlled trial comparing vitamin E-diffused HXLPE liner (E1™, Biomet Orthopedics, Warsaw, IN) and medium cross-linked polyethylene liner (ArComXL™, Biomet Orthopedics, Warsaw, IN). Their study involved 54 patients and radio-stereometry was used to measure the liner wear. At postoperative 5 years, median femoral head penetration into the liner was 0.05 mm in the vitamin E-diffused group and 0.07 mm in the medium cross-linked group. Takada et al. [61] compared penetration of 32 mm alumina head into second-generation annealed HXLPE liner (X3™, Stryker Orthopaedics, Mahwah, NJ) versus first-generation remelted HXLPE liner (Longevity™, Zimmer Inc., Warsaw, IN). The linear wear of the second-generation group was significantly lower than that of the first-generation group (0.045 ± 0.023 versus 0.076 ± 0.031 mm/year, $P < 0.001$). However, no osteolysis was detected on radiographs in both groups.

14.5 Summary

THA remains the most effective treatment for patients with late-stage ONFH. Most patients are young or middle aged and the outcome of THA is

Table 14.1 Long-term results of first-generation HXLPE liners with cobalt-chromium bearings

Authors	HXLPE	Hips	Age years	FU (years)	Head (mm) (%)	Wear rate[a] (mm/year)	Osteolysis %	Osteolysis Method
Lachiewicz et al. [48]	Longevity®[b]	84	61	11	26–40	0.024	14	XR
Babovic and Trousdale [51]	Longevity®[b]	54	39	10	22–32	0.02 ± 0.005	0	XR
Bragdon et al. [53]	Longevity®[b]	174	60	7–13	28 (57%) 32 (43%)	0.010 ± 0.056	0	XR
Bedard et al. [52]	Marathon®[c]	150	56	10[d]	28 (99%) 32 (1%)	0.05[e]	0.7	XR
Engh et al. [54]	Marathon®	79	63	10	28	0.04 ± 0.06	0	XR
Greiner et al. [56]	Marathon®	89	42	10	20–32	0.049 ± 0.19	0	XR
Garcia-Rey et al. [55]	Durasul®[f]	42	67	10[d]	28	0.02 ± 0.016	0	XR
Johanson et al. [57]	Durasul®	25	56	10	28	0.005 ± 0.002	20[g]	XR
Snir et al. [58]	Crossfire®[h]	48	60	11	28	0.122	4.6	XR

HXLPE highly cross-linked polyethylene, *FU* follow-up duration, *CT* computed tomography, *XR* simple radiographs
[a]Expressed as mean ± standard deviation
[b]10 Mrad of gamma beam irradiation and remelted; sterilized with gas plasma
[c]5 Mrad of gamma irradiation and remelted; sterilized with gas plasma
[d]Minimum follow-up duration
[e]Includes bedding-in period
[f]9.5 Mrad of electron beam irradiation and remelted; sterilized with ethylene oxide
[g]Cemented stem
[h]7.5 Mrad of gamma irradiation and annealed; sterilized with 3 Mrad nitrogen irradiation

not satisfactory. The most common cause of failure is wear of bearing surface and wear-related osteolysis. In the literature, HXLPE bearing provided promising results with minimal wear and osteolysis. Nevertheless, long-term results are unknown and further studies are warranted.

References

1. Saito S, Saito M, Nishina T, Ohzono K, Ono K. Long-term results of total hip arthroplasty for osteonecrosis of the femoral head. A comparison with osteoarthritis. Clin Orthop Relat Res. 1989;(244):198–207.
2. Berry DJ, Harmsen WS, Cabanela ME, Morrey BF. Twenty-five-year survivorship of two thousand consecutive primary Charnley total hip replacements: factors affecting survivorship of acetabular and femoral components. J Bone Joint Surg Am. 2002;84-A:171–7.
3. Mont MA, Hungerford DS. Non-traumatic avascular necrosis of the femoral head. J Bone Joint Surg Am. 1995;77:459–74.
4. Kim YH, Oh JH, Oh SH. Cementless total hip arthroplasty in patients with osteonecrosis of the femoral head. Clin Orthop Relat Res. 1995;(320):73–84.
5. Hernigou P, Beaujean F. Abnormalities in the bone marrow of the iliac crest in patients who have osteonecrosis secondary to corticosteroid therapy or alcohol abuse. J Bone Joint Surg Am. 1997;79:1047–53.
6. Hernigou P, Beaujean F, Lambotte JC. Decrease in the mesenchymal stem-cell pool in the proximal femur in corticosteroid-induced osteonecrosis. J Bone Joint Surg Br. 1999;81:349–55.
7. Lee JS, Lee JS, Roh HL, Kim CH, Jung JS, Suh KT. Alterations in the differentiation ability of mesenchymal stem cells in patients with nontraumatic osteonecrosis of the femoral head: comparative analysis according to the risk factor. J Orthop Res. 2006;24:604–9.
8. Gangji V, Hauzeur JP, Schoutens A, Hinsenkamp M, Appelboom T, Egrise D. Abnormalities in the replicative capacity of osteoblastic cells in the proximal femur of patients with osteonecrosis of the femoral head. J Rheumatol. 2003;30:348–51.
9. Tian L, Baek SH, Jang J, Kim SY. Imbalanced bone turnover markers and low bone mineral density in patients with osteonecrosis of the femoral head. Int Orthop. 2018;42:1545–9.
10. Kim YH, Kim JS. Histologic analysis of acetabular and proximal femoral bone in patients with osteonecrosis of the femoral head. J Bone Joint Surg Am. 2004;86-A:2471–4.
11. Yoo JJ, Song WS, Koo KH, Yoon KS, Kim HJ. Osteogenic abilities of bone marrow stromal cells are not defective in patients with osteonecrosis. Int Orthop. 2009;33:867–72.
12. Tingart M, Beckmann J, Opolka A, Matsuura M, Schaumburger J, Grifka J, Grassel S. Analysis of bone matrix composition and trabecular microarchitecture of the femoral metaphysis in patients with osteonecrosis of the femoral head. J Orthop Res. 2009;27:1175–81.
13. Calder JD, Pearse MF, Revell PA. The extent of osteocyte death in the proximal femur of patients with osteonecrosis of the femoral head. J Bone Joint Surg Br. 2001;83:419–22.
14. Chiu KH, Shen WY, Ko CK, Chan KM. Osteonecrosis of the femoral head treated with cementless total hip arthroplasty. A comparison with other diagnoses. J Arthroplast. 1997;12:683–8.
15. Ortiguera CJ, Pulliam IT, Cabanela ME. Total hip arthroplasty for osteonecrosis: matched-pair analysis of 188 hips with long-term follow-up. J Arthroplast. 1999;14:21–8.
16. Cornell CN, Salvati EA, Pellicci PM. Long-term follow-up of total hip replacement in patients with osteonecrosis. Orthop Clin North Am. 1985;16:757–69.
17. Salvati EA, Cornell CN. Long-term follow-up of total hip replacement in patients with avascular necrosis. Instr Course Lect. 1988;37:67–73.
18. Piston RW, Engh CA, De Carvalho PI, Suthers K. Osteonecrosis of the femoral head treated with total hip arthroplasty without cement. J Bone Joint Surg Am. 1994;76:202–14.
19. Stulberg BN, Singer R, Goldner J, Stulberg J. Uncemented total hip arthroplasty in osteonecrosis: a 2- to 10-year evaluation. Clin Orthop Relat Res. 1997;(334):116–23.
20. Brinker MR, Rosenberg AG, Kull L, Galante JO. Primary total hip arthroplasty using noncemented porous-coated femoral components in patients with osteonecrosis of the femoral head. J Arthroplast. 1994;9:457–68.
21. Fye MA, Huo MH, Zatorski LE, Keggi KJ. Total hip arthroplasty performed without cement in patients with femoral head osteonecrosis who are less than 50 years old. J Arthroplast. 1998;13:876–81.
22. Kim YG, Kim SY, Park BC, Kim PT, Ihn JC, Kim ID. Uncemented Harris-Galante total hip arthroplasty in patients with osteonecrosis of the femoral head. A 10-16-year follow-up study. Acta Orthop. 2005;76:42–8.
23. Xenakis TA, Beris AE, Malizos KK, Koukoubis T, Gelalis J, Soucacos PN. Total hip arthroplasty for avascular necrosis and degenerative osteoarthritis of the hip. Clin Orthop Relat Res. 1997;(341):62–8.
24. Johannson HR, Zywiel MG, Marker DR, Jones LC, McGrath MS, Mont MA. Osteonecrosis is not a predictor of poor outcomes in primary total hip arthroplasty: a systematic literature review. Int Orthop. 2011;35:465–73.
25. Issa K, Naziri Q, Maheshwari AV, Rasquinha VJ, Delanois RE, Mont MA. Excellent results and minimal complications of total hip arthroplasty in sickle cell hemoglobinopathy at mid-term follow-up using

cementless prosthetic components. J Arthroplast. 2013;28:1693–8.
26. Ha YC, Kim HJ, Kim SY, Kim TY, Koo KH. THA using an anatomic stem in patients with femoral head osteonecrosis. Clin Orthop Relat Res. 2008;466:1141–7.
27. Kim YH, Kim JS, Park JW, Joo JH. Contemporary total hip arthroplasty with and without cement in patients with osteonecrosis of the femoral head: a concise follow-up, at an average of seventeen years, of a previous report. J Bone Joint Surg Am. 2011;93:1806–10.
28. Min BW, Song KS, Bae KC, Cho CH, Lee KJ, Kim HJ. Second-generation cementless total hip arthroplasty in patients with osteonecrosis of the femoral head. J Arthroplast. 2008;23:902–10.
29. Baek SH, Kim SY. Cementless total hip arthroplasty with alumina bearings in patients younger than fifty with femoral head osteonecrosis. J Bone Joint Surg Am. 2008;90:1314–20.
30. Baek SH, Kim WK, Kim JY, Kim SY. Do alumina matrix composite bearings decrease hip noises and bearing fractures at a minimum of 5 years after THA? Clin Orthop Relat Res. 2015;473:3796–802.
31. Kim SY, Kyung HS, Ihn JC, Cho MR, Koo KH, Kim CY. Cementless Metasul metal-on-metal total hip arthroplasty in patients less than fifty years old. J Bone Joint Surg Am. 2004;86-A:2475–81.
32. Brodner W, Bitzan P, Meisinger V, Kaider A, Gottsauner-Wolf F, Kotz R. Serum cobalt levels after metal-on-metal total hip arthroplasty. J Bone Joint Surg Am. 2003;85-A:2168–73.
33. Willert HG, Buchhorn GH, Fayyazi A, Flury R, Windler M, Koster G, Lohmann CH. Metal-on-metal bearings and hypersensitivity in patients with artificial hip joints. A clinical and histomorphological study. J Bone Joint Surg Am. 2005;87:28–36.
34. Ha YC, Kim SY, Kim HJ, Yoo JJ, Koo KH. Ceramic liner fracture after cementless alumina-on-alumina total hip arthroplasty. Clin Orthop Relat Res. 2007;458:106–10.
35. Howard DP, Wall PDH, Fernandez MA, Parsons H, Howard PW. Ceramic-on-ceramic bearing fractures in total hip arthroplasty: an analysis of data from the National Joint Registry. Bone Joint J. 2017;99-B:1012–9.
36. Walter WL, Waters TS, Gillies M, Donohoo S, Kurtz SM, Ranawat AS, Hozack WJ, Tuke MA. Squeaking hips. J Bone Joint Surg Am. 2008;90(Suppl 4):102–11.
37. Lee YK, Yoo JJ, Koo KH, Yoon KS, Kim HJ. Metal neck and liner impingement in ceramic bearing total hip arthroplasty. J Orthop Res. 2011;29:218–22.
38. Baek SH, Kim JY, Han JW, Kim SY. Potential risk of AMC ceramic liner for dissociation after square seating. J Orthop Sci. 2018;23:600–3.
39. Kurtz SM, Gawel HA, Patel JD. History and systematic review of wear and osteolysis outcomes for first-generation highly crosslinked polyethylene. Clin Orthop Relat Res. 2011;469:2262–77.
40. Campbell P, Shen FW, McKellop H. Biologic and tribologic considerations of alternative bearing surfaces. Clin Orthop Relat Res. 2004;(418):98–111.
41. Kurtz SM, Muratoglu OK, Evans M, Edidin AA. Advances in the processing, sterilization, and crosslinking of ultra-high molecular weight polyethylene for total joint arthroplasty. Biomaterials. 1999;20:1659–88.
42. Sakoda H, Voice AM, McEwen HM, Isaac GH, Hardaker C, Wroblewski BM, Fisher J. A comparison of the wear and physical properties of silane cross-linked polyethylene and ultra-high molecular weight polyethylene. J Arthroplast. 2001;16:1018–23.
43. Rohrl SM, Li MG, Nilsson KG, Nivbrant B. Very low wear of non-remelted highly cross-linked polyethylene cups: an RSA study lasting up to 6 years. Acta Orthop. 2007;78:739–45.
44. Tower SS, Currier JH, Currier BH, Lyford KA, Van Citters DW, Mayor MB. Rim cracking of the cross-linked longevity polyethylene acetabular liner after total hip arthroplasty. J Bone Joint Surg Am. 2007;89:2212–7.
45. Furmanski J, Kraay MJ, Rimnac CM. Crack initiation in retrieved cross-linked highly cross-linked ultrahigh-molecular-weight polyethylene acetabular liners: an investigation of 9 cases. J Arthroplast. 2011;26:796–801.
46. Kim YH, Choi Y, Kim JS. Cementless total hip arthroplasty with alumina-on-highly cross-linked polyethylene bearing in young patients with femoral head osteonecrosis. J Arthroplast. 2011;26:218–23.
47. Mall NA, Nunley RM, Zhu JJ, Maloney WJ, Barrack RL, Clohisy JC. The incidence of acetabular osteolysis in young patients with conventional versus highly crosslinked polyethylene. Clin Orthop Relat Res. 2011;469:372–81.
48. Lachiewicz PF, Soileau ES, Martell JM. Wear and osteolysis of highly crosslinked polyethylene at 10 to 14 years: the effect of femoral head size. Clin Orthop Relat Res. 2016;474:365–71.
49. Lee JH, Lee BW, Lee BJ, Kim SY. Midterm results of primary total hip arthroplasty using highly cross-linked polyethylene: minimum 7-year follow-up study. J Arthroplast. 2011;26:1014–9.
50. Min BW, Lee KJ, Song KS, Bae KC, Cho CH. Highly cross-linked polyethylene in total hip arthroplasty for osteonecrosis of the femoral head: a minimum 5-year follow-up study. J Arthroplast. 2013;28:526–30.
51. Babovic N, Trousdale RT. Total hip arthroplasty using highly cross-linked polyethylene in patients younger than 50 years with minimum 10-year follow-up. J Arthroplast. 2013;28:815–7.
52. Bedard NA, Callaghan JJ, Stefl MD, Willman TJ, Liu SS, Goetz DD. Fixation and wear with a contemporary acetabular component and cross-linked polyethylene at minimum 10-year follow-up. J Arthroplast. 2014;29:1961–9.
53. Bragdon CR, Doerner M, Martell J, Jarrett B, Palm H, Multicenter Study Group, Malchau H. The 2012

John Charnley Award: clinical multicenter studies of the wear performance of highly crosslinked remelted polyethylene in THA. Clin Orthop Relat Res. 2013;471:393–402.
54. Engh CA Jr, Hopper RH Jr, Huynh C, Ho H, Sritulanondha S, Engh CA Sr. A prospective, randomized study of cross-linked and non-cross-linked polyethylene for total hip arthroplasty at 10-year follow-up. J Arthroplast. 2012;27:2–7.e1.
55. Garcia-Rey E, Garcia-Cimbrelo E, Cruz-Pardos A. New polyethylenes in total hip replacement: a ten- to 12-year follow-up study. Bone Joint J. 2013;95-B:326–32.
56. Greiner JJ, Callaghan JJ, Bedard NA, Liu SS, Gao Y, Goetz DD. Fixation and wear with contemporary acetabular components and cross-linked polyethylene at 10-years in patients aged 50 and under. J Arthroplast. 2015;30:1577–85.
57. Johanson PE, Digas G, Herberts P, Thanner J, Karrholm J. Highly crosslinked polyethylene does not reduce aseptic loosening in cemented THA 10-year findings of a randomized study. Clin Orthop Relat Res. 2012;470:3083–93.
58. Snir N, Kaye ID, Klifto CS, Hamula MJ, Wolfson TS, Schwarzkopf R, Jaffe FF. 10-year follow-up wear analysis of first-generation highly crosslinked polyethylene in primary total hip arthroplasty. J Arthroplast. 2014;29:630–3.
59. Stambough JB, Pashos G, Bohnenkamp FC, Maloney WJ, Martell JM, Clohisy JC. Long-term results of total hip arthroplasty with 28-millimeter cobalt-chromium femoral heads on highly cross-linked polyethylene in patients 50 years and less. J Arthroplast. 2016;31:162–7.
60. Nebergall AK, Greene ME, Laursen MB, Nielsen PT, Malchau H, Troelsen A. Vitamin E diffused highly cross-linked polyethylene in total hip arthroplasty at five years: a randomised controlled trial using radiostereometric analysis. Bone Joint J. 2017;99-B:577–84.
61. Takada R, Jinno T, Koga D, Miyatake K, Muneta T, Okawa A. Comparison of wear rate and osteolysis between second-generation annealed and first-generation remelted highly cross-linked polyethylene in total hip arthroplasty. A case control study at a minimum of five years. Orthop Traumatol Surg Res. 2017;103:537–41.

Metal-on-Metal Total Hip Arthroplasty

15

Jun-Ki Moon, Jun-Il Yoo, Yeesuk Kim, and Young-Ho Kim

15.1 Introduction

Young active patients with painful arthritis of the hip need durable hip implant and want a high level of activity postoperatively. Polyethylene wear was a major concern of THA with the use of metal-on-conventional polyethylene bearing. To address this concern, highly cross-linked polyethylene and metal-on-metal (MoM) bearings were developed [1]. The MoM bearing has lower wear rates than metal-on-conventional polyethylene bearing.

It has an ability of self-polishing and self-healing of surface scratches [2, 3]. This bearing had been popularized since early 1990s. This bearing was used in 35% of all THAs in the United States in 2006 and 16% of all THAs in Australia from 1999 to 2007.

However, in midterm follow-up studies, THAs and resurfacings with MoM bearings had unacceptably high rates of revision [4]. Adverse reactions to metal debris (ARMD), a unique mode of failure of MoM THAs, included metallosis, pseudotumors, and aseptic lymphocyte-dominated vasculitis-associated lesions (ALVAL) [4]. Although the etiology of ARMD is not clear, it is affected by patient-specific sensitivity to metal and may differ according to the implant type or head size of the MoM bearings [5].

Several studies reported early failure of MoM bearings in hip resurfacing and large-diameter THA [4, 6, 7]. Other studies reported that ARMD is not exclusive to large MoM bearings in THA, and a small-diameter MoM bearing may also trigger metal hypersensitivity reactions leading to ARMD [8, 9].

In this chapter, we present the clinical performance of MoM THAs according to femoral head size. We also reviewed the history and tribological characteristics of MoM bearings, wear and corrosion in MoM bearings, metal ion levels, and ARMD.

15.2 History of MoM Bearings

The MoM bearing was first used by Wiles in 1938 with a stainless steel implant, but the clinical results were not known due to breakout of World War II [10].

In the early 1960s, McKee and Farrar [11] developed a cemented metal-on-metal THA using a cobalt-chromium-molybdenum alloy. However, failures developed in 50% during the

J.-K. Moon · Y.-H. Kim (✉)
Department of Orthopaedic Surgery, Hanyang University Guri Hospital, Guri-si, South Korea
e-mail: kimyh1@hanyang.ac.kr

J.-I. Yoo
Department of Orthopaedic Surgery, Gyeongsang National University Hospital, Jinju-si, South Korea

Y. Kim
Department of Orthopaedic Surgery, Hanyang University Seoul Hospital, Seoul, South Korea

W. R. Drescher et al. (eds.), *Advances in Specialist Hip Surgery*,
https://doi.org/10.1007/978-3-030-61830-8_15

14-year follow-up [12] and prosthesis was abandoned. Another version of MoM THA was developed by Ring in 1979. But it was abandoned due to high failure rates (32%) at 15-year follow-up [13]. Since then, the low-friction arthroplasty with the use of metal-on-polyethylene (MoP) bearing became the most popular option of THA [14]. However, wear of polyethylene liner and wear-related osteolysis appeared as major concerns of MoP bearings [15–17] and MoM articulation was reintroduced by Weber in 1988 as an alternative articulation to MoP articulations [18]. Some studies reported that a proportion of first-generation McKee THAs survived more than 20 years [19–21] and have driven to the development of second-generation MoM bearings [22]. In the second-generation MoM bearings, a forged alloy containing high carbon content (0.20–0.25%) was adopted [23]. With better metallurgy and improved dimensional control over clearance, a new 28 mm second-generation MoM bearing was developed. Then, second-generation MoM bearings evolved to larger diameter heads (>36 mm), which afforded better stability, increased mobility, and lower friction [24].

15.3 Clinical Results of Large-Diameter (>36 mm) MoM THA

The first-generation McKee-Farrar MoM prosthesis had a large-diameter femoral head and a broad neck. The broad neck of the McKee-Farrar femoral component posed an impingement against the rim of the acetabular component. Curved sharp corner of the McKee-Farrar stem posed varus stem insertion, which resulted in excessive stress concentration within the cement mantle and early failure [25, 26]. Several studies reported that equatorial bearing and increased frictional torque due to inadequate manufacturing caused early failures of McKee-Farrar prostheses [19, 25, 26].

Large-diameter second-generation MoM bearings were expected to have better long-term outcomes and better stability than 28 mm MoM bearings. However, several studies revealed that the use of large-head MoM bearings increases metallic wear and frequently induces metal debris-related complications [4, 27–31]. Langton et al. [7] reported a high failure rate of 49% in patients who underwent MoM THAs with a large-diameter head due to "metal disease." In the study of Matharu et al. [6] the 10-year failure rate was 27.1% following 36 mm MoM THA. In the study of Langton et al. [32] involving 95 MoP and 249 MoM THAs, the median volumetric loss from the MoM cohort was over four times larger than that from the MoP cohort (1.01 mm^3 vs. 0.23 mm^3, $p < 0.001$). Several studies indicated a poor performance of large-head MoM THAs including significant incidences of ARMDs (Table 15.1). In a recent Finnish registry study, Seppanen et al. [16] reported that the 10-year survivorship free from all-cause revisions was lower in large-head MoM THAs than in conventional THAs.

15.4 Clinical Results of 28 mm Second-Generation MoM THA

Second-generation MoM THAs with small-diameter heads are recognized to have lower frictional torques, better metallurgy, and greater control over dimensional clearance due to improved manufacturing compared to earlier generation implants. Eswaramoorthy et al. [33] report the 10-year outcome of 85 primary THAs using the Metasul MoM bearing. Six hips (7.1%) required revision surgery. Histological examination showed an ALVAL-type tissue response in two of the six hips. In 2108, Moon et al. reported 20-year follow-up study of 28 mm Metasul MoM bearings. In their study, the implant survival rate was 90.1% with favorable clinical outcomes and low rate of osteolysis [34]. Other long-term follow-up studies on the 28 mm MoM bearings reported favorable results and similar survival rates (Table 15.2).

Holloway et al. examined the long-term results of 29 MoM THAs using a polyethylene sandwich liner design and reported a high rate (17.2%, 5/29) of osteolysis [35]. Delaunay et al. [36]

Table 15.1 Clinical results of THA with large-head (>36 mm) MoM articulation

Author	Prosthesis	Number of hips	Length of follow-up (years)	Mean age at THA (years)	Survivorship for revision	ARMD
Berton et al. [28]	Durom cups Alloclassic-SL stem large-head Metasul bearing	100	4.8	50 (18–70)	93%	0%
Langton et al. [7]	ASR THR 30 hips with Corail stem and 57 hips with S-ROM stem	87	6	NA	51%	25%
Althuizen et al. [75]	Durom cups	64 (60 pts)	3.1	NA	86%	5%
Hosny et al. [27]	Birmingham hip resurfacing cup Synergy stem	44 (41 pts)	5 (3.3–7)	49.9 (25–71)	93%	5%
Levy and Ezzet [30]	Conserve/Profemur renaissance	66	2.1	NA	86%	11%
Lombardi et al. [29]	M2a-38	636	8	58 (19–91)	91%	4%
	Magnum	804	6	58 (19–91)	94%	1%

NA not available, *MoM* metal-on-metal, *THR* total hip replacement, *ARMD* adverse reactions to metal debris, *ASR* articular surface replacement, *THA* total hip arthroplasty

Table 15.2 Clinical results of second-generation MoM THA with small head

Author	Prosthesis	Number of hips	Length of follow-up (years)	Mean age at THA (years)	Survivorship for revision
Eswaramoorthy et al. [33]	52 hips with cemented Stuehmer-Weber cups and 52 hips with Allofit uncemented cups 28 mm Metasul bearing	85 (82 pts)	10.8 (10.2–12.2)	61.6 (44–84)	Cup and stem 94%
Randelli et al. [76]	Alloclassic CSF cups 83 hips with Alloclassic SL stems, 37 hips with custom-made stems, and 18 hips with Wagner cone stems 28 mm Metasul bearing	138 (100 pts)	13 (11.2–14.1)	50 (19–74)	Cup 97% Cup and stem 94%
Dastane et al. [77]	28 hips with cemented Weber cups and 41 hips with cementless APR cups 28 mm Metasul bearing	69 (66 pts)	13 (8–16.4)	62.5 (27–85)	Cup 97.3% Cup and stem 92.2%
Innmann et al. [78]	Cementless cup and stem 28 mm Metasul bearing	79	12 (10–15)	42 (21–50)	Cup and stem 90.9%
Lass et al. [37]	Alloclassic CSF cups Zweymüller Alloclassic stems 28 mm Metasul bearing	52 (49 pts)	17.9	56 (22–79)	Cup 95% Cup and stem 93%
Delaunay et al. [36]	59 hips with Armor-Allofit cups and 24 Alloclassic CSF cups Alloclassic SL stems 28 mm Metasul bearing	83 (68 pts)	13	42 (24–50)	Cup and stem 96%
Kim et al. [34]	Wagner standard cup and CLS titanium alloy stem 28 mm Metasul bearing	114 (92 pts)	20 (17–23)	46.2 (25–52)	Cup 91% Cup and stem 90.1%

APR anatomical porous replacement, *MoM* metal-on-metal, *THA* total hip arthroplasty reported one revision surgery due to asymptomatic osteolysis above the acetabular cup. The authors suspected backside wear of polyethylene as the cause of osteolysis. Another long-term study by Moon et al. suggested that polyethylene particles from backside wear might be one of the main causes of these implant failures [34].

Several studies showed that early implant failures from ARMDs were rare in MoM THAs with small-head Metasul bearings [34, 36, 37]. However, in a multicenter study involving 300 THAs using small-diameter head MoM devices, ARMD developed in 5% and represented 70% of revisions during a mean of 11 years [8]. The bearing used in that study was the M2a Taper (Biomet, Warsaw, IN, USA), which had Co-Cr tapered insert that was secured within a titanium porous plasma spray-coated outer shell. Ultima bearing (DePuy International Ltd), another design of small-head second-generation MoM articulation, also showed different outcomes compared with Metasul MoM bearings. Donell et al. [38] reported a high revision rate (13.8%) at 5 years for the Ultima MoM bearings. This prosthesis had an acetabular insert manufactured from a high-carbon Co-Cr-Mo alloy with a 28 mm diameter hemispherical articular surface secured in the titanium shell. Unlike Metasul MoM bearings, these implants have no polyethylene sandwich between the articulating metal liner and the outer metal shell. Therefore, various second-generation small-head MoM articulations should be differentiated, when interpreting the results according to each implant design.

15.5 Wear and Corrosion in MoM THA

15.5.1 Wear

The wear rates in retrieved large-diameter, first-generation MoM bearings tended to increase when the clearance is large over the range of 127–386 μm [39]. This excessive clearance leads to an increase of contact pressure within the bearing, which results in an increase in volumetric wear [40]. On the other hand, a too small clearance leads to an equatorial contact and increases frictional torque and jamming, which might lead to loosening of acetabular component [24]. Optimal clearance to obtain sufficient lubrication and minimize wear is mandatory. In a retrieval study of first-generation MoM bearings by McKellop et al. [41] the long-term linear wear rate was 6 μm/year and the volumetric wear rate was 6 mm^3/year. The linear wear rates for the first-generation MoM bearings ranged from 1 to 4.2 μm in previous retrieval studies [39, 42].

The second-generation Metasul MoM bearing had a clearance of 100 μm because a hip simulator study using polyethylene sandwich liner design revealed that the optimal diametral clearance for 28 and 32 mm bearings was 100 μm [39]. Wrought-forged Co-Cr alloys were harder and had better abrasive and adhesive wear characteristics than cast alloys [39]. High-carbon (0.20–0.25%) Co-Cr alloys were developed to reduce the wear rate than low-carbon (0.05–0.08%) alloys [39]. In the retrieval study of second-generation Metasul MoM bearings, an annual linear wear rate was 5 μm/year and a volumetric wear rate was 0.3 mm^3/year. These wear rates were at least 20 times smaller than those of MoP bearings [43]. Rieker et al. [44] reported an annual linear wear rate of 6.2 μm in their study of 172 Metasul MoM THAs. Reportedly, the wear rates of the first- and second-generation MoM bearings were much less than the wear rate of MoP bearings.

However, the inflammatory response to wear particle depends on the number of wear particles as well as total volume of wear. Because the size of metal wear particles (<0.1 μm) is much smaller compared to polyethylene particles (approximately 0.5 μm), a much more number of metal particles can be generated in MoM bearings compared to the same volume of polyethylene wear [45, 46]. The lower incidence of osteolysis in second-generation MoM implants than MoP implants can be explained by renal excretion of the small-size metallic particles [34]. Macrophage phagocytosis occurs predominantly when the particle size is 0.5–10 μm. The metal wear particles are too small (<0.1 μm) to induce a phagocytosis and activate interleukin-6 in macrophages

[45, 47]. Unphagocytized metallic particles are excreted by the kidney or captured in the reticuloendothelial system [48].

On the other hand, nanometer-sized metal particles can also induce a profound innate and adaptive immune response. These particles might elevate the level of metal ions, which are cytotoxic and induce apoptosis of macrophages resulting in the release of lysosomal enzymes into tissues [49]. Metal ions can induce a cell-mediated delayed immune response, T lymphocyte perivascular infiltration [50, 51].

15.5.2 Taper Corrosion

Catelas and Wimmer [52] brought a new concept of "tribocorrosion" to explain the wear mechanism of MoM articulations. It is a thought that wear and corrosion synergistically interact to generate metallic wear debris. The metallic particles can complex with proteins and may lead to a T lymphocyte-mediated hypersensitivity response [52].

Significant forces can be loaded at the modular junction of the prosthetic head and stem-neck taper, resulting in fretting and corrosion at this junction [53, 54]. Various designs of taper shape, head length, and head diameter may affect fretting and corrosion at the modular taper junction [55, 56].

Dyrkacz et al. compared the corrosion at the head-neck interface between 36 and 28 mm MoM bearing and reported that large-diameter heads increased corrosion compared with small-diameter heads [57]. The authors speculated that the greater torque of the larger head caused increased corrosion. These findings were supported by later studies by Del Balso et al. [58] and by Langton et al. [32].

15.6 Metal Ion Levels

There are some controversies involving the influence of head size of MoM bearings on serum metal ion levels. The variations in modular taper junction designs among manufacturers may contribute to the metal ion levels as well as the head size. Nonetheless, several studies showed consistent outcomes of increased metal ion levels for large-head MoM THAs (Table 15.3). Malviya et al. [59] reported high metal ion levels in patients with large-head MoM THAs and con-

Table 15.3 Summary of the literature evaluating ARMD and metal ion levels in large-head MoM THA

Author	Prosthesis	Number of hips	Length of follow-up (years)	ARMD	Metal ion levels (μg/L) Co	Cr
Matthies et al. [67]	6 hips with Adept implants, 19 hips with ASR implants, 51 hips with Birmingham hip resurfacing implants, 15 hips with Cormet, 7 hips with Durom implants, and 7 hips with M2a-Magnum implants	105	NA	69%	8.45 (0.5–386.5)	5.6 (0.4–179)
Bosker et al. [66]	M2a-Magnum femoral head ReCap acetabular component	108 (107 pts)	3.6 (2.1–4.5)	39%	9.2 (1–139)	7.5 (0.7–90)
Bayley et al. [65]	M2a-Magnum acetabular component and Mallory-Head stem	191	4.5 (2–8)	20%	0.87 (0.28–201.82)	1.12 (0.23–79.36)
Malviya et al. [59]	Birmingham hip modular head system	50	2	NA	5.21 (1.2–14.2)	2.78 (0.3–7.85)
Sutphen et al. [68]	Durom MoM articulation	113 (102 pts)	4.94	68.6%	NA	NA
Konan et al. [31]	Durom MoM articulation and a M/L Taper stem	71	7 (6.5–9)	32%	5 (0.5–11)	3 (0.4–12)

NA not available, *MoM* metal-on-metal, *ARMD* adverse reactions to metal debris, *THA* total hip arthroplasty cluded that the use of large modular heads was associated with a risk of increased metal ion level. Garbuz et al. [60] reported higher metal ion levels in patients with large-head MoM THAs compared with hip resurfacings in a randomized controlled trial, and suggested that the cause of high metal ions in the MoM THA group was related to the modularity of the metallic head and stem trunnion. Other studies reported that a higher Co/Cr ratio in blood was associated with the high prevalence of severe taper corrosion and an increased risk for ARMDs in large-head MoM THAs [61, 62]. The high Co/Cr ratio may be explained by different solubility of Co and Cr ions. Co ions are more soluble, whereas Cr ions tend to be retained in surrounding soft tissue.

Several studies reported lower metal ion levels in small-head MoM THAs compared with large-head MoM THAs (Table 15.4), and this may be explained by a difference of torque on the taper interface according to the head size [57]. In a long-term follow-up study on metal ion level in patients with MoM THAs with 28 mm Metasul bearings, median Co level peaked at a value of 2.87 μg/L at 4 years and then decreased to 2.0 μg/L at 9 years, and median Cr level increased up to 0.75 μg/L after 5 years and then decreased to 0.56 μg/L at 7 years [63]. In the minimum of 17-year follow-up study by Lass et al. [37], the median serum Co ion level was 0.75 μg/L at 10 years and decreased to 0.70 μg/L, and the median serum Cr ion level was 0.95 μg/L at 10 years and decreased to 0.70 μg/L. In the study of Kim et al. [64], the mean serum metal ion levels were 0.92 μg/L for serum Co and 0.71 μg/L for serum Cr at an average of 20-year follow-up. The authors suggested that lower levels of metal ion may be the reason for less frequent development of pseudotumors in small-head MoM THAs compared to large-head MoM THAs.

15.7 Adverse Reaction to Metal Debris in MoM THA

Langton et al. classified metal debris-related complications after MoM bearing resurfacing arthroplasties and THAs [4]. ARMDs have been reported to occur in high frequencies in large-head MoM THAs [65]. Bosker et al. [66] reported a higher incidence of pseudotumor formation after large-diameter MoM THAs. At a mean follow-up of 3.6 years, 42 (39%) out of 108 patients were diagnosed as having a pseudotumor on CT scans. In the study of Matthies et al. [67], 69% of patients undergoing large-head MoM THAs had a pseudotumor on metal artifact reduction sequence-magnetic resonance imaging (MARS-MRI). Sutphen et al. [68] reported a high prevalence (60.9%) of asymptomatic pseudotumors after large-head MoM THAs in their MRI study of 102 patients. Konan et al. [31] reported the

Table 15.4 Summary of the literature evaluating ARMD and metal ion levels in small-head MoM THA

Author	Prosthesis	Number of hips	Length of follow-up (years)	ARMD	Metal ion levels (μg/L) Co	Cr
Reiner et al. [9]	56 hips with CLS Spotorno stem, 9 hips with G2 stem, 1 hip with Vision femoral stem 28 mm Metasul bearing	66 (53 pts)	15.5 (10.6–19.3)	41%	1.52 (0.24–13.58)	2.5 (0.21–22.69)
Lombardi et al. [8]	M2a Taper MoM bearings	300 (258 pts)	10 (2–19)	5%	NA	NA
Lass et al. [37]	Alloclassic CSF cups Zweymüller Alloclassic stems 28 mm Metasul bearing	52 (49 pts)	17.9	NA	0.7 (0.4–5.1)	0.7 (0.4–2.1)
Kim et al. [64]	Wagner standard cup and CLS titanium alloy stem 28 mm Metasul bearing	91 (72 pts)	20.3 (18–24)	27.9%	0.92 (0.06–5.8)	0.71 (0.02–0.96)

NA not available, *MoM* metal-on-metal, *ARMD* adverse reactions to metal debris, *THA* total hip arthroplasty, *Co* cobalt, *Cr* chromium natural history of asymptomatic pseudotumors in 71 large-head MoM THAs. The authors found that 35% of patients with an early pseudotumor underwent revision arthroplasty, one-third of pseudotumors showed volumetric increase, and new pseudotumors developed in 8% during mid-term follow-up. Large-diameter heads were more likely to develop pseudotumors [65].

However, the occurrence of ARMD was reported and raised a concern that small-head MoM articulations may also trigger metal hypersensitivity reactions and result in failure. In a recent MRI study of small-head MoM THAs, pseudotumors were found in 41% at a minimum follow-up of 10 years and most of them were asymptomatic [9]. Ando et al. [69] reported that the incidence of pseudotumors was 20.6% at a mean 5-year follow-up after small-head MoM THAs.

In a recent study on the prevalence and natural course of pseudotumors after small-head MoM THA, Moon et al. followed 72 patients undergoing 28 mm diameter MoM THA. At a mean 20 years of follow-up, pseudotumors were observed in 26/91 hips (28.6%). Volume of the pseudotumor increased in four hips (15.4%), did not change in 21 hips (80.8%), and decreased in one hip (3.8%). There was no case of new-onset pseudotumor. At the final follow-up, mean serum Co ion levels and median Co/Cr ratios were significantly greater in patients with pseudotumors, but the serum Cr ion levels were similar [64]. One patient with mild groin pain showed markedly increased pseudotumor volume with elevated serum metal ion levels. The authors suggested that the metal debris derived from taper corrosion might have induced the formation of pseudotumor, but pseudotumor would not commonly result in late implant failure although this can be affected by patient-specific sensitivity to metal debris. Delaunay et al. [36] supported these findings by reporting that none of the complications, failures, or revisions were directly related to the metallic nature of the 28 mm Metasul bearings. Nonetheless, surveillance of serum metal ion levels should be monitored in symptomatic patients with small-head MoM bearings.

15.8 Carcinogenic Risk

As Cr and Ni have been known to be carcinogenic compounds [70], a concern remains that the risk of malignancies such as lymphoma and leukemia will be increased in patients undergoing MoM THAs [71, 72]. However, Mathiesen et al. [73] reported that the incidence of leukemia and lymphoma did not increase after MoM THAs. Visuri et al. [71] reported no significant difference in the tumor incidence between MoMs and MoPs. In addition, the incidences of sarcoma other tumors did not differ between the two. In a recent population study reported by Makela et al. [74], MoM hip arthroplasties were not associated with an increased overall risk of cancer during a mean follow-up of 4 years. Therefore, the evidence of MoM-induced carcinogenicity is vague.

15.9 Conclusions

In conclusion, both first- and second-generation MoM bearings showed much lower wear rates than MoP bearings. Low rates of osteolysis were observed in the second-generation MoM bearings. This low rate can be explained by the smaller size of metal wear particles and renal excretion of the small particles. Increased torques acting along the taper interface may explain the increased metal ion levels, ARMD, and early failures of large-head MoM bearings. Second-generation MoM THAs with a 28 mm head, confined to Metasul, seem to be a useful option owing to the low rates of cup loosening, osteolysis, pseudotumor formation, and later normalization of serum metal ion levels. Nevertheless, even in second-generation MoM THAs with small heads, serial surveillance of metal ions is mandatory in symptomatic patients.

References

1. Wroblewski BM, Siney PD, Fleming PA. Charnley low-frictional torque arthroplasty: follow-up for 30 to 40 years. J Bone Joint Surg Br. 2009;91:447–50.
2. Anissian HL, Stark A, Gustafson A, Good V, Clarke IC. Metal-on-metal bearing in hip prosthesis generates

100-fold less wear debris than metal-on-polyethylene. Acta Orthop Scand. 1999;70:578–82.
3. Fisher J, Jin Z, Tipper J, Stone M, Ingham E. Tribology of alternative bearings. Clin Orthop Relat Res. 2006;453:25–34.
4. Langton DJ, Jameson SS, Joyce TJ, Hallab NJ, Natu S, Nargol AV. Early failure of metal-on-metal bearings in hip resurfacing and large-diameter total hip replacement: a consequence of excess wear. J Bone Joint Surg Br. 2010;92:38–46.
5. Williams DH, Greidanus NV, Masri BA, Duncan CP, Garbuz DS. Prevalence of pseudotumor in asymptomatic patients after metal-on-metal hip arthroplasty. J Bone Joint Surg Am. 2011;93:2164–71.
6. Matharu GS, Nandra RS, Berryman F, Judge A, Pynsent PB, Dunlop DJ. Risk factors for failure of the 36 mm metal-on-metal Pinnacle total hip arthroplasty system: a retrospective single-centre cohort study. Bone Joint J. 2017;99-B:592–600.
7. Langton DJ, et al. Accelerating failure rate of the ASR total hip replacement. J Bone Joint Surg Br. 2011;93:1011–6.
8. Lombardi AV Jr, Berend KR, Adams JB, Satterwhite KL. Adverse reactions to metal-on-metal are not exclusive to large heads in total hip arthroplasty. Clin Orthop Relat Res. 2016;474:432–40.
9. Reiner T, et al. MRI findings in patients after small-head metal-on-metal total hip arthroplasty with a minimum follow-up of 10 years. J Bone Joint Surg Am. 2017;99:1540–6.
10. Wiles P. The surgery of the osteoarthritic hip. Br J Surg. 1958;45:488–97.
11. McKee GK, Watson-Farrar J. Replacement of arthritic hips by the McKee-Farrar prosthesis. J Bone Joint Surg Br. 1966;48:245–59.
12. August AC, Aldam CH, Pynsent PB. The McKee-Farrar hip arthroplasty. A long-term study. J Bone Joint Surg Br. 1986;68:520–7.
13. Bryant MJ, Mollan RA, Nixon JR. Survivorship analysis of the ring hip arthroplasty. J Arthroplast. 1991;6:5–10.
14. Charnley J. The long-term results of low-friction arthroplasty of the hip performed as a primary intervention. J Bone Joint Surg Br. 1972;54:61–76.
15. Oparaugo PC, Clarke IC, Malchau H, Herberts P. Correlation of wear debris-induced osteolysis and revision with volumetric wear-rates of polyethylene: a survey of 8 reports in the literature. Acta Orthop Scand. 2001;72:22–8.
16. Wroblewski BM. Osteolysis due to particle wear debris following total hip arthroplasty: the role of high-density polyethylene. Instr Course Lect. 1994;43:289–94.
17. Jasty M, Bragdon C, Jiranek W, Chandler H, Maloney W, Harris WH. Etiology of osteolysis around porous-coated cementless total hip arthroplasties. Clin Orthop Relat Res. 1994;308:111–26.
18. Weber BG. Experience with the Metasul total hip bearing system. Clin Orthop Relat Res. 1996;329: 69–77.
19. Schmalzried TP, Szuszczewicz ES, Akizuki KH, Petersen TD, Amstutz HC. Factors correlating with long term survival of McKee-Farrar total hip prostheses. Clin Orthop Relat Res. 1996;329:S48–59.
20. Clarke MT, Darrah C, Stewart T, Ingham E, Fisher J, Nolan JF. Long-term clinical, radiological and histopathological follow-up of a well-fixed McKee-Farrar metal-on-metal total hip arthroplasty. J Arthroplast. 2005;20:542–6.
21. Jacobsson SA, Djerf K, Wahlstrom O. Twenty-year results of McKee-Farrar versus Charnley prosthesis. Clin Orthop Relat Res. 1996;329:S60–8.
22. Amstutz HC, et al. Metal-on-metal total hip replacement workshop consensus document. Clin Orthop Relat Res. 1996;329:S297–303.
23. Triclot P. Metal-on-metal: history, state of the art (2010). Int Orthop. 2011;35:201–6.
24. Rieker CB, et al. Influence of the clearance on in-vitro tribology of large diameter metal-on-metal articulations pertaining to resurfacing hip implants. Orthop Clin North Am. 2005;36:135–42, vii.
25. Zahiri CA, et al. Lessons learned from loosening of the McKee-Farrar metal-on-metal total hip replacement. J Arthroplast. 1999;14:326–32.
26. Amstutz HC, Grigoris P. Metal on metal bearings in hip arthroplasty. Clin Orthop Relat Res. 1996;329:S11–34.
27. Hosny HA, Srinivasan SC, Keenan J, Fekry H. Midterm results with Birmingham hip resurfacing/synergy stem modular metal-on-metal total hip arthroplasty. Acta Orthop Belg. 2013;79:386–91.
28. Berton C, Girard J, Krantz N, Migaud H. The Durom large diameter head acetabular component: early results with a large-diameter metal-on-metal bearing. J Bone Joint Surg Br. 2010;92:202–8.
29. Lombardi AV Jr, Berend KR, Morris MJ, Adams JB, Sneller MA. Large-diameter metal-on-metal total hip arthroplasty: dislocation infrequent but survivorship poor. Clin Orthop Relat Res. 2015;473:509–20.
30. Levy YD, Ezzet KA. Poor short term outcome with a metal-on-metal total hip arthroplasty. J Arthroplast. 2013;28:1212–7.
31. Konan S, Duncan CP, Masri BS, Garbuz DS. What is the natural history of asymptomatic pseudotumors in metal-on-metal THAs at mid-term follow-up? Clin Orthop Relat Res. 2017;475:433–41.
32. Langton DJ, et al. Material loss at the femoral head taper: a comparison study of the Exeter metal-on-polyethylene and contemporary metal-on-metal total hip arthroplasty. Bone Joint J. 2018;100-B:1310–9.
33. Eswaramoorthy V, Moonot P, Kalairajah Y, Biant LC, Field RE. The Metasul metal-on-metal articulation in primary total hip replacement: clinical and radiological results at ten years. J Bone Joint Surg Br. 2008;90:1278–83.
34. Moon JK, Kim Y, Hwang KT, Yang JH, Oh YH, Kim YH. Long-term outcomes after metal-on-metal total hip arthroplasty with a 28-mm head: a 17- to 23-year follow-up study of a previous report. J Arthroplast. 2018;33:2165–72.

35. Holloway I, Walter WL, Zicat B, Walter WK. Osteolysis with a cementless second generation metal-on-metal cup in total hip replacement. Int Orthop. 2009;33:1537–42.
36. Delaunay CP, Putman S, Puliero B, Begin M, Migaud H, Bonnomet F. Cementless total hip arthroplasty with Metasul bearings provides good results in active young patients: a concise follow-up. Clin Orthop Relat Res. 2016;474:2126–33.
37. Lass R, et al. Primary cementless total hip arthroplasty with second-generation metal-on-metal bearings: a concise follow-up, at a minimum of seventeen years, of a previous report. J Bone Joint Surg Am. 2014;96:e37.
38. Donell ST, et al. Early failure of the Ultima metal-on-metal total hip replacement in the presence of normal plain radiographs. J Bone Joint Surg Br. 2010;92:1501–8.
39. Rieker CB, Schon R, Kottig P. Development and validation of a second-generation metal-on-metal bearing: laboratory studies and analysis of retrievals. J Arthroplast. 2004;19:S5–11.
40. Chan FW, Bodyn JD, Medley JB, Krygier JJ, Tanzer M. The Otto Aufranc Award. Wear and lubrication of metal-on-metal hip implants. Clin Orthop Relat Res. 1999;369:10–24.
41. McKellop H, et al. In vivo wear of three types of metal on metal hip prostheses during two decades of use. Clin Orthop Relat Res. 1996;329:S128–40.
42. Schmalzried TP, Peters PC, Maurer BT, Bragdon CR, Harris WH. Long-duration metal-on-metal total hip arthroplasties with low wear of the articulating surfaces. J Arthroplast. 1996;11:322–31.
43. Sieber HP, Rieker CB, Kottig P. Analysis of 118 second-generation metal-on-metal retrieved hip implants. J Bone Joint Surg Br. 1999;81:46–50.
44. Rieker C, Kottig P. In vivo tribological performance of 231 metal-on-metal hip articulations. Hip Int. 2002;12:73–6.
45. Doorn PF, Mirra JM, Campbell PA, Amstutz HC. Tissue reaction to metal on metal total hip prostheses. Clin Orthop Relat Res. 1996;329:S187–205.
46. Athanasou NA. The pathobiology and pathology of aseptic implant failure. Bone Joint Res. 2016;5:162–8.
47. Green TR, Fisher J, Stone M, Wroblewski BM, Ingham E. Polyethylene particles of a 'critical size' are necessary for the induction of cytokines by macrophages in vitro. Biomaterials. 1998;19:2297–302.
48. Cobb AG, Schmalzreid TP. The clinical significance of metal ion release from cobalt-chromium metal-on-metal hip joint arthroplasty. Proc Inst Mech Eng H. 2006;220:385–98.
49. Mahendra G, Pandit H, Kliskey K, Murray D, Gill HS, Athanasou N. Necrotic and inflammatory changes in metal-on-metal resurfacing hip arthroplasties. Acta Orthop. 2009;80:653–9.
50. Davies AP, Willert HG, Campbell PA, Learmonth ID, Case CP. An unusual lymphocytic perivascular infiltration in tissues around contemporary metal-on-metal joint replacements. J Bone Joint Surg Am. 2005;87:18–27.
51. Willert HG, et al. Metal-on-metal bearings and hypersensitivity in patients with artificial hip joints. A clinical and histomorphological study. J Bone Joint Surg Am. 2005;87:28–36.
52. Catelas I, Wimmer MA. New insights into wear and biological effects of metal-on-metal bearings. J Bone Joint Surg Am. 2011;93:S76–83.
53. Jacobs JJ, et al. Local and distant products from modularity. Clin Orthop Relat Res. 1995;319:94–105.
54. Gilbert JL, Buckley CA, Jacobs JJ. In vivo corrosion of modular hip prosthesis components in mixed and similar metal combinations. The effect of crevice, stress, motion, and alloy coupling. J Biomed Mater Res. 1993;27:1533–44.
55. Del Balso C, Teeter MG, Tan SC, Lanting BA, Howard JL. Taperosis: does head length affect fretting and corrosion in total hip arthroplasty? Bone Joint J. 2015;97-B:911–6.
56. Tan SC, Teeter MG, Del Balso C, Howard JL, Lanting BA. Effect of taper design on trunnionosis in metal-on-polyethylene total hip arthroplasty. J Arthroplast. 2015;30:1269–72.
57. Dyrkacz RM, Brandt JM, Ojo OA, Turgeon TR, Wyss UP. The influence of head size on corrosion and fretting behaviour at the head-neck interface of artificial hip joints. J Arthroplast. 2013;28:1036–40.
58. Del Balso C, Teeter MG, Tan SC, Howard JL, Lanting BA. Trunnionosis: does head size affect fretting and corrosion in total hip arthroplasty? J Arthroplast. 2016;31:2332–6.
59. Malviya A, et al. What advantage is there to be gained using large modular metal-on-metal bearings in routine primary hip replacement? A preliminary report of a prospective randomised controlled trial. J Bone Joint Surg Br. 2011;93:1602–9.
60. Garbuz DS, Tanzer M, Greidanus NV, Masri BA, Duncan CP. The John Charnley Award: metal-on-metal hip resurfacing versus large-diameter head metal-on-metal total hip arthroplasty: a randomized clinical trial. Clin Orthop Relat Res. 2010;468:318–25.
61. Hothi HS, Berber R, Whttaker RK, Blunn GW, Skinner JA, Hart AJ. The relationship between cobalt/chromium ratios and the high prevalence of head-stem junction corrosion in metal-on-metal total hip arthroplasty. J Arthroplast. 2016;31:1123–7.
62. Laaksonen I, Galea VP, Donahue GS, Matuszak SJ, Muratoglu O, Malchau H. The cobalt/chromium ratio provides similar diagnostic value to a low cobalt threshold in predicting adverse local tissue reactions in patients with metal-on-metal hip arthroplasty. J Arthroplast. 2018;33:3020–4.
63. Bernstein M, Desy NM, Petit A, Zukor DJ, Huk OL, Antoniou J. Long-term follow-up and metal ion trend of patients with metal-on-metal total hip arthroplasty. Int Orthop. 2012;36:1807–12.
64. Moon JK, Kim Y, Hwang KT, Yang JH, Ryu JA, Kim YH. Prevalence and natural course of pseudotumours after small-head metal-on-metal total hip arthro-

plasty: a minimum 18-year follow-up study of a previous report. Bone Joint J. 2019;101-B:317–24.
65. Bayley N, et al. What are the predictors and prevalence of pseudotumor and elevated metal ions after large-diameter metal-on-metal THA? Clin Orthop Relat Res. 2015;473:477–84.
66. Bosker BH, Ettema HB, Boomsma MF, Kollen BJ, Maas M, Verheyen CC. High incidence of pseudotumour formation after large-diameter metal-on-metal total hip replacement: a prospective cohort study. J Bone Joint Surg Br. 2012;94:755–61.
67. Matthies AK, Skinner JA, Osmani H, Henckel J, Hart AJ. Pseudotumors are common in well-positioned low-wearing metal-on-metal hips. Clin Orthop Relat Res. 2012;470:1895–906.
68. Sutphen SA, MacLaughlin LH, Madsen AA, Russell JH, McShane MA. Prevalence of pseudotumor in patients after metal-on-metal hip arthroplasty evaluated with metal ion analysis and MARS-MRI. J Arthroplast. 2016;31:260–3.
69. Ando W, et al. A comparison of the effect of large and small metal-on-metal bearings in total hip arthroplasty on metal ion levels and the incidence of pseudotumour: a five-year follow-up of a previous report. Bone Joint J. 2018;100-B:1018–24.
70. Chervona Y, Arita A, Costa M. Carcinogenic metals and the epigenome: understanding the effect of nickel, arsenic, and chromium. Metallomics. 2012;4:619–27.
71. Visuri T, Koskenvuo M. Cancer risk after McKee-Farrar total hip replacement. Orthopedics. 1991;14:137–42.
72. Swierenga SH, Gilman JP, McLean JR. Cancer risk from inorganics. Cancer Metastasis Rev. 1987;6:113–54.
73. Mathiesen EB, Ahlbom A, Bermann G, Lindgren JU. Total hip replacement and cancer. A cohort study. J Bone Joint Surg Br. 1995;77:345–50.
74. Makela KT, et al. Risk of cancer with metal-on-metal hip replacements: population based study. BMJ. 2012;345:e4646.
75. Althuizen MN, van Hooff ML, van den Berg-van Erp SH, van Limbeek J, Nihof MW. Early failures in large head metal-on-metal total hip arthroplasty. Hip Int. 2012;22:641–7.
76. Randelli F, Banci L, D'Anna A, Visentin O, Randelli G. Cementless Metasul metal-on-metal total hip arthroplasties at 13 years. J Arthroplast. 2012;27:186–92.
77. Dastane M, Wan Z, Deshmane P, Long WT, Dorr LD. Primary hip arthroplasty with 28-mm Metasul articulation. J Arthroplast. 2011;26:662–4.
78. Innmann MM, et al. Minimum ten-year results of a 28-mm metal-on-metal bearing in cementless total hip arthroplasty in patients fifty years of age and younger. Int Orthop. 2014;38:929–34.

16 Early Experience with Ceramic-on-Ceramic Resurfacing

Justin Cobb

16.1 20 Years of Modern Resurfacing

Metal-on-metal (MoM) hip resurfacing has been known as an effective option of hip arthroplasty, especially in young and active patients [1–4]. Patients with resurfaced hips have superior clinical function over patients with total hip replacements, with little or no wear at the bearing surface in comparison to hard-on-soft bearings [5]. Both of the two most serious complications following hip replacement, death and infection are substantially rarer in patients undergoing hip resurfacing when compared to those undergoing conventional total hip arthroplasty [6, 7], which is often presented as the gold standard of hip replacement [8]. However, resurfacing patients with poorly positioned implants, poorly designed implants and undersized implant have reported progressive pain leading to early revision [9–11]. This pain was prominent especially in female patients and was thought to be caused by either of the two problems: metal ion particles generated by excessive wear associated with adverse soft-tissue reactions to metal debris [12] or soft-tissue impingement on the hard metal edges of the components [13]. Despite these two problems, hip resurfacing is easy to revise and hip registries continue to show superior survivorship of hip resurfacing in young and active males, if done using a well-designed device when compared to conventional total hip arthroplasty [8, 14]. However, a concern has been raised regarding high circulating levels of both cobalt (Co) and chromium (Cr) and this concern has made the MoM resurfacing a less attractive option and reduced the global usage of this procedure.

16.1.1 Modern Bearing Couples

BIOLOX® *delta* (CeramTec, Plochingen, Germany) is a zirconia-toughened alumina (ZTA) with enhanced resistance to fracture. The use of BIOLOX® *delta* has virtually eliminated the already low fracture risk of the third-generation ceramic bearings [14–16]. The fracture risk of the delta ceramic in the arthroplasty registries and assessment by the manufacturer are now estimated at <0.001%. Most of the delta ceramic factures involve the liner due to malseating in the inner taper of the metal shell. Along with alumina (Al) and zirconia (Zr), delta ceramic also contains traces of chromium (Cr), strontium (Sr) and very low amounts of yttrium (Y). This ceramic has a 15-year history of worldwide use and has showed the lowest wear rate among all bearing couples used in hip arthroplasty [15]. The very low wear rate of delta ceramic and absence of elevated metal ion levels in the bloodstream [17]

J. Cobb (✉)
Imperial College London, London, UK
e-mail: j.cobb@imperial.ac.uk

W. R. Drescher et al. (eds.), *Advances in Specialist Hip Surgery*,
https://doi.org/10.1007/978-3-030-61830-8_16

virtually abolish the risk of adverse local tissue reactions (ALTR), allergic reactions and systemic cobalt toxicity, which can complicate some MoM hip replacements. BIOLOX® *delta* contains very small amount of Cr, and Cr level remains below the detection limit in the blood [18]. Strontium ions are found in the blood of control patients without any implant and remain at similar background level in patients with BIOLOX® *delta* ceramic implants [18]; yttrium ions are not detected [18].

The use of BIOLOX® *delta* ceramic-on-ceramic bearings may also minimise the risk of periprosthetic infection, a serious complication associated with THA. A significant reduction in biofilm formation and minimal adherence of microorganisms on the ceramic surface compared to metal and highly cross-linked polyethylene (HXL PE) may be the reason for the low risk of periprosthetic joint infection (PJI) in ceramic-on-ceramic hip arthroplasty. Reportedly, the PJI incidence of ceramic THA was <0.5% at 10 years compared to >1% with polyethylene bearings including HXL PE [14, 16, 19].

16.1.2 Fixation Surfaces

The uncemented fixation of the H1 hip resurfacing is not novel. The rough coating of plasma-sprayed titanium and hydroxyapatite (HA) has been applied by an implant coating specialist (Medicoat AG, Mägenwil, Switzerland) with more than 30 years of experience. Acetabular cups using these coatings have been standard designs for more than 25 years [14, 16]. Several MoM hip resurfacing designs for non-cemented use have successfully been implanted in a large series of patients [20, 21]. Titanium (Ti) ions may be released during the bone on-growth process of the non-cemented hip of knee prosthesis [22], but Ti ions from titanium dioxide (TiO_2) coatings or titanium-aluminium-vanadium (TiAlV) hip or knee arthroplasty components are not associated with toxic or carcinogenic reactions [23]. Bonding between the ceramic liner and metal shell was examined by shear fatigue and pull-off testing. The strength of the bond exceeded expectations, while masking of the devices at the edge of the bonded surface was challenging, requiring further close development work between the manufacturers.

16.1.3 The H1 Design

The contours of the H1 were identified as part of Wael Dandachli's thesis, and patented in 2006. We were investigating the position and orientation of the acetabulum in the pelvis at that time, and noticed the shapes of the contours in three dimensions. After collecting a number of these contours in healthy hips, we were able to describe the contours of the articular surfaces of the acetabulum as well as the femoral head. These contours were consistent in healthy individuals and in patients with early-stage osteoarthritis, although osteophytic development and erosion distorted the contours in later stages. The version and inclination of the acetabulum, which were measured from CT scans, were fairly constant. By treating the acetabular rim as a plane, with deviations above and beneath that plane, a rim contour was established with iliac, pubic and ischial eminences, and troughs between them. Importantly, the length of the trough between the iliac and ischial eminence was substantially longer than the ilio-pubic trough. The length of the ischio-pubic trough, comprising the transverse acetabular ligament, was similar to the ilio-pubic trough, allowing the H1 acetabular component to be symmetric, reducing inventory.

On the femoral head side, the margin of the articular surface was also found to be constant in healthy controls, with a more prominent flexion and extension facet, reaching up to the equator, while the medial and lateral extents were substantially less than this. In normal hips, the extent of both the anterior and posterior facets was similar, once again allowing for a symmetric design (Fig. 16.1).

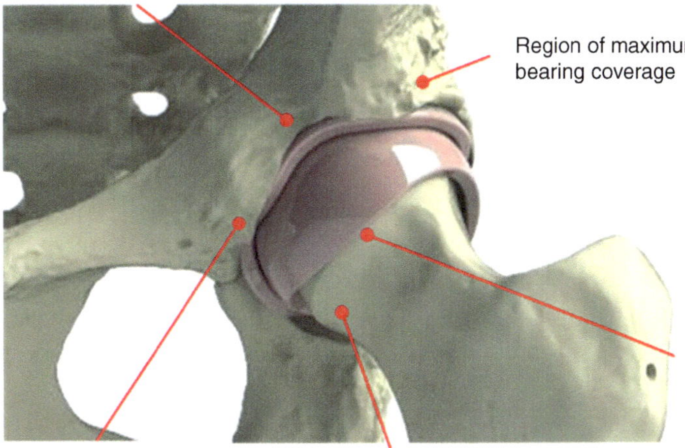

Fig. 16.1 The anatomic features of the H1 ceramic-on-ceramic resurfacing

16.1.4 Optimising for Ceramic Manufacture

The contours were 'optimised' for ceramic manufacture, by reducing their depth slightly. Substantial time had to be devoted to the blending of the radius of the acetabular articular surface with the rim on the acetabular component, to ensure that no sharp edges remained. This posed a technical problem, as the ceramic manufacturers had only used symmetric designs before—an example of the close relationship needed between the design team and the manufacturers. A short stem was needed to hold the head during machining. Diameter of the stem was only 7 mm and it was not designed to endure excessive loading. The stem does aid the proper insertion and perfect fit of the H1 head onto the machined surfaces (Fig. 16.2).

16.2 Implant Sizes and Range

16.2.1 H1 Femoral Head

Diameter of the H1 head components ranges from 40 to 58 mm. These correspond directly to the labelled size and match the internal diameter of the compatible cup. The internal diameter of the device is designed to be just over 1 mm smaller than the machined diameter of the sleeve and chamfer cutter. This difference in diameter is sufficient to ensure that a press fit exists at the extreme values of the tolerance stack of the instruments. Further primary fixation is obtained by longitudinal fins. Each H1 head has a single compatible cup, which is larger than the femoral head by 7 mm.

16.2.2 H1 Cup

The true external diameter of the H1 cup component is approximately 0.5 mm greater than the labelled size. This size includes the average thickness of the VPS coating. The true internal diameter of the H1 cup component corresponds directly to the labelled size and is 7 mm less than the labelled external diameter. For example, a 57/50 mm cup as labelled has a nominal 57.5 mm external diameter and a nominal 50 mm internal diameter (the bearing surface). Under-reaming is required for adequate press fit. It is recommended to under-ream by 1 mm from the labelled cup size (Fig. 16.3). Optimal press fit will be achieved by careful acetabular bone preparation and implant placement. The cup trial does not give an indication of press fit, but is intended to advise the user on cup orientation and depth.

The cup design has subs.

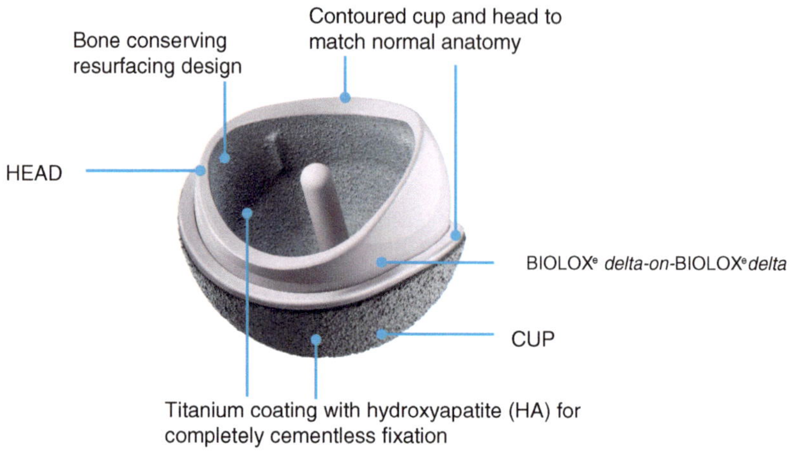

Fig. 16.2 The H1 resurfacing prostheses

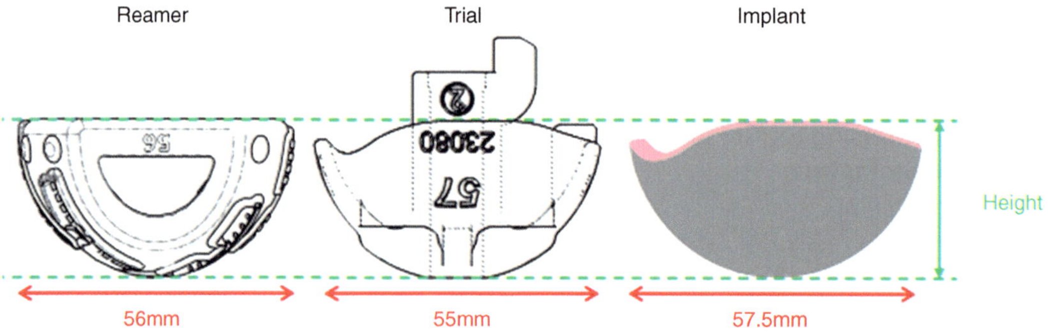

Fig. 16.3 Dimensions of the H1 acetabular component, trial, and single-use reamer

16.2.3 Instrumentation

The instrumentation is all size specific and single use, to maximise the quality of the bone preparation, and minimise the number of instruments needed intraoperatively. Three trays of instruments are used: a generic set, which includes the sizing tool, with two further size-specific trays, one for the femoral head, and the other for the acetabular instruments (Fig. 16.4).

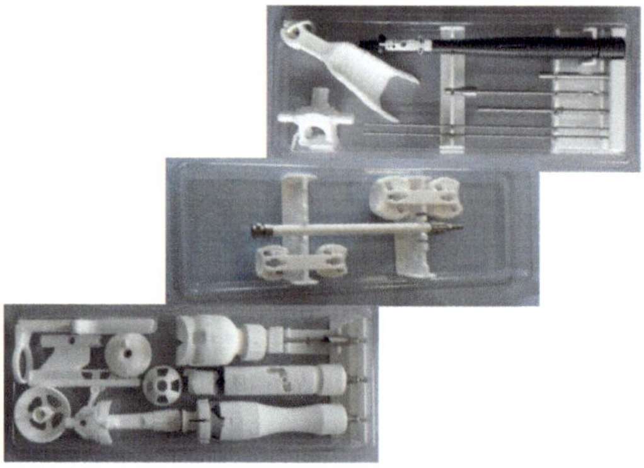

Fig. 16.4 Three trays of single-use instruments

16.2.4 Clinical Experience

Prior to starting the MHRA-approved study, a single test case was undertaken in a 37-year-old man with psoriatic arthritis who had received a Birmingham hip resurfacing 8 years earlier, rendering him ineligible for the safety study. The procedure went smoothly, confirming that the instrumentation was indeed fit for the trial, and the postoperative follow-up has been satisfactory (Fig. 16.5).

Following this 'pilot study' every patient who was eligible for the trial was offered access to the study, and a log kept of those who both wanted to join the study or refused. Owing to substantial delays with the regulatory processes involved, the trial did not start until September of 2017. The first 20 cases were completed within 4 months, all with CTRSA. Since then an additional 75 cases have been undertaken in 4 centres around the UK, with centres in Belgium and Germany following in 2020.

16.2.5 Operations

No major operative issues have been experienced: the operations have all been completed successfully as planned. The Oxford Hip Scores (OHSs) have improved as expected, with a median score of 46/48 at 6 months. As predicted in this group of patients, several have returned to very high levels of activity, recording fast running speeds at only 6 months following surgery.

16.2.6 Clinical Outcomes

On the trial protocol, outcome is measured using patient-reported outcome measures (PROMs). Preoperative scores increased substantially by 6 weeks, and again significantly at 3 months (Fig. 16.6). The improvement in scores seen after this time point failed to reach significance owing to the ceiling effect of these scores.

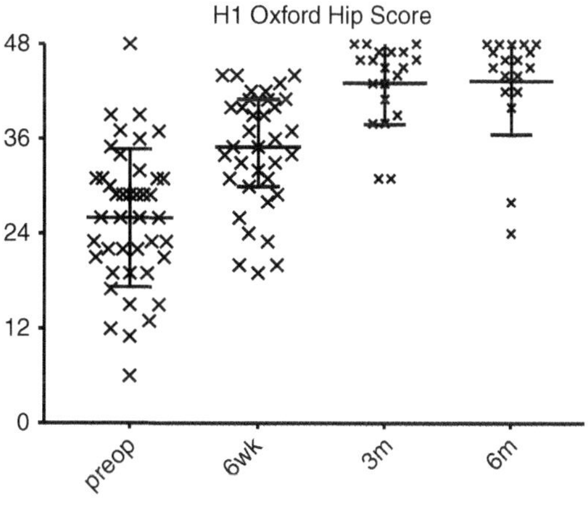

Fig. 16.6 Oxford Hip Scores of H1 safety study

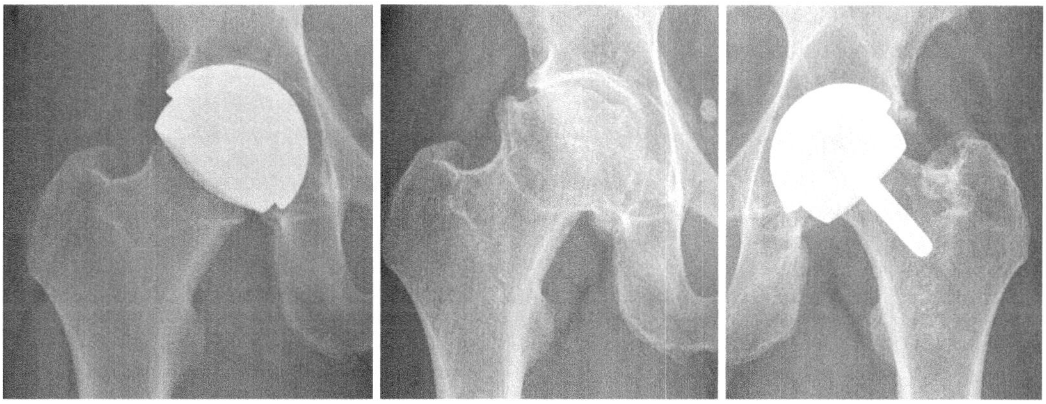

Fig. 16.5 A 37-year-old man had been operated with Birmingham resurfacing on the left hip due to osteoarthritis. Eight years later, he underwent H1 resurfacing on the right hip. Postoperative 2-year radiograph after the H1 resurfacing

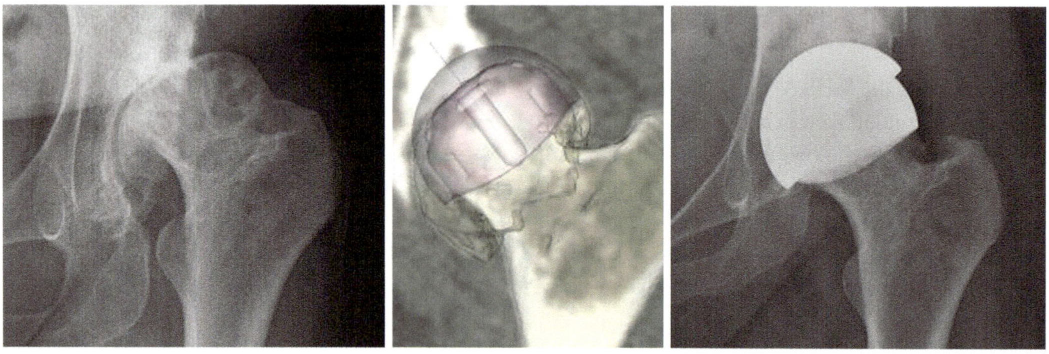

Fig. 16.7 A 50-year-old woman had painful osteoarthritis secondary to Crowe II DDH. Preoperative radiograph. Planning with acrylic templates of H1 resurfacing. Post-operative 6-month radiograph

16.2.7 Case Study

A 50-year-old woman with painful arthrosis secondary to DDH consented to join the trial. Imaging studies confirmed that her Crowe II dysplasia was suitable for H1 if the femoral bone stock was adequate. At operation, the bone quality was good and the femoral head was resurfaced (Fig. 16.7). At 18 months after surgery, OHS was 48 points.

16.2.8 Morbidity and Mortality

After 95 cases, two patients have had to undergo further surgery: one who sustained an impacted fracture slipping in her bathroom, and another who sustained a displaced subcapital fracture at 3 months post-op playing tennis. Both have had uneventful revision using primary cementless hip prostheses.

16.3 Conclusions

It is still early in the evolution of this clinical study to reach any major conclusions. Early results suggest that the device is fit for purpose, and that the entire clinical study should be completed. To date, our results are favourable and we continue the clinical trial of the resurfacing.

Acknowledgements This work has been carried out by the Embody Orthopaedic team, led by Susannah Clarke, Camilla Halewood and Rob Wozencroft.

References

1. Amstutz HC, Le Duff MJ, Campbell PA, Gruen TA, Wisk LE. Clinical and radiographic results of metal-on-metal hip resurfacing with a minimum ten-year follow-up. J Bone Joint Surg Am. 2010;92:2663–71.
2. Daniel J, Pradhan C, Ziaee H, Pynsent P, McMinn D. Results of Birmingham hip resurfacing at 12 to 15 years. Bone Joint J. 2014;96:1298–306.
3. Treacy R, McBryde C, Shears E, Pynsent P. Birmingham hip resurfacing. Bone Joint J. 2011;93:27–33.
4. Van Der Straeten C, Van Quickenborne D, De Roest B, Calistri A, Victor J, De Smet K. Metal ion levels from well-functioning Birmingham Hip Resurfacings decline significantly at ten years. Bone Joint J. 2013;95:1332–8.
5. Clarke I, Good V, Williams P, Schroeder D, Anissian L, Stark A, et al. Ultra-low wear rates for rigid-on-rigid bearings in total hip replacements. Proc Inst Mech Eng H. 2000;214:331–47.
6. Berstock J, Beswick A, Lenguerrand E, Whitehouse M, Blom A. Mortality after total hip replacement surgery. Bone Joint Res. 2014;3:175–82.
7. McMinn D, Snell K, Daniel J, Treacy R, Pynsent P, Riley R. Mortality and implant revision rates of hip arthroplasty in patients with osteoarthritis: registry based cohort study. BMJ. 2012;344:e3319.
8. Seppänen M, Mäkelä K, Virolainen P, Remes V, Pulkkinen P, Eskelinen A. Hip resurfacing arthroplasty: short-term survivorship of 4,401 hips from the Finnish Arthroplasty Register. Acta Orthop. 2012;83:207–13.

9. Langton D, Jameson S, Joyce T, Hallab N, Natu S, Nargol A. Early failure of metal-on-metal bearings in hip resurfacing and large-diameter total hip replacement. Bone Joint J. 2010;92:38–46.
10. Langton D, Joyce T, Jameson S, Lord J, Van Orsouw M, Holland J, et al. Adverse reaction to metal debris following hip resurfacing. Bone Joint J. 2011;93:164–71.
11. Van Der Straeten C, Grammatopoulos G, Gill HS, Calistri A, Campbell P, De Smet KA. The 2012 Otto Aufranc Award: the interpretation of metal ion levels in unilateral and bilateral hip resurfacing. Clin Orthop Relat Res. 2013;471:377–85.
12. Willert H-G, Buchhorn GH, Fayyazi A, Flury R, Windler M, Köster G, et al. Metal-on-metal bearings and hypersensitivity in patients with artificial hip joints. J Bone Joint Surg Am. 2005;87:28–36.
13. Cobb JP, Davda K, Ahmad A, Harris SJ, Masjedi M, Hart AJ. Why large-head metal-on-metal hip replacements are painful: the anatomical basis of psoas impingement on the femoral head-neck junction. J Bone Joint Surg Br. 2011;93:881–5.
14. AOA. Australian Orthopaedic Association National Joint Replacement Registry. 2015.
15. Beraudi A, Stea S, De Pasquale D, Bordini B, Catalani S, Apostoli P, et al. Metal ion release: also a concern for ceramic-on-ceramic couplings? Hip Int. 2014;24:321–6.
16. NJR. National Joint Registry. National Joint Registry for England and Wales. 2015.
17. Sargeant A, Goswami T, Swank M. Ion concentrations from hip implants. J Surg Orthop Adv. 2005;15:113–4.
18. Kretzer JP, Sonntag R, Kiefer H, Reinders J. Ion release in ceramic and metal-on-metal bearings. Bone Joint J. 2016;98:122.
19. Trampuz A, Maiolo EM, Winkler T, Perka C. Biofilm formation on ceramic, metal and polyethylene bearing components from hip joint replacement systems. Bone Joint J Orthop Proc. 2016;98-B:80.
20. Girard J. Is it time for cementless hip resurfacing? HSS J. 2012;8:245–50.
21. Gross TP, Liu F. Current status of modern fully porous coated metal-on-metal hip resurfacing arthroplasty. J Arthroplast. 2014;29:181–5.
22. Hutt J, Lavigne M, Lungu E, Belzile E, Morin F, Vendittoli P-A. Comparison of whole-blood metal ion levels among four types of large-head, metal-on-metal total hip arthroplasty implants. A concise follow-up, at five years, of a previous report. J Bone Joint Surg Am. 2016;98:257–66.
23. BEIs ACoGIHTa. Threshold limit values for chemical substances and physical agents and biological exposure indices. Paper presented at: American Conference of Governmental Industrial Hygienists TLVs and BEIs, Cincinnati, OH. 2010.

17 Cup Positioning Using Anatomical Landmarks of the Acetabulum

Jeong Joon Yoo, Young-Kyun Lee, Jae-Hwi Nho, Jun-Il Yoo, Woo-Lam Jo, and Kyung-Hoi Koo

17.1 Introduction

Optimal cup positioning is important to prevent dislocation and wear-related problems after total hip arthroplasty (THA) [1–3]. Contemporary bearings with the use of highly cross-linked polyethylene and newest ceramic composites have been shown to reduce wear and wear-related osteolysis. Even with the use of contemporary bearings, malposition of the acetabular cup remains a major concern of THA [4, 5]. Optimal cup positioning during THA is challenging [1–3], and it needs a substantial learning period [6–8].

In 1978, Lewinnek suggested a safe zone of cup position: 30°–50° of abduction and 5°–25° of anteversion [9]. The positioning of an acetabular cup can be influenced by several factors, such as underlying pathologies of affected hips, surgical approach, change of patient's position during the operation, soft-tissue tension, and implant design [10–14]. To obtain proper cup position, mechanical guides and computer-assisted navigation systems have been developed. However, the use of mechanical guides still results in large variations of cup position [15, 16], and clinical use of the hip navigation system is not validated yet [17–19].

In a previous study, we introduced a method to optimize the cup position using anatomical bony landmarks: transverse acetabular notch (TAN) and anterior acetabular notch (AAN) of the acetabulum [20]. Although this method requires preoperative CT scan, it is highly reproducible and easily applicable.

17.2 Preoperative Planning Using Reconstructed CT Scan

Preoperative CT scan is mandated for the measurement of acetabular abduction and anteversion.

J. J. Yoo
Department of Orthopedic Surgery, Seoul National University College of Medicine, Seoul, South Korea
e-mail: jjyos@snu.ac.kr

Y.-K. Lee
Department of Orthopedic Surgery, Seoul National University Bundang Hospital, Seongnam, South Korea

J.-H. Nho
Department of Orthopedic Surgery, Soonchunhyang University Hospital, Seoul, South Korea

J.-I. Yoo
Department of Orthopedic Surgery, Gyeongsang National University Hospital, Jinju, South Korea

W.-L. Jo
Department of Orthopedic Surgery, Seoul St. Mary's Hospital, Seoul, South Korea

K.-H. Koo (✉)
Department of Orthopaedic Surgery, Seoul National University Bundang Hospital, Seongnam, South Korea

Department of Orthopedic Surgery, Seoul National University College of Medicine, Seoul, South Korea
e-mail: khkoo@snu.ac.kr

W. R. Drescher et al. (eds.), *Advances in Specialist Hip Surgery*,
https://doi.org/10.1007/978-3-030-61830-8_17

In the normal pelvis, there are two notches at the rim of the acetabulum. One is TAN at the lower margin and the other is at the anterior margin, which we have named AAN (Fig. 17.1). The TAN is at the vicinity of the inferior pole of the acetabulum and the AAN is at the vicinity of the anterior pole of acetabulum (Fig. 17.2).

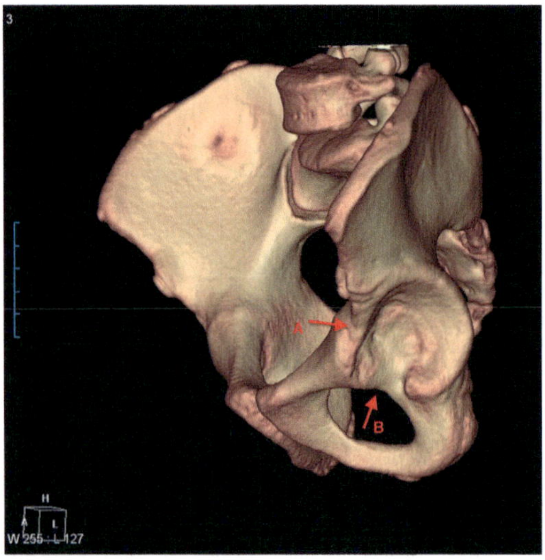

Fig. 17.1 (A) Anterior acetabular notch (AAN) is at the middle of the anterior rim and the (B) transverse acetabular notch (TAN) is at the lower margin of the cotyloid fossa

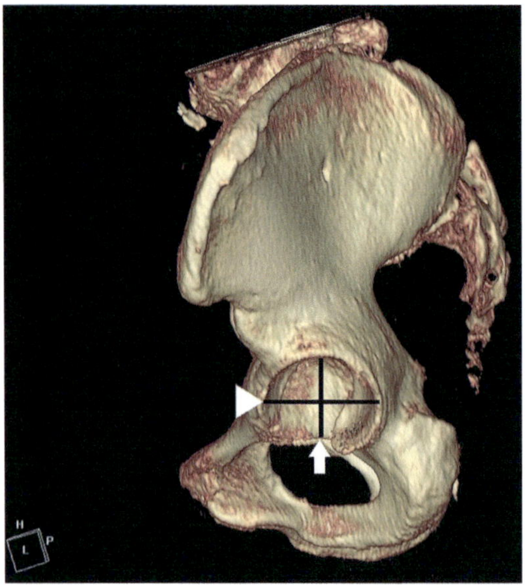

Fig. 17.2 The AAN (arrowhead) is at the vicinity of the anterior pole of the acetabulum and the TAN (arrow) is at the vicinity of the inferior pole

On the anteroposterior radiograph of the hip, the TAN appears at the lowest point of the teardrop and the AAN appears at the middle of the anterior acetabular margin. On a CT scan, the TAN appears as the teardrop in the mid-coronal image of the acetabulum, and the AAN at the anterior point in the mid-axial image.

We use the TAN as a landmark to align cup abduction, and the AAN as a landmark to align cup anteversion (Fig. 17.1) [20].

The acetabular abduction is the angle between a line drawn from the teardrop to the lateral acetabular margin and the inter-teardrop line on the mid-coronal CT image (Fig. 17.3a). The acetabular anteversion is obtained on the mid-axial image by measuring the angle between a line drawn from the anterior acetabular margin to the posterior acetabular margin and a line perpendicular to the line connecting the centers of both femoral heads (Fig. 17.3b) [21].

If the surgeon sets the target of cup position at 40° abduction and 15° anteversion as suggested by Lewinnek et al. [9], the acetabular abduction is used as a reference to adjust cup abduction, and acetabular anteversion as a reference to adjust cup anteversion, as below.

A circumferential length of an arc (α) in a circle of a radius (R) can be calculated by the formula

$$2 \times \pi \times R \times \frac{\alpha^{\circ}}{360}$$

Reportedly, the mean diameter of the normal acetabulum is 52 mm (range 43.4–57.4 mm [22]). When acetabular abduction is a α° and 52 mm sized cup is used, the distance ($D1$) between the inferior point of 40° abduction and the TAN can be calculated by the formula

$$D1 = \left| 2 \times \pi \times 52\,\text{mm} \times \frac{\left(\alpha^{\circ} - 40^{\circ}\right)}{360} \right|$$
$$= \left|0.91 \times (\alpha - 40)\right| \text{mm} \fallingdotseq \left|\alpha - 40\right| \text{mm}$$

When the acetabular abduction is greater than 40°, the inferior point is inside the TAN. On the other hand, when the acetabular abduction is less than 40°, the inferior point is outside the TAN (Fig. 17.4).

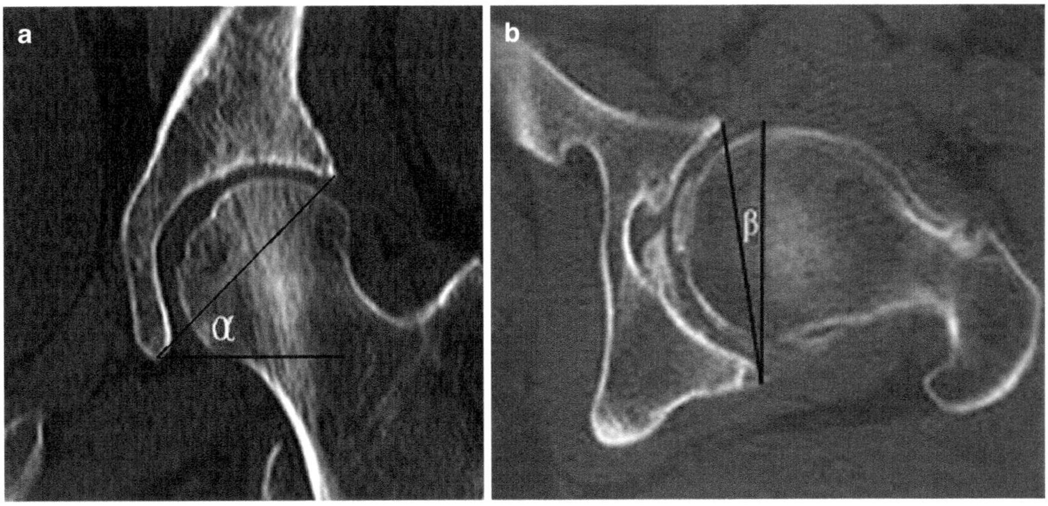

Fig. 17.3 (**a**) Acetabular abduction angle (α) is measured on a mid-coronal CT image. (**b**) Acetabular anteversion angle (β) is measured on a mid-axial CT image

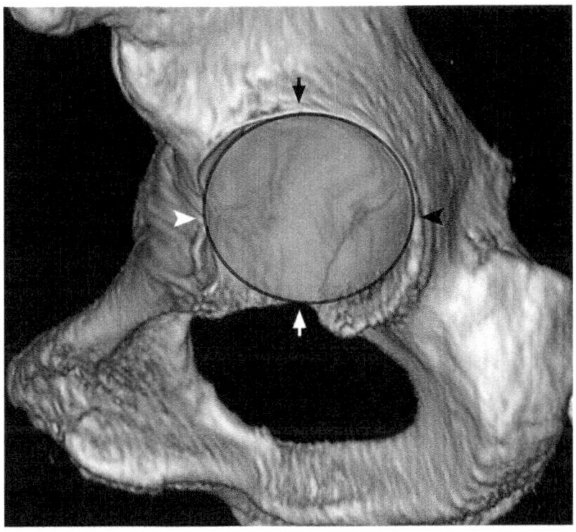

Fig. 17.4 When the acetabular abduction is 40° and anteversion is 15°, the cup is aligned to the native acetabular abduction and anteversion. The cup abduction is aligned to the superior point (black arrow) and the TAN (white arrow) and cup anteversion are aligned to the posterior point (black arrowhead) and the AAN (white arrowhead). When acetabular abduction is greater than 40°, the cup inferior point is inside the TAN and when less than 40°, it is outside the TAN. Likewise, when acetabular anteversion is greater than 15°, the cup anterior point is outside the AAN and when less than 15°, it is inside the AAN

Likewise, when acetabular anteversion is $\beta°$, the distance ($D2$) between the anterior point of 15° anteversion and the AAN can also be calculated by the formula

$$D2 \fallingdotseq |\beta - 15| \text{mm}$$

When the acetabular anteversion is greater than 15°, the anterior point is outside the AAN and when the acetabular anteversion is less than 15°, the anterior point is inside the AAN (Fig. 17.4).

When 50–54 mm sized cups, which are common in use, are inserted, the difference of the distance (0.03–0.11 mm per 1°) according to the cup size is negligible in this calculation.

A preoperatively calculated $D1$ and $D2$ can be used to adjust cup abduction and cup anteversion during the insertion of the acetabular cup.

17.3 Surgical Technique

The acetabulum is exposed by retraction of the femur anteriorly or posteriorly, depending on the approach. First and foremost, appropriate exposure of the acetabulum is essential to obtain optimal cup positioning, and meticulous removal of the labrum and any overhanging capsule eases component insertion.

We use the posterior approach, which will provide the basis of our description. To obtain complete exposure of the acetabulum, the superior and inferior portions of the capsule should be incised vertically and the capsule flaps should be retracted sufficiently.

Following hip dislocation and femoral neck osteotomy, the acetabulum should be exposed completely along its entire circumference. If difficulty is encountered with anterior retraction of the femur, the surgeon should release the anterior-superior capsule and the reflected head of the rectus muscle; this will facilitate the maneuver of retraction.

Once the acetabulum is fully visualized by retracting capsule flaps, labrum, transverse acetabular ligament, ligamentum teres, and pulvinar should be removed to expose bony acetabulum, cotyloid fossa, TAN, and AAN (Fig. 17.5a). Care must be taken to cauterize the acetabular branches of the obturator artery, which can lead to bleeding postoperatively.

The acetabulum is reamed down to the cotyloid fossa until the acetabular cartilage is completely removed. Depending on the used implant system, under-reaming by 1 or 2 mm is performed.

Afterwards, the surgeon should identify four points: the superior and inferior points for 40° cup abduction, and the anterior and posterior points for 15° cup anteversion (Fig. 17.5b). The inferior point is adjacent to the TAN as calculated by the above formula for abduction, the superior point is the opposite point of the TAN, the anterior point is adjacent to the AAN as calculated by the above formula for anteversion, and the posterior point is the opposite point of the AAN.

These four points are marked with electrocautery. The cup is inserted by repeated tapping until obtaining a secure press fit. The cup abduction should be adjusted to the line between the superior and inferior points, and the cup anteversion to the line between the anterior and posterior points. During insertion, the cup alignment should be repeatedly assessed and the cup handle should be manipulated to adjust cup position. After implantation of cup, osteophytes should be trimmed around the acetabular component to avoid impingement between acetabular osteophytes and femoral component [23].

The liner, femoral stem, and head are inserted. After reduction of the femoral head, the hip capsule and short external rotators should be repaired tightly with the use of trans-osseous suture to restore soft-tissue tension [24].

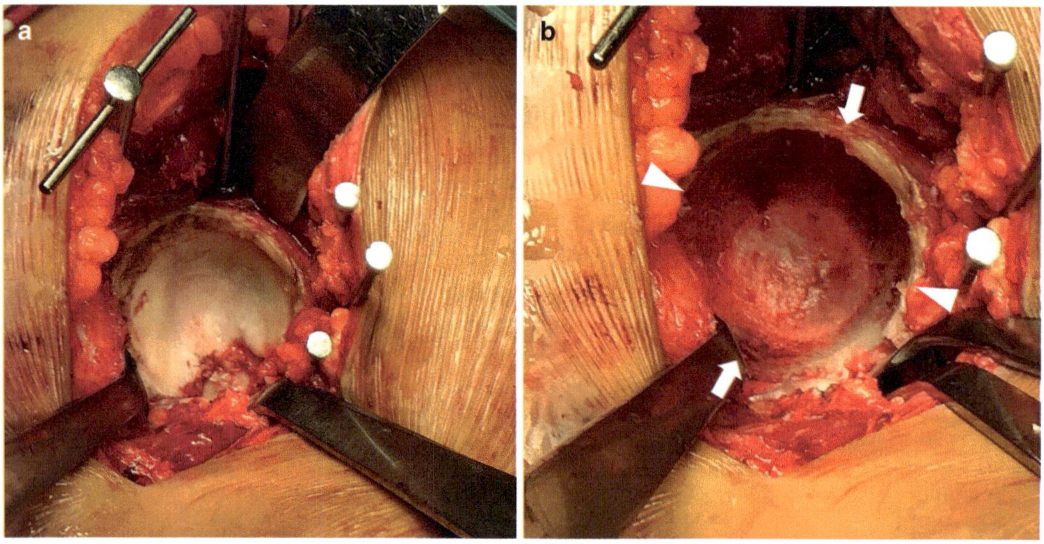

Fig. 17.5 (**a**) The acetabular labrum and transverse acetabular ligament are removed to obtain complete exposure of the acetabulum. (**b**) After reaming, the TAN (lower arrow) and AAN (right arrowhead) are identified. Then, four landmarks for cup alignment—the superior (upper arrow), inferior (lower arrow), anterior (right arrowhead), and posterior (left arrowhead) points—are marked

17.4 Simplified Four Steps for Practical Use

The current method requires comprehensive knowledge of acetabular anatomy, CT imaging, and mathematical formulas. Thus, it might be practically difficult. Thus, we simplified the method into four steps for practical use:

1. Measure acetabular abduction ($\alpha°$) and anteversion ($\beta°$) on preoperative CT scans.
2. Calculate $|\alpha - 40|$ and $|\beta - 15|$.
3. During the operation, locate the TAN and AAN, and mark four reference points at the rim of the acetabulum: superior point, opposite point of TAN; inferior point, $|\alpha - 40|$ mm inside (when α was <40) or outside the TAN (when α was >40); posterior point, the opposite point of AAN; and anterior point, $|\beta - 15|$ mm inside (when β was <15) or outside the AAN (when β was >15).
4. During press-fitting of the cup, adjust the cup abduction to the line between the superior and inferior points and cup anteversion to the line between the anterior and posterior points.

17.5 Postoperative Cup Position

In a previous study with the use of this technique in 50 THAs, we reported actual cup position and subsequent dislocation rate. The mean cup abduction was 40° (range 32°–47°) and the mean cup anteversion was 17° (range 8°–25°) (Fig. 17.6). The mean difference of cup abduction from the target abduction of 40° was 1.76° (SD, 1.84°; range 0.0°–8.4°) and the mean difference of cup anteversion from the target anteversion of 15° was 3.47° (SD, 2.83°; range 0.1°–8.8°). In all 50 hips, cup abduction and anteversion were within the safe zone.

During the follow-up of 5 years, no hip dislocated [20].

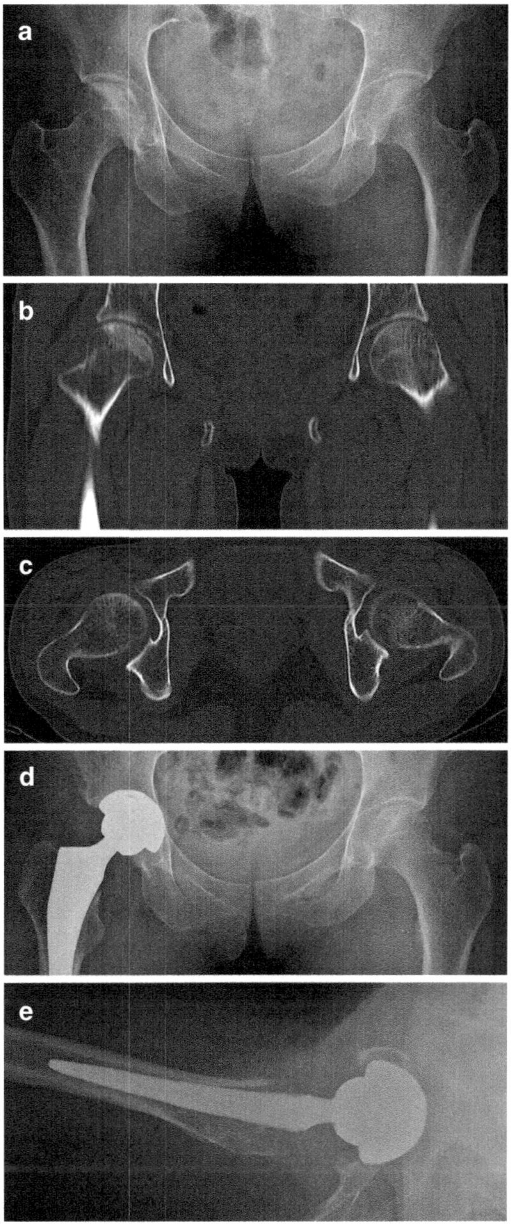

Fig. 17.6 (**a**–**e**) A 36-year-old man had osteonecrosis in the right femoral head as seen on his (**a**) preoperative AP radiograph. (**b**) The acetabular abduction is 44.6 as measured on the preoperative mid-coronal CT scan. (**c**) On the preoperative mid-axial CT scan, the acetabular anteversion is 13.7. (**d**) The 6-week postoperative AP radiograph shows that the cup abduction is 37.1. (**e**) On the lateral radiograph, the cup anteversion is 14.4

17.6 Limitations of Our Method

First, our method necessitates preoperative CT scanning, which is costly and associated with a risk of radiation exposure. Second, our method is not applicable when the acetabulum is not identifiable, such as with a fused hip or severely dysplastic hip. Third, to use our method, the surgeon should identify the landmarks, measure and mark the calculated distances, and then align the cup to the marks, which necessitates a learning curve.

References

1. Paterno SA, Lachiewicz PF, Kelley SS. The influence of patient-related factors and the position of the acetabular component on the rate of dislocation after total hip replacement. J Bone Joint Surg Am. 1997;8:1202.
2. Turner RS. Postoperative total hip prosthetic femoral head dislocations. Incidence, etiologic factors, and management. Clin Orthop Relat Res. 1994;301:196.
3. Dorr LD, Wolf AW, Chandler R, Conaty JP. Classification and treatment of dislocations of total hip arthroplasty. Clin Orthop Relat Res. 1983;173:151.
4. Lee YK, Ha YC, Yoo JI, Jo WL, Kim KC, Koo KH. Mid-term results of the BIOLOX delta ceramic-on-ceramic total hip arthroplasty. Bone Joint J. 2017;6:741.
5. Kim YH, Park JW, Kim JS. Long-term results of third-generation ceramic-on-ceramic bearing cementless total hip arthroplasty in young patients. J Arthroplast. 2016;11:2520.
6. Callaghan JJ, Heekin RD, Savory CG, Dysart SH, Hopkinson WJ. Evaluation of the learning curve associated with uncemented primary porous-coated anatomic total hip arthroplasty. Clin Orthop Relat Res. 1992;282:132.
7. Romanowski JR, Swank ML. Imageless navigation in hip resurfacing: avoiding component malposition during the surgeon learning curve. J Bone Joint Surg Am. 2008;90(Suppl 3):65–70.
8. Thorey F, Klages P, Lerch M, Florkemeier T, Windhagen H, von Lewinski G. Cup positioning in primary total hip arthroplasty using an imageless navigation device: is there a learning curve? Orthopedics. 2009;32(10 Suppl):14–7.
9. Lewinnek GE, Lewis JL, Tarr R, Compere CL, Zimmerman JR. Dislocations after total hip-replacement arthroplasties. J Bone Joint Surg Am. 1978;2:217.
10. McCollum DE, Gray WJ. Dislocation after total hip arthroplasty. Causes and prevention. Clin Orthop Relat Res. 1990;261:159.
11. Steppacher SD, Kowal JH, Murphy SB. Improving cup positioning using a mechanical navigation instrument. Clin Orthop Relat Res. 2011;2:423.
12. Zhu J, Wan Z, Dorr LD. Quantification of pelvic tilt in total hip arthroplasty. Clin Orthop Relat Res. 2010;2:571.
13. Ryan JA, Jamali AA, Bargar WL. Accuracy of computer navigation for acetabular component placement in THA. Clin Orthop Relat Res. 2010;1:169.
14. Olsen M, Chiu M, Gamble P, Boyle RA, Tumia N, Schemitsch EH. A comparison of conventional guidewire alignment jigs with imageless computer navigation in hip resurfacing arthroplasty. J Bone Joint Surg Am. 2010;9:1834.
15. Digioia AM 3rd, Jaramaz B, Plakseychuk AY, Moody JE Jr, Nikou C, Labarca RS, Levison TJ, Picard F. Comparison of a mechanical acetabular alignment guide with computer placement of the socket. J Arthroplast. 2002;3:359.
16. Hassan DM, Johnston GH, Dust WN, Watson G, Dolovich AT. Accuracy of intraoperative assessment of acetabular prosthesis placement. J Arthroplast. 1998;1:80.
17. DiGioia AM, Jaramaz B, Blackwell M, Simon DA, Morgan F, Moody JE, Nikou C, Colgan BD, Aston CA, Labarca RS, Kischell E, Kanade T. The Otto Aufranc Award. Image guided navigation system to measure intraoperatively acetabular implant alignment. Clin Orthop Relat Res. 1998;355:8.
18. Jolles BM, Genoud P, Hoffmeyer P. Computer-assisted cup placement techniques in total hip arthroplasty improve accuracy of placement. Clin Orthop Relat Res. 2004;426:174.
19. Nogler M, Kessler O, Prassl A, Donnelly B, Streicher R, Sledge JB, Krismer M. Reduced variability of acetabular cup positioning with use of an imageless navigation system. Clin Orthop Relat Res. 2004; 426:159.
20. Ha YC, Yoo JJ, Lee YK, Kim JY, Koo KH. Acetabular component positioning using anatomic landmarks of the acetabulum. Clin Orthop Relat Res. 2012; 12:3515.
21. Stem ES, O'Connor MI, Kransdorf MJ, Crook J. Computed tomography analysis of acetabular anteversion and abduction. Skelet Radiol. 2006;6:385.
22. Murtha PE, Hafez MA, Jaramaz B, DiGioia AM 3rd. Variations in acetabular anatomy with reference to total hip replacement. J Bone Joint Surg Br. 2008;3:308.
23. Kim JT, Lee J, Lee YK, Ha YC, Won YY, Lee K, Khanduja V, Koo KH. What is the tolerated width of periacetabular osteophytes to avoid impingement in cementless THA?: a three-dimensional simulation study. Arch Orthop Trauma Surg. 2018;138:1165.
24. Ji HM, Kim KC, Lee YK, Ha YC, Koo KH. Dislocation after total hip arthroplasty: a randomized clinical trial of a posterior approach and a modified lateral approach. J Arthroplast. 2012;3:378.

18 Intraoperative Measurement of Cementless Stem Anteversion

Tae-Young Kim, Chan-Ho Park, Jung-Taek Kim, Jin-Woo Kim, and Kyung-Hoi Koo

18.1 Introduction

During total hip arthroplasty (THA), the femoral stem as well as acetabular cup should be placed in optimal position to minimize impingement and dislocation after surgery [1–3]. Several methods have been introduced to optimize the position of the acetabular cup [1, 4–8]. Since cementless THAs are popularized, anteversion of the femoral stem as well as the cup position has become a matter of concern [3, 9–11]. To prevent dislocation and impingement, femoral stem should be anteverted to 10°–30° [12]. However, it is difficult to manipulate the stem anteversion during the operation, if a cementless stem is used. The geometry of the medullary canal of the proximal canal is different in each individual and cementless stems slide into the femoral canal during press fitting of cementless stem. To address this problem of cementless THA, the concept of combined anteversion was introduced. According to this concept, the stem anteversion should be measured first, and then the target anteversion of the cup is calculated and the cup should be anteverted to the target [3, 9, 10, 13].

In this chapter, we discuss the accuracy of the intraoperative measurement of stem anteversion and the knee problem affecting the discrepancy between the surgeon's estimation and the real stem anteversion.

18.2 Measurement of Stem Anteversion

Stem anteversion is defined as the angle between the axis of the stem-neck and the trans-epicondylar axis of the distal femur (Fig. 18.1) [14, 15]. It cannot be measured exactly during the operation because surgeons cannot define the trans-epicondylar axis. Instead of the trans-epicondylar axis, surgeons usually use the axis of the tibia as a surrogate reference to measure the stem version, with the assumption that tibial axis is vertical to the trans-epicondylar axis [14, 15].

T.-Y. Kim (✉)
Department of Orthopaedic Surgery, Konkuk University Medical Center, School of Medicine, Konkuk University, Seoul, South Korea
e-mail: tykim@kuh.ac.kr

C.-H. Park
Department of Orthopedic Surgery, Yeungnam University Medical Center, Daegu, South Korea

J.-T. Kim
Department of Orthopaedic Surgery, Ajou University Hospital, Suwon-si, Gyeonggi-do, South Korea

J.-W. Kim
Department of Orthopaedic Surgery, Eulji Medical Center, Eulji University College of Medicine, Seoul, South Korea

K.-H. Koo
Department of Orthopaedic Surgery, Seoul National University Bundang Hospital, Seongnam, South Korea

Department of Orthopedic Surgery, Seoul National University College of Medicine, Seoul, South Korea
e-mail: khkoo@snu.ac.kr

W. R. Drescher et al. (eds.), *Advances in Specialist Hip Surgery*,
https://doi.org/10.1007/978-3-030-61830-8_18

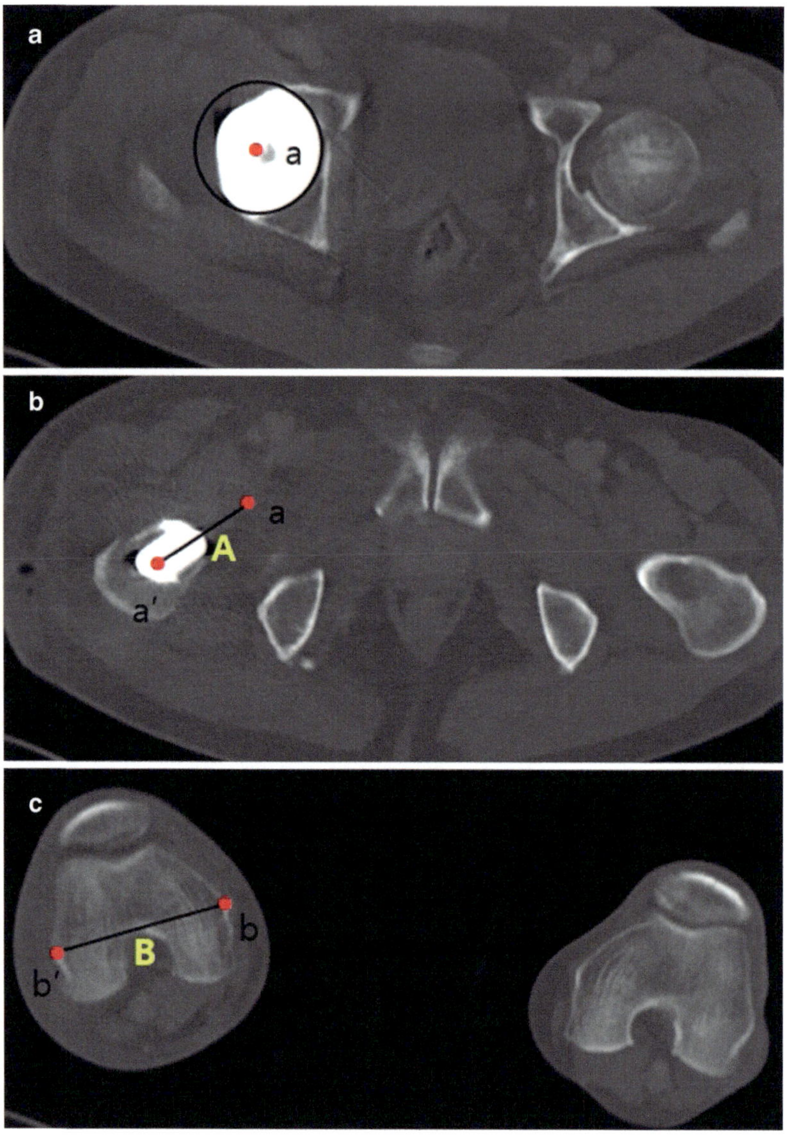

Fig. 18.1 CT measurement of stem anteversion. (**a**) CT scan showing the largest diameter of the acetabular component, the center of the modular head (a) is marked; (**b**) CT scan showing the largest width of the stem-neck, the center of the base of the trunnion (a') is marked. A line (A) is drawn between the two centers, which is the stem-neck axis; (**c**) CT scan showing the most prominent point of the lateral and medial femoral epicondyles (b and b') is marked. A line (B) is drawn between these two points, which is the trans-epicondylar line of the femur. The angle between the axis of the stem-neck and the trans-epicondylar line is the CT anteversion of the stem

Dorr et al. [14] measured the anteversion of 109 cementless stems on postoperative CT scan, and the measurement ranged from 8.6° retroversion to 27.1° anteversion. Only 45% of femoral stems had optimal anteversion of 10°–30°. The authors described that the cementless stems slide into the medullary canal of the proximal femur during press fitting, and different shapes of the femoral canal account for the wide range of stem anteversion. Other authors reported similar findings in their measurements of cementless stems [11, 16].

In the literature, the surgeons' measurement of stem anteversion was reported to be greater than real stem anteversion by 2°–7°. Tibia should be rotated internally to place the lower leg vertically and the stem anteversion is overestimated, if posterior approach is used and hip is dislocated posteriorly. In the study of Dorr et al., intraoperative measurement of stem anteversion was smaller by 1.5° than the real stem anteversion, which was measured on postoperative CT scan [14]. Wines and McNicol also reported an underestimation of the intraoperative measurement by 1.1° [11]. On the other hand, Hirata et al. reported a significant overestimation [15]. In their study, the surgeons' estimation was greater than real stem anteversion by a mean of 5.8° (range 11° underestimation to 25° overestimation), and the mean absolute discrepancy between the intraoperative measurement and real stem anteversion was 7.3°. In a previous study [17], we also showed that the intraoperative measurement overestimated stem anteversion by a mean of 2.0°. However, the absolute discrepancy was <5° in most of the cases (72%).

18.3 Intraoperative Measurement of Stem Anteversion in the Presence of Knee Problem

The prevalence of osteoarthritis of ipsilateral hip and knee has been estimated to be 11% in senile population (>65 years of age) [18]. It is projected that the incidence of ipsilateral knee and hip osteoarthritis will increase in the future [9].

In patients with a varus deformity of the knee, the tibial axis is not vertical to the trans-epicondylar axis of the distal femur. The presence of genu varum or tibia vara deformity would result in an apparent decrease in the measurement of femoral stem anteversion. When the patient has such deformities, surgeons should consider the possible underestimation of their measurement of stem anteversion.

Hirata et al. compared the intraoperatively estimated stem anteversion (estimated prosthetic anteversion) to stem anteversion measured by postoperative CT scan (true anteversion) in 73 THAs. In their study, the estimated prosthetic anteversion was significantly greater than the true anteversion by 5.8°. The mean absolute value of the measurement error was 7.3° ranging from 11° underestimation to 25° overestimation. There was a tendency of overestimation when the true anteversion was smaller and presence of knee osteoarthritis significantly increased the erroneous measurement [15].

Previously, we performed a study to determine the accuracy of the intraoperative measurement of stem anteversion and to investigate factors affecting the discrepancy between the intraoperative measurement and the real stem anteversion measured on CT scan [17].

Our study involved 67 cementless THAs in 65 patients who did not have ipsilateral total knee arthroplasty. The intraoperative measurement of stem anteversion (mean 21.5° ± 8.5°; range 5.0°–39.0°) was greater than the CT measurement (mean 19.5° ± 8.7°; range 4.5°–38.5°) by 2.0°. The absolute value of discrepancy averaged 4.5° and the correlation coefficient between intraoperative and CT measurements was 0.837. When there was a genu varum deformity, the intraoperative measurement underestimated the stem anteversion.

In the absence of varus deformity of the knee, the axis of the tibia is perpendicular to the trans-epicondylar axis, when lower leg is placed vertically. However, in the presence of genu varum deformity, the lower leg should be rotated more internally to place the lower leg vertically. This would result in an apparent decrease of femoral stem anteversion (Fig. 18.2). When the patient

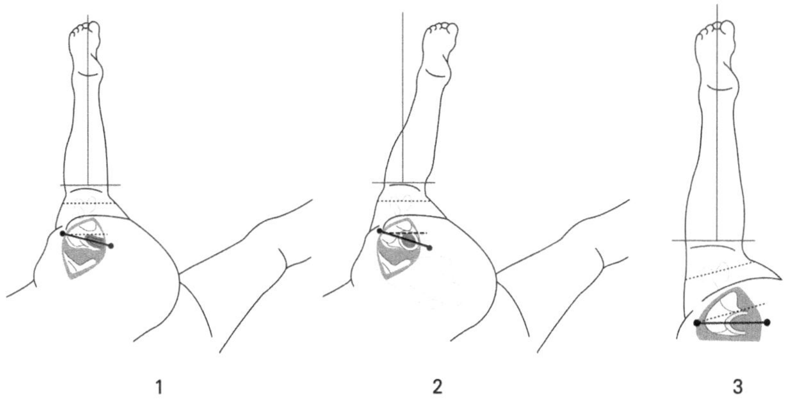

Fig. 18.2 Long axis of the lower leg as the reference for determination of femoral stem anteversion during posterior approach in total hip arthroplasty. (1) Long axis of the lower leg in normal knee; (2) long axis of the lower leg with varus deformity of the knee; (3) to place the lower leg vertically, the lower leg should be rotated more internally. Solid long lines = long axis of the lower leg; dotted lines = trans-epicondylar axis; black line connecting solid circles = femoral neck axis

has a varus deformity of the knee, surgeons should consider the possible underestimation of their measurement of stem anteversion. The real anteversion of stem is greater than the intraoperative measurement.

However, it should be noted that our results cannot be applied to patients who underwent ipsilateral total knee arthroplasty and we used only posterior approach in our patients. Our results might be otherwise, if different approaches were used.

References

1. Stefl M, Lundergan W, Heckmann N, McKnight B, Ike H, Murgai R, Dorr LD. Spinopelvic mobility and acetabular component position for total hip arthroplasty. Bone Joint J. 2017;99-B(1 Suppl A):37.
2. Trousdale RT, Cabanela ME, Berry DJ. Anterior iliopsoas impingement after total hip arthroplasty. J Arthroplast. 1995;10(4):546.
3. Yoshimine F. The safe-zones for combined cup and neck anteversions that fulfill the essential range of motion and their optimum combination in total hip replacements. J Biomech. 2006;39(7):1315.
4. Beverland DE, O'Neill CK, Rutherford M, Molloy D, Hill JC. Placement of the acetabular component. Bone Joint J. 2016;98-B(1 Suppl A):37.
5. Kennedy JG, Rogers WB, Soffe KE, Sullivan RJ, Griffen DG, Sheehan LJ. Effect of acetabular component orientation on recurrent dislocation, pelvic osteolysis, polyethylene wear, and component migration. J Arthroplast. 1998;13(5):530.
6. Phan D, Bederman SS, Schwarzkopf R. The influence of sagittal spinal deformity on anteversion of the acetabular component in total hip arthroplasty. Bone Joint J. 2015;97-B(8):1017.
7. Pierrepont JW, Feyen H, Miles BP, Young DA, Bare JV, Shimmin AJ. Functional orientation of the acetabular component in ceramic-on-ceramic total hip arthroplasty and its relevance to squeaking. Bone Joint J. 2016;98-B(7):910.
8. Spencer-Gardner L, Pierrepont J, Topham M, Bare J, McMahon S, Shimmin AJ. Patient-specific instrumentation improves the accuracy of acetabular component placement in total hip arthroplasty. Bone Joint J. 2016;98-B(10):1342.
9. Dorr LD, Malik A, Dastane M, Wan Z. Combined anteversion technique for total hip arthroplasty. Clin Orthop Relat Res. 2009;467(1):119.
10. Pierchon F, Pasquier G, Cotten A, Fontaine C, Clarisse J, Duquennoy A. Causes of dislocation of total hip arthroplasty. CT study of component alignment. J Bone Joint Surg Br. 1994;76(1):45.
11. Wines AP, McNicol D. Computed tomography measurement of the accuracy of component version in total hip arthroplasty. J Arthroplast. 2006;21(5):696.
12. D'Lima DD, Urquhart AG, Buehler KO, Walker RH, Colwell CW Jr. The effect of the orientation of the acetabular and femoral components on the range of motion of the hip at different head-neck ratios. J Bone Joint Surg Am. 2000;82(3):315.
13. Dorr LD, Malik A, Wan Z, Long WT, Harris M. Precision and bias of imageless computer navigation and surgeon estimates for acetabular component position. Clin Orthop Relat Res. 2007;465:92.
14. Dorr LD, Wan Z, Malik A, Zhu J, Dastane M, Deshmane P. A comparison of surgeon estimation and computed tomographic measurement of femoral component anteversion in cementless total hip arthroplasty. J Bone Joint Surg Am. 2009;91(11):2598.
15. Hirata M, Nakashima Y, Ohishi M, Hamai S, Hara D, Iwamoto Y. Surgeon error in performing intraoperative estimation of stem anteversion in cementless total hip arthroplasty. J Arthroplast. 2013;28(9):1648.
16. Reikeras O, Gunderson RB. Components anteversion in primary cementless THA using straight stem and hemispherical cup: a prospective study in 91 hips using CT-scan measurements. Orthop Traumatol Surg Res. 2011;97(6):615.
17. Lee YK, Kim JW, Kim TY, Ha YC, Koo KH. Validity of the intra-operative measurement of stem anteversion and factors for the erroneous estimation in cementless total hip arthroplasty using postero-lateral approach. Orthop Traumatol Surg Res. 2018;104(3):341.
18. Dawson J, Linsell L, Zondervan K, Rose P, Randall T, Carr A, Fitzpatrick R. Epidemiology of hip and knee pain and its impact on overall health status in older adults. Rheumatology (Oxford). 2004;43(4):497.

Part VI

Revision Hip Arthroplasty

Triflange Cup and 3-D Printing in THA

19

Ajay Premkumar, Cynthia Kahlenberg, Kyle Morse, Victoria X. Wang, and Michael B. Cross

19.1 Introduction

This chapter focuses on strategies to appropriately manage pelvic discontinuity in the revision arthroplasty setting, with special attention on the use of custom triflange implants and the emerging role of 3-D printing technologies. Pelvic discontinuity refers to a form of bone loss in which the superior aspect of the pelvis is separated from the inferior aspect through the acetabulum [1]. The management of pelvic discontinuity in revision total hip arthroplasty can be challenging and requires a thorough understanding of the bone loss pattern as well as available treatment options. The goal of the treatment for large acetabular defects and pelvic discontinuity is to create a unitized hemipelvis by either biological healing of the discontinuity or mechanically fixing the superior and inferior aspects of the pelvis with rigid and durable fixation. The Paprosky classification for acetabular bone loss helps provide a framework to approach, classify, and plan for revision total hip arthroplasty in cases of pelvic discontinuity. This classification uses an anteroposterior radiograph to evaluate the integrity of major anatomic landmarks, including the teardrop, ilioischial line, and degree of cup migration, and has been shown to correlate highly with subsequent intraoperative findings [2]. Specifically, obturator ring asymmetry, medial migration of the inferior hemipelvis with disruption of the ilioischial line, and a visible fracture line on an AP pelvis have all been associated with pelvic discontinuity [3]. According to the Paprosky classification, pelvic discontinuity occurs in a type IIC or type IIIB acetabular defect, depending on whether the cup has migrated less than or more than 2 cm, respectively. As imaging modalities have evolved since the creation of this classification system in the 1990s, the addition of the Judet views, inlet/outlet views, and three-dimensional computed tomography (CT) scans can all be used to better understand the acetabular defect morphology preoperatively [2].

19.2 Approach and Treatment Options for Managing Pelvic Discontinuity

When approaching revision arthroplasty cases involving pelvic discontinuity, a surgeon should carefully plan for how to address the discontinuity itself, through either distraction or compression, as well as select the optimal implant to manage the acetabular defect. One must assess intraoperatively whether an adequate press fit can

A. Premkumar · C. Kahlenberg · K. Morse
V. X. Wang · M. B. Cross (✉)
Department of Orthopaedic Surgery, Hospital for Special Surgery, New York, NY, USA
e-mail: premkumara@HSS.EDU; KahlenbergC@hss.edu; MorseK@hss.edu; wangv@hss.edu; CrossM@HSS.EDU

W. R. Drescher et al. (eds.), *Advances in Specialist Hip Surgery*,
https://doi.org/10.1007/978-3-030-61830-8_19

be obtained with a trial acetabular shell, and consider the potential for long-term biologic fixation with the use of a hemispherical cup. Furthermore, an evaluation of the chronicity of the discontinuity as well as the quantity and quality of the remaining host bone is essential.

Acute pelvic discontinuities, such as from an intraoperative fracture during noncemented cup insertion, often heal using compression plating. Specifically, for Paprosky type IIIB defects with acute discontinuity, the typical treatment options include posterior compression plating, often with a 3.5 mm pelvic reconstruction plate, and bone grafting or additional fixation of the anterior column, followed by insertion of a multi-hole porous coated noncemented acetabular component using multiple screws for additional construct stability. It should be noted that while a traditional approach prioritizes posterior column fixation and bone grafting of the anterior column, recent studies have suggested that bicolumnar fixation, including the use of a 4.5 mm antegrade screw for anterior column fixation, provides increased biomechanical stability compared to posterior plating alone [4]. This approach has shown most promise in patients with modest bone loss and large bony surfaces amenable to compression. On the other hand, chronic discontinuities, due to local factors, abundant fibrous tissue, and poor host bone vascularity, are known to have poor bone healing potential and a poor likelihood of successful management with compression plating.

In the setting of chronic discontinuities with adequate bone stock, a distraction technique may be employed, followed by sequential reaming until rim contact is obtained. If there is a type III defect and rim deficiencies, highly porous augments may be sized and placed around the trial cup to fill the specific acetabular defects. Trabecular metal augments can be fixed to host bone using cancellous screws, and a highly porous coated acetabular shell can be impacted into position, and cemented to the metal augments. Highly porous metals maximize bony ingrowth by improving initial stability and minimizing stress shielding. In the setting of discontinuity, jumbo cups (sizes >62 mm in women or >66 mm in men) are usually required to increase bone contact with the deficient acetabulum, with the increased surface area of larger porous cups increasing the likelihood of osseointegration [5–7]. Additional fixation can then be obtained using cancellous screws through cup screw holes. Long-term outcomes for the distraction technique are limited given its relatively recent introduction; however one study of 20 patients revealed that 75% had radiographic cup stability at a mean follow-up of 4.5 years, with another showing 83.3% survivorship of 32 patients at a mean of 5.2 years [8, 9].

In cases where bone quantity and/or quality do not allow for biologic fixation, acetabular cages with bulk allograft may be used. Advantages of large surface area cages are to dissipate hip forces across a large amount of damaged bone and decrease the risk of future cup protrusion into the true pelvis. Disadvantages of this construct are a lack of biologic fixation and subsequent reliance on multiple screws for mechanical stability, with several series describing significantly high rates of mechanical loosening (up to 31% at 5 years), as well as early mechanical failure (up to 15%) [10–12]. Another strategy in this setting is the use of a cup-cage technique, in which the acetabular defect can be filled with allograft, then a hemispherical shell is placed to provide potential long-term biologic fixation, and then a cage is cemented into the acetabular shell and fixed with screws to allow for initial mechanical stability. In this situation, a liner is cemented into the cage. Early and midterm results for cup-cage constructs are very promising, with 5–10-year survivorship being approximately 85–90% in small series of patients [13–15]. However, long-term data is still lacking.

19.3 Custom Triflange

Another option for the treatment of pelvic discontinuities is the use of a patient-specific acetabular component with ileal, ischial, and often pubic flanges, known as a custom triflange implant. The three rigid flanges emanating from the acetabular cup provide areas for contact with intact bone of the ilium, ischium, and pubis, and also allow for custom placement of screw holes to achieve ideal purchase in these areas. In smaller sized defects with better bone quality and quantity, a biflange component with ischial and ileal flanges only can be alternatively used. While the number and location of screws available depend on the size of the patient and amount of bone remaining, typically, the smallest flange is the pubic flange, while the ischial flange has 3–6 screw holes which typically accommodate 6.5 mm acetabular screws and rest on the posterior surface of the ischial tuberosity, and the largest ileal flange has two rows of three or four screw holes which accommodate 6.5 mm screws. Screw fixation through the flanges allows for initial rigid stability, until biologic fixation is achieved through implant coating, if possible. However, due to the nature of the sclerotic bone, limited vascularity, and limited bony contact, biologic fixation is often not achieved.

Given some of the considerations and disadvantages noted previously of various treatment options for severe acetabular bone loss, custom triflanges are growing in popularity as an effective alternative to distraction arthroplasty in the setting of pelvic discontinuity, especially for type IIIB acetabular defects [16]. While indications are evolving, custom triflange components are currently used for cases with known discontinuity, large contained defects with possible discontinuity, and complex revision cases with insufficient bone stock.

Typically after a surgeon suspects or diagnoses a pelvic discontinuity on plain radiographs, three-dimensional imaging (usually CT) with thin cuts through the acetabulum is sent to the manufacturer, who then creates an accurate model of the patient's anatomy and acetabular defect for the surgeon. Some manufacturers deliver a physical model of the hemipelvis in addition to a digital model. After evaluating this model, the surgeon may decide that the particular pattern of acetabular bone loss may not be sufficiently treated with traditional methods, and a custom implant prototype is then created by the manufacturer and shared digitally and adjusted as needed by the surgeon. It should be noted that the surgeon is an active participant in this process, and must indicate the preferred size and location of ileal, ischial, and often pubic flanges for screw fixation, as well as note the areas of overhanging bone which can be removed to allow the flanges to rest appropriately on host bone. Further, the surgeon will choose the desired correction of the leg length inequality, acetabular anteversion and inclination, and medial position of the cup. The implant hip center of rotation, cup anteversion, and cup abduction are created using anatomic landmarks of the model such as the obturator foramen, iliac wing, and pubic ramus [17]. In general, the best results and lowest failure rates occur with medialization of the acetabular component, and thus the most medial location of the hip center of rotation is often desired. Once approved, the custom implant is manufactured and sent to the surgeon. Various manufacturers offer different triflange features; however, the implants are usually composed of titanium and include porous as well as hydroxyapatite-coated options.

Regarding surgical technique, usage of a triflange involves an extensive exposure of the ilium, ischium, and pubis. Temporary fixation usually begins with the ischium and care must be taken to release enough tissue distally off the femur including the gluteus maximus tendon to avoid stretch or retraction injury to the sciatic nerve when placing the ischial flange. Similarly, dissection over the ilium should avoid injury to the superior gluteal nerve, because good bone is often seen in the ilium; thus, dissection and screw placement through the ileal flange should not be carried too proximal on the ilium to limit the injury to the abductors. Finally, subperiosteal dissection and extreme care should be used to avoid anterior neurovascular structures during exposure of the pubis. The final construct often has 9–15 screws for fixation. Various polyethylene liners are available, with lateralized, elevated, and constrained options; however specific types of liners vary between implant companies and the surgeon should have a firm understanding of available options prior to surgery.

Some disadvantages of using this technique are patient exposure to increased radiation during a CT scan, delay in time for implant fabrication, implant cost, and inability to modify the implant/surgical plan intraoperatively. However, to date, costs and implant manufacturing time may be decreasing with increasing volume of production, and clinical results using this technique for this challenging problem have been promising.

19.4 Triflange Outcomes

While known to have a higher complication rate and poorer survivorship than primary hip implants, some authors have reported excellent midterm survivorship of custom triflange components. Tauton et al. reported 95% revision-free rate of a custom triflange component in a series of 57 hips at a mean of 65-month follow-up while DeBoer et al. reported 100% survivorship with explantation as the primary endpoint at a mean follow-up of 123 months [18, 19].

Common complications associated with triflange components include deep infection, dislocation, sciatic nerve injury, and aseptic loosening. Infection rates have been reported to range from 0 to 11% for custom triflange components, while dislocation rates have been reported up to 21% [18, 20–23].

Despite relatively high complication rates, patients do well clinically with studies often reporting significant improvement in mean Harris Hip Score, and one study even reported a mean Harris Hip Score of 90 postoperatively (Table 19.1) [24]. Further, in terms of function, Christie et al. reported that in a series of 67 patients who all required walking aids preoperatively, 54% were able to walk with no walking aid at a mean of 53-month follow-up [22].

Radiographically, triflange outcomes are difficult to assess given that the metal implant often obscures bony apposition; further, the sclerotic bone in the remaining acetabulum often does not allow bone on-growth to occur. Thus, radiolucencies are often seen postoperatively, even at early follow-up [22]. Still discontinuity union rates continue to be high at medium-term follow-up [19, 23]. Thus, radiolucencies themselves are not useful to evaluate fixation of triflange implants. Instead, change in implant position over time on serial radiographs, and radiolucencies around the screws, may be more useful to evaluate long-term

Table 19.1 Patient-reported outcome scores for custom triflange components

Author	PMID	Number of hips	Mean duration of follow-up	Patient-reported outcome scores
Christie	11764351	67	53 months (range, 24–107)	HHS pre-op: 33.3 HHS post-op: 82.1
Tauton	21997785	57	65 months (range, 24–215)	HHS pre-op: not reported HHS post-op: 74.8
Barlow	26742903	63	4.32 years	WOMAC pre-op: 38.94 WOMAC post-op: 71.35
Berasi	25315276	23	57 months (range, 28–108 months)	HHS pre-op: 42 HHS post-op: 65
Berend	29292340	95	3.5 years (range, 1–11 years)	HHS pre-op: 46 HHS post-op: 75
DeBoer	17403808	20	123 months (range, 89–157 months)	HHS pre-op: 41 HHS post-op: 80
Myncke	30423635	22	25 months	HHS pre-op: not reported HHS post-op: 68
Gladnick	29033157	73	7.5 years (range, 5–12 years)	HOOS Jr pre-op: not reported HOOS Jr post-op: 85
Moore	29451937	35	Minimum 10 years	HHS pre-op: 28 HHS post-op: 90
Wind	23464943	19	31 months (range, 16–59)	HHS pre-op: 38 HHS post-op: 63 WOMAC pre-op: 43 WOMAC post-op: 26

fixation of a custom triflange implant. Cross-sectional imaging may be helpful in assessing bony healing after triflange implantation, though this too can be obscured by artifact. Additionally, the lack of radiographic healing is less important than patient symptoms as multiple authors have reported cases of asymptomatic aseptic loosening with custom triflanges [22, 25, 26].

Reported costs of custom triflange components are in the range of $11,000–$12,500 [18, 21]. While significantly more expensive than primary hip components, these costs are in line with the costs of cup-cage constructs which have been reported to cost around $11,250 [27]. Thus, for cases of massive bone loss requiring advanced reconstruction techniques, custom triflange components may be a reasonable cost-effective option.

19.5 The Evolution of 3-D Printing

The use of 3-D printing technology is rapidly expanding within hip arthroplasty, and orthopedics in general. While initially used to develop physical models to better understand patient anatomy and aid in both diagnosis and surgical planning, with the ability to print metals, patient-specific instrumentation (PSI) and personalized implants are now being made and applied to solve a wide variety of previously challenging problems within orthopedic surgery, including the development of custom triflange components.

3-D printing has often been referred to as "additive manufacturing" as the end product is produced by adding layers sequentially. This type of manufacturing is in contrast to subtractive techniques, such as machining, and in particular milling, in which material is removed from stock to create the final product. As a computer-controlled process, 3-D printing can produce extraordinarily complex designs with precise detail. Initially referred to as "rapid prototyping," early 3-D printing technologies were harnessed to quickly build model prototypes, as the manufacturing of limited production prototypes with more traditional methods such as molding, casting, or machining was more expensive and time consuming due to the requisite development of tooling, jig, or mold creation. Perhaps the most important advantage of 3-D printing and additive manufacturing is that it is unconstrained by design complexity and allows for continual production of unique designs to develop personalized instrumentation and implants, thus allowing for "mass personalization" [28].

The origin of modern 3-D printing technologies traces its foundation to Charles Hull, a co-founder of 3D Systems, when he patented the stereolithography (STL) file format in 1984, now the common file format for 3-D printers [29]. The process he envisioned was to create an object's cross-sectional area to build a three-dimensional object. This process was later developed into one of the major types of 3-D printing techniques, stereolithography, which utilizes an ultraviolet laser to pattern and cure photopolymers into a solid three-dimensional object by adding the material in cross-sectional layers. In 1986, Carl Deckard patented selective laser sintering (SLS) [30, 31]. This process involves sequentially adding powder layers of plastic, metal, ceramic, or glass in a cross section and the use of a computer-controlled laser to sinter or harden the powder into the final shape. The laser is able to scan over the entire layer of powder from a programed three-dimensional shape and selectively sinter the desired cross section only. This is similar to other processes: direct metal laser sintering (DMLS) and selective laser melting (SLM), in which the cross-sectional area is melted instead of sintered. Lastly, in 1988, Scott Crump helped develop the second technique: fused deposition modeling (FDM), a process by which thermoplastic beads or streams are extruded through a nozzle and immediately hardened to form solid layers [32]. The part is built sequentially by a moving printer head over the desired shape forming the cross section in the horizontal plane and then moving vertically.

19.6 Use of 3-D Printing in Orthopedic Surgery and Revision THA

In 1990, Mankovich et al. described the application of 3-D printing technology in medicine by utilizing CT imaging data to construct a physical model of cranial bony anatomy [17, 33, 34]. Today, this principle can be applied in orthopedics to develop a better understanding of patient anatomy and for surgical planning. In orthopedics, CT is generally preferred as the imaging modality of choice as bone has a higher contrast and exposure compared to MRI [34]. Following image acquisition, the original file format, DICOM (Digital Imaging and Communications in Medicine), is uploaded into a software processing program to create a 3-D reconstruction of the images. The processed 3-D image is then exported to STL format and sent to the printer for manufacturing. The transformation of medical imaging into 3-D printed models has several applications. The first is a more accurate understanding of anatomical landmarks and pathology [35–37]. 3-D printing can also be used to create PSI and custom implants. Within total hip arthroplasty, PSI can be used to accurately size and position the acetabular and femoral components during surgery [38]. Similar to other medical applications of 3-D printing, advanced imaging is used to develop a 3-D model of the patient's anatomy. Guides are then created utilizing selective laser sintering and are of two broad types: constrained and non-constrained. A constrained guide shows the correct direction of implantation while a non-constrained design assists in the physical insertion of the implant.

The development of custom implants is applicable to complex reconstruction surgery where generic components may not be well suited. Selective laser melting is used to build implants from a titanium alloy powder, and has been used to create various constructs, including custom triflange implants. Given the precision and accuracy inherent in selective laser melting, various meshes can be added within the implant's microstructure to aid osseointegration [39]. Utilizing computer-aided design, the cup's design can be altered in several ways to optimize its biomechanical properties and ensure a precise fit and optimal restoration of hip mechanics. Finite element analysis can be performed to reduce the amount of stress shielding experienced by the cup during loading and minimize the risk of peri-prosthetic fractures while maintaining implant strength to avoid implant failure. The iliac, ischial, and pubic flanges can be designed to accurately match the patient's anatomy to reduce the amount of bone removed and optimize fixation as the screw placement can be varied to gain maximal purchase. Lastly, varying surface finishes can be applied such as porous surface finishes or hydroxyapatite to increase bone on-growth, silver finishing to decrease infection, and smooth finishing to decrease soft-tissue irritation [39].

Case Example 1

Eighty-year-old female presented with left-hip pain, shortening of the left lower extremity, and chronic peri-prosthetic hip dislocation (Fig. 19.1a, b). The patient had a history of

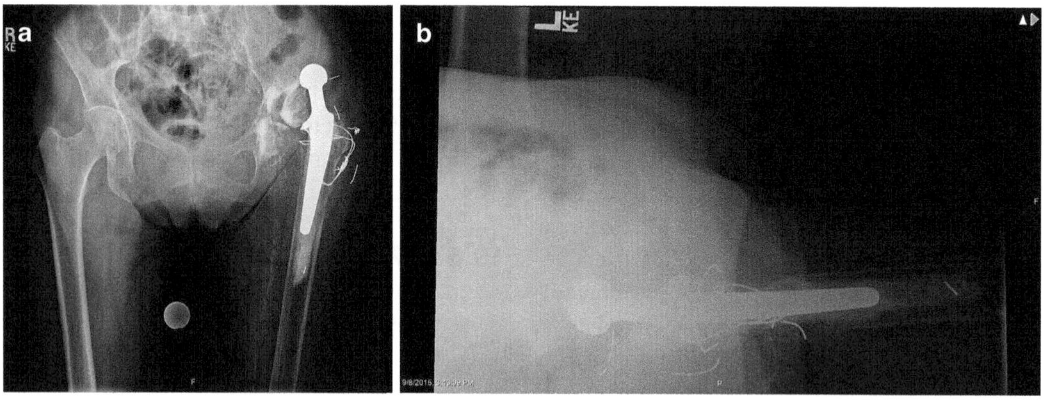

Fig. 19.1 (**a**, **b**) AP pelvis and L hip cross-table lateral radiographs taken on initial presentation, demonstrating failure of the left acetabular component with dislocation and superior migration of the femoral head

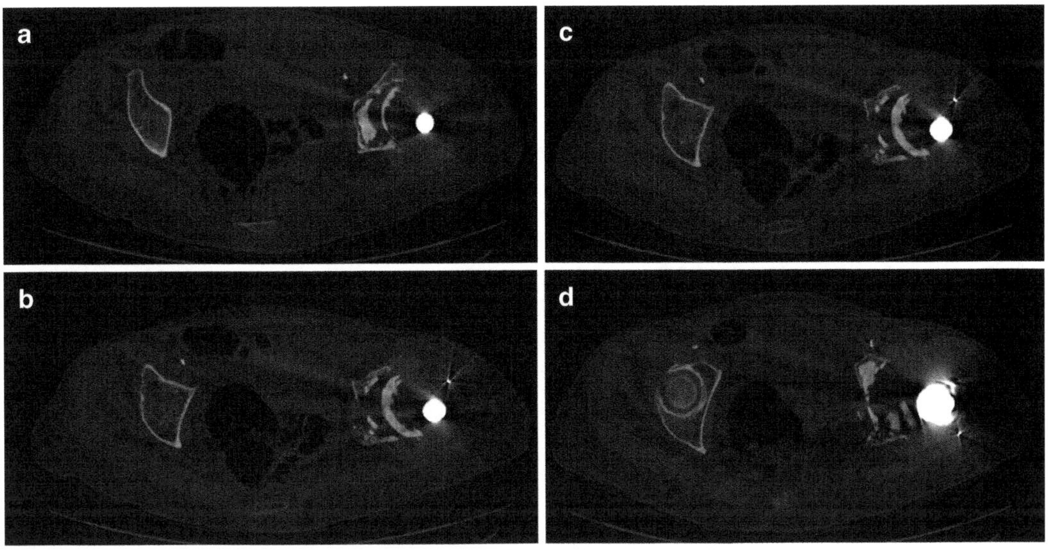

Fig. 19.2 (**a**–**d**) Preoperative computed tomography (CT) showed extensive acetabular osteolysis with disruption of the medial wall

left-hip surgery as a child for hip dysplasia. She underwent primary left total hip replacement with cemented polyethylene acetabular component 40 years prior to presentation. Preoperative X-rays on presentation showed failure of the acetabular component with dislocation and superior migration of the femoral head. Preoperative computed tomography (CT) showed extensive acetabular osteolysis with disruption of the medial wall (Fig. 19.2a–d). Given her pattern of osteolysis, as well as her remaining bone stock, a decision to proceed with revision hip arthroplasty with a custom triflange implant was made.

Intraoperatively, extensive osteolysis was noted. The polyethylene cup was found to be fragmented and was removed, along with remaining cement within the acetabulum. Exposure was obtained for implantation of the custom-made triflange component. The component was fixed with non-locking and locking screws in the ilium and ischium, including a large "home-run" screw in the ischium. The femoral stem was noted to be well fixed and ultimately was maintained. Upon reduction in the operating room, the hip was noted to be stable through range of motion (Fig. 19.3a, b).

Postoperatively, the patient's pain resolved. She walked with a cane with no limp and was able to go up and downstairs normally and walk 2–3 blocks at a time. She suffered a dislocation which was treated with closed reduction and no further surgery.

Case Example 2

A 60-year-old female presented with 1 year of left-hip pain. The patient had a history of left total hip arthroplasty for avascular necrosis that required revision 14 years prior to presentation, due to severe polyethylene wear. She subsequently developed debilitating groin pain and inability to bear weight. Upon presentation, radiographs revealed a cage construct, severe polyethylene wear, and aseptic loosening with superior migration of the femoral head (Fig. 19.4a, b). A preoperative CT (Fig. 19.5a–c) was performed and showed extensive acetabular osteolysis as well as loosening and superolateral migration of the acetabular component. Given her specific pattern of acetabular osteolysis, a biflange construct was selected.

Intraoperatively, the fibrous tissue surrounding the cage was freed and the cage and all screws were removed without complication. The ilium and ischium were exposed and a custom biflange component was positioned as templated preoperatively. All screw holes were filled and excel-

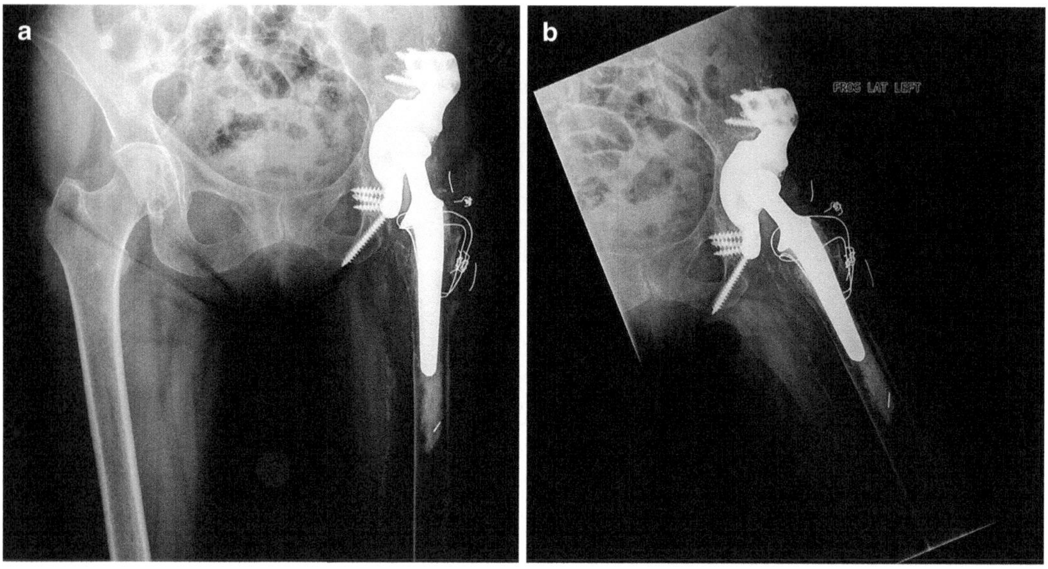

Fig. 19.3 (**a**, **b**) Postoperative AP pelvis and frog lateral radiographs demonstrating revision THA using a custom tri-flange implant for acetabular reconstruction, and retention of the original femoral stem

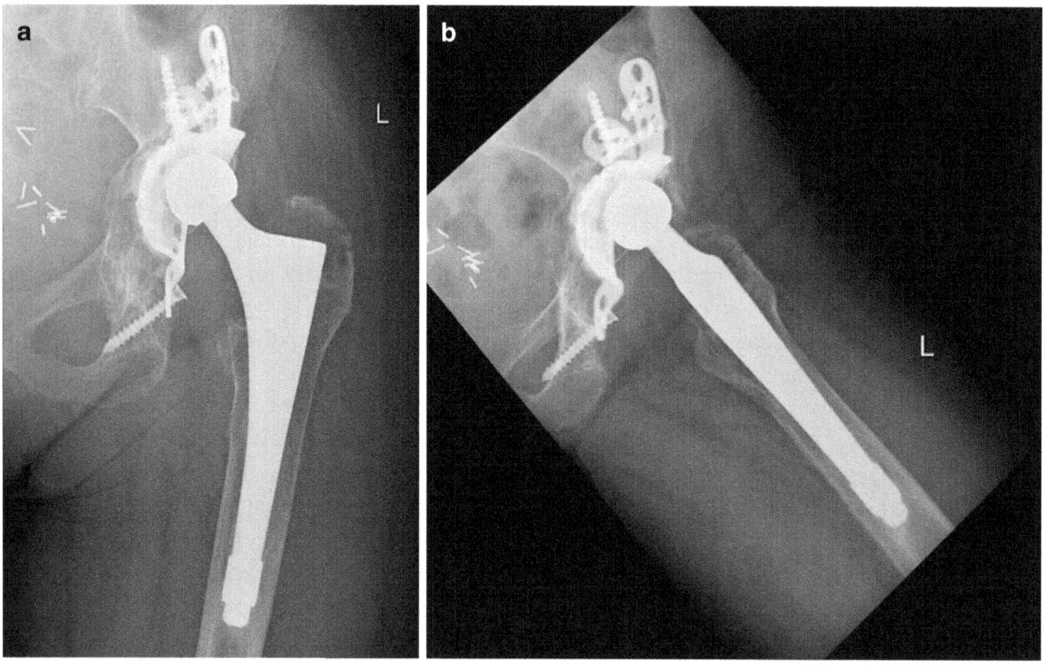

Fig. 19.4 (**a**, **b**) AP pelvis and frog lateral left-hip radiographs taken on initial presentation, demonstrating severe polyethylene wear, evidence of revision acetabular component loosening, and superior migration of the femoral head

lent fixation was noted. A liner was placed, the components were trialed, and the hip was noted to have excellent stability (Fig. 19.6a, b).

Postoperatively, the patient was initially made toe-touch weight bearing and ambulated with a cane up and down stairs. She had mild or occasional pain but was able to perform all activities of daily living. She was progressed to weight bearing as tolerated after 6 weeks and was doing very well when seen at the 1-year

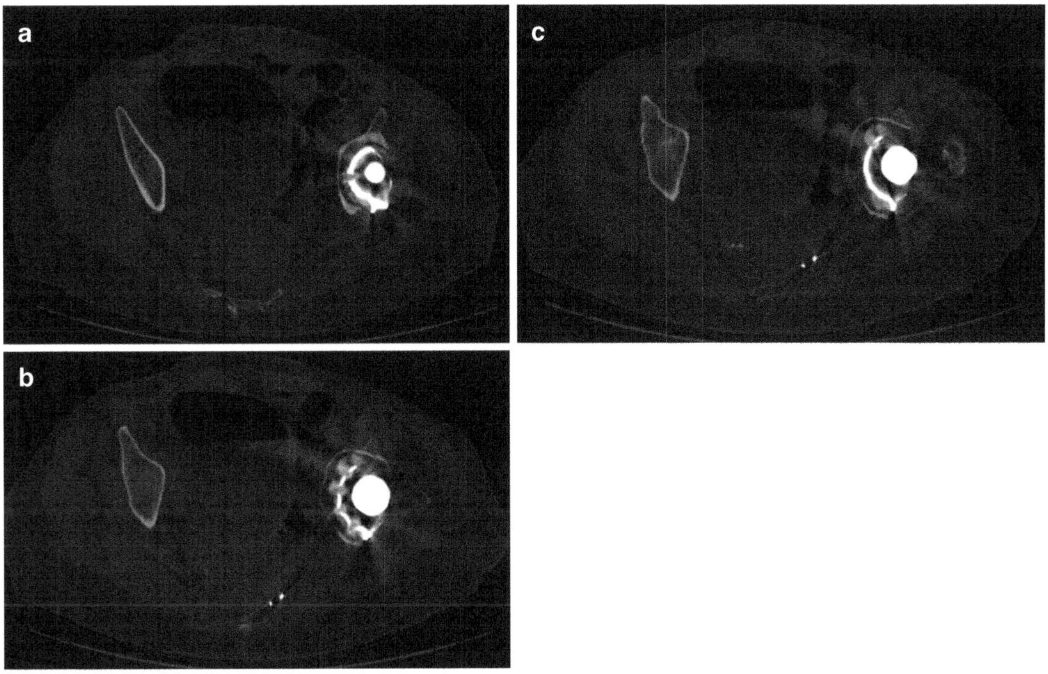

Fig. 19.5 (a–c) Preoperative computed tomography (CT) further demonstrated extensive acetabular osteolysis with superolateral migration of the revision acetabular component

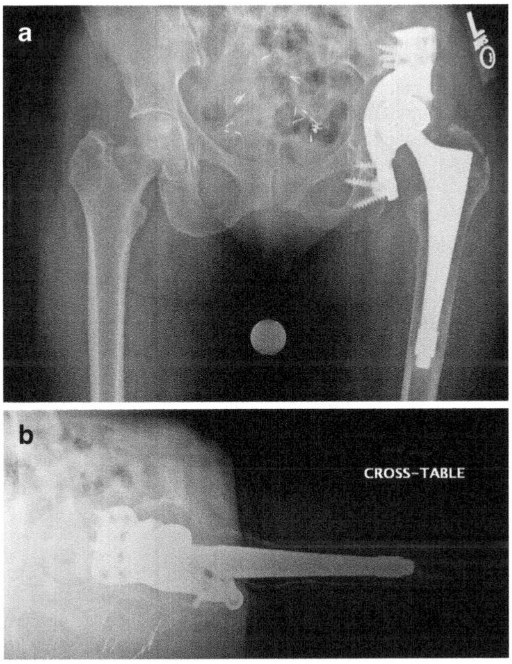

Fig. 19.6 (a, b) Postoperative AP pelvis and cross-table lateral radiographs demonstrating revision THA using a custom biflange implant for acetabular reconstruction, and retention of the original femoral stem

postoperative visit. She is back to work and ambulates without walking aids.

19.7 Summary

Large acetabular defects and pelvic discontinuity are challenging to manage in the revision hip arthroplasty setting. The goal of the treatment for large acetabular defects and pelvic discontinuity is to create a unitized hemipelvis by either biological healing of the discontinuity or mechanically fixing the superior and inferior aspects of the pelvis with rigid and durable fixation. Custom triflanges are growing in popularity as an effective alternative to other implant options in the setting of the large acetabular defects and pelvic discontinuity. Advanced imaging such as CT is used to identify scenarios where custom triflange implants may be most useful and as a basis for creating bony models; through dialogue between the surgeon and manufacturer, 3-D printing technologies then allow for the creation of customized patient-specific implants to best accommodate the remaining host bone and optimize screw purchase. In general, screw fixation through the flanges allows for initial rigid stability until biologic fixation is achieved through implant coating. Several authors have reported excellent midterm survivorship of custom triflange components; however long-term data is needed to further evaluate this promising treatment strategy.

References

1. Berry DJ, Lewallen DG, Hanssen AD, Cabanela ME. Pelvic discontinuity in revision total hip arthroplasty. J Bone Joint Surg Am. 1999;81:1692–702. https://doi.org/10.2106/00004623-199912000-00006.
2. Paprosky WG, Cross MB. CORR Insights®: validity and reliability of the Paprosky acetabular defect classification. Clin Orthop Relat Res. 2013;471:2266. https://doi.org/10.1007/s11999-013-2938-2.
3. Abdel MP, Trousdale RT, Berry DJ. Pelvic discontinuity associated with total hip arthroplasty: evaluation and management. J Am Acad Orthop Surg. 2017;25:330–8. https://doi.org/10.5435/JAAOS-D-15-00260.
4. Gililland JM, Anderson LA, Henninger HB, Kubiak EN, Peters CL. Biomechanical analysis of acetabular revision constructs: is pelvic discontinuity best treated with bicolumnar or traditional unicolumnar fixation? J Arthroplast. 2013;28:178–86. https://doi.org/10.1016/j.arth.2012.04.031.
5. Lakstein D, Backstein D, Safir O, Kosashvili Y, Gross AE. Trabecular metal cups for acetabular defects with 50% or less host bone contact. Clin Orthop Relat Res. 2009;467:2318–24. https://doi.org/10.1007/s11999-009-0772-3.
6. von Roth P, Abdel MP, Harmsen WS, Berry DJ. Uncemented jumbo cups for revision total hip arthroplasty: a concise follow-up, at a mean of twenty years, of a previous report. J Bone Joint Surg Am. 2015;97:284–7. https://doi.org/10.2106/JBJS.N.00798.
7. Whaley AL, Berry DJ, Harmsen WS. Extra-large uncemented hemispherical acetabular components for revision total hip arthroplasty. J Bone Joint Surg Am. 2001;83-A:1352–7. https://doi.org/10.2106/00004623-200109000-00010.
8. Sheth NP, Melnic CM, Brown N, Sporer SM, Paprosky WG. Two-centre radiological survivorship of acetabular distraction technique for treatment of chronic pelvic discontinuity. Bone Joint J. 2018;100-B:909–14. https://doi.org/10.1302/0301-620X.100B7.BJJ-2017-1551.R1.
9. Sporer SM, Bottros JJ, Hulst JB, Kancherla VK, Moric M, Paprosky WG. Acetabular distraction: an alternative for severe defects with chronic pelvic discontinuity? Clin Orthop Relat Res. 2012;470:3156–63. https://doi.org/10.1007/s11999-012-2514-1.
10. Berry DJ. Antiprotrusio cages for acetabular revision. Clin Orthop Relat Res. 2004;(420):106–12. https://doi.org/10.1097/00003086-200403000-00015.
11. Regis D, Sandri A, Bonetti I, Bortolami O, Bartolozzi P. A minimum of 10-year follow-up of the Burch-Schneider cage and bulk allografts for the revision of pelvic discontinuity. J Arthroplast. 2012;27:1057–1063.e1. https://doi.org/10.1016/j.arth.2011.11.019.
12. Saleh KJ, Jaroszynski G, Woodgate I, Saleh L, Gross AE. Revision total hip arthroplasty with the use of structural acetabular allograft and reconstruction ring: a case series with a 10-year average follow-up. J Arthroplast. 2000;15:951–8. https://doi.org/10.1054/arth.2000.9055.
13. Amenabar T, Rahman WA, Hetaimish BM, Kuzyk PR, Safir OA, Gross AE. Promising mid-term results with a cup-cage construct for large acetabular defects and pelvic discontinuity. Clin Orthop Relat Res. 2016;474:408–14. https://doi.org/10.1007/s11999-015-4210-4.
14. Eggli S, Müller C, Ganz R. Revision surgery in pelvic discontinuity: an analysis of seven patients. Clin Orthop Relat Res. 2002;398:136–45. https://doi.org/10.1097/00003086-200205000-00020.
15. Rogers BA, Whittingham-Jones PM, Mitchell PA, Safir OA, Bircher MD, Gross AE. The reconstruction of periprosthetic pelvic discontinuity. J Arthroplast. 2012;27:1499–1506.e1. https://doi.org/10.1016/j.arth.2011.12.017.
16. Goodman GP, Engh CA. The custom triflange cup: build it and they will come. Bone Joint J. 2016;98-B:68–72. https://doi.org/10.1302/0301-620X.98B.36354.
17. Mankovich NJ, Robertson DR, Cheeseman AM. Three-dimensional image display in medicine. J Digit Imaging. 1990;3:69–80.
18. Taunton MJ, Fehring TK, Edwards P, Bernasek T, Holt GE, Christie MJ. Pelvic discontinuity treated with custom triflange component: a reliable option. Clin Orthop Relat Res. 2012;470:428–34. https://doi.org/10.1007/s11999-011-2126-1.
19. DeBoer DK, Christie MJ, Brinson MF, Morrison JC. Revision total hip arthroplasty for pelvic discontinuity. J Bone Joint Surg Am. 2007;89:835–40. https://doi.org/10.2106/JBJS.F.00313.
20. Berasi CC, Berend KR, Adams JB, Ruh EL, Lombardi AV. Are custom triflange acetabular components effective for reconstruction of catastrophic bone loss? Clin Orthop Relat Res. 2015;473:528–35. https://doi.org/10.1007/s11999-014-3969-z.
21. Berend ME, Berend KR, Lombardi AV, Cates H, Faris P. The patient-specific triflange acetabular implant for revision total hip arthroplasty in patients with severe acetabular defects: planning, implantation, and results. Bone Joint J. 2018;100-B:50–4. https://doi.org/10.1302/0301-620X.100B1.BJJ-2017-0362.R1.
22. Christie MJ, Barrington SA, Brinson MF, Ruhling ME, DeBoer DK. Bridging massive acetabular

defects with the triflange cup: 2- to 9-year results. Clin Orthop Relat Res. 2001;393:216–27. https://doi.org/10.1097/00003086-200112000-00024.
23. Gladnick BP, Fehring KA, Odum SM, Christie MJ, DeBoer DK, Fehring TK. Midterm survivorship after revision total hip arthroplasty with a custom triflange acetabular component. J Arthroplast. 2018;33:500–4. https://doi.org/10.1016/j.arth.2017.09.026.
24. Moore KD, McClenny MD, Wills BW. Custom triflange acetabular components for large acetabular defects: minimum 10-year follow-up. Orthopedics. 2018;41:e316–20. https://doi.org/10.3928/01477447-20180213-11.
25. Myncke I, van Schaik D, Scheerlinck T. Custom-made triflanged acetabular components in the treatment of major acetabular defects. Short-term results and clinical experience. Acta Orthop Belg. 2017;83:341–50.
26. Barlow BT, Oi KK, Lee Y-Y, Carli AV, Choi DS, Bostrom MP. Outcomes of custom flange acetabular components in revision total hip arthroplasty and predictors of failure. J Arthroplast. 2016;31:1057–64. https://doi.org/10.1016/j.arth.2015.11.016.
27. Schwarzkopf R, Ihn HE, Ries MD. Pelvic discontinuity: modern techniques and outcomes for treating pelvic disassociation. Hip Int. 2015;25:368–74. https://doi.org/10.5301/hipint.5000270.
28. Trauner KB. The emerging role of 3D printing in arthroplasty and orthopedics. J Arthroplast. 2018;33:2352–4. https://doi.org/10.1016/j.arth.2018.02.033.
29. Bagaria V, Bhansali R, Pawar P. 3D printing- creating a blueprint for the future of orthopedics: current concept review and the road ahead! J Clin Orthop Trauma. 2018;9:207–12. https://doi.org/10.1016/j.jcot.2018.07.007.
30. Deckard CR, inventor; University of Texas System, assignee. Method and apparatus for producing parts by selective sintering. US patent 5597589. 28 Jan 1997.
31. Hull CW, inventor; 3D Systems Inc, assignee. Apparatus for production of three-dimensional objects by stereolithography. US patent 4575330. 19 Dec 1989.
32. Crump SS, inventor; Stratasys Inc, assignee. Apparatus and method for creating three-dimensional objects. US patent 5,121,329. 9 June 1992.
33. Mankovich NJ, Cheeseman AM, Stoker NG. The display of three-dimensional anatomy with stereolithographic models. J Digit Imaging. 1990;3:200–3.
34. Wong TM, Jin J, Lau TW, Fang C, Yan CH, Yeung K, To M, Leung F. The use of three-dimensional printing technology in orthopaedic surgery. J Orthop Surg (Hong Kong). 2017;25:1–7. https://doi.org/10.1177/2309499016684077.
35. Bizzotto N, Tami I, Santucci A, Adani R, Poggi P, Romani D, Carpeggiani G, Ferraro F, Festa S, Magnan B. 3D Printed replica of articular fractures for surgical planning and patient consent: a two years multi-centric experience. 3D Print Med. 2015;2:2. https://doi.org/10.1186/s41205-016-0006-8.
36. Zerr J, Chatzinoff Y, Chopra R, Estrera K, Chhabra A. Three-dimensional printing for preoperative planning of total hip arthroplasty revision: case report. Skelet Radiol. 2016;45:1431–5. https://doi.org/10.1007/s00256-016-2444-1.
37. Xu J, Li D, Ma R, Barden B, Ding Y. Application of rapid prototyping pelvic model for patients with DDH to facilitate arthroplasty planning: a pilot study. J Arthroplast. 2015;30:1963–70. https://doi.org/10.1016/j.arth.2015.05.033.
38. Henckel J, Holme TJ, Radford W, Skinner JA, Hart AJ. 3D-printed patient-specific guides for hip arthroplasty. J Am Acad Orthop Surg. 2018;26:e342–8. https://doi.org/10.5435/JAAOS-D-16-00719.
39. Wyatt MC. Custom 3D-printed acetabular implants in hip surgery—innovative breakthrough or expensive bespoke upgrade? Hip Int. 2015;25:375–9. https://doi.org/10.5301/hipint.5000294.

Trochanteric Osteotomy

20

Mathias P. G. Bostrom, Branden R. Sosa, and Kevin Staats

20.1 Introduction

Trochanteric osteotomies (TO) were commonly used for primary total hip arthroplasty (THA) as advocated by Sir John Charnley in the 1960s and 1970s [1]. The advantages of conducting a TO for primary THA were the exact component positioning through an extensive surgical approach and the possibility to address abductor laxity by tightening the abductor muscles through distal trochanteric advancement. Through precise preoperative planning tools and development of modern implant designs and less invasive surgical approaches, the use of TO has declined dramatically in primary THA. Currently, TO is only used in revision arthroplasty or complex primary THA, such as congenital hip diseases (e.g., dysplasia, high hip dislocation, post-Perthes), posttraumatic arthritis (± retained hardware), or severe deformity [2, 3]. This chapter gives an overview of the most common types of TO with an emphasis on indications, technique, and complications.

M. P. G. Bostrom (✉) · B. R. Sosa
Hospital for Special Surgery, Weill Medical College of Cornell University, New York, NY, USA
e-mail: bostromm@hss.edu; sosab@hss.edu

K. Staats
Division of Orthopedics, Department of Orthopedics and Trauma Surgery, Medical University of Vienna, Vienna, Austria
e-mail: kevin.staats@meduniwien.ac.at

20.2 Preoperative Considerations

Preoperative planning of revision THA or complex primary THA is crucial for successful postoperative outcomes. A meticulous physical examination should include gait analysis, muscle function evaluation, limb length assessment, and sources of pain. Analyzing the gait of the patient is necessary for the determination of abductor laxity and weakness. Preoperative abductor muscle strength is an important factor when performing TO; it gives substantial information about possible pathomechanisms (e.g., recurrent dislocations), but it is particularly useful to determine the tensile strength of the soft-tissue reconstruction after TO. Additionally, surgeons should be aware of the characteristics of the implants and hardware to have all tools available when performing surgery. Particularly in revision THA, it is vital to get information on the retained implant such as the surface of the stem, presence and extent of coatings, and mode of fixation. In addition if information on the retained implant is available then implant-specific extraction tools can be obtained.

Preoperative radiographic evaluation should include anteroposterior (AP) standing pelvis X-ray and AP and lateral X-rays of the entire femur to evaluate the following points [4]:

- Curvature of the femur
- Axis, centering, and shape of femoral implant

W. R. Drescher et al. (eds.), *Advances in Specialist Hip Surgery*,
https://doi.org/10.1007/978-3-030-61830-8_20

- Presence of osteolysis
- Presence of additional hardware
- Condition of a cement plug when present

Templating is crucial for the surgeon to have a comprehensive plan including the length of the TO (measured from the tip of the greater trochanter), modality, and position of the new implant. Computed tomography (CT) is essential since it gives useful additional information about bone quality, osseointegration, and position of the retained implant. Magnetic resonance imaging (MRI) may be indicated to assess the condition of the surrounding muscular structures and soft tissue.

In most cases, the final decision to perform the TO is made intraoperatively, but preoperatively the patients should be informed about the possibility that the procedure may be necessary since subsequent postoperative rehabilitation and mobilization are different if a TO is performed.

20.3 Sliding Trochanteric Osteotomy

20.3.1 Introduction

The sliding TO was first described by English [5] and refined by Glassman [6]. The technique used in a sliding TO allows for an intact vastus lateralis origin to prevent proximal trochanteric migration and an improved compression after refixation due to medial directed forces through gluteus medius and vastus lateralis [7].

Indications for sliding TO are:

- Challenging dislocation due to protrusion, scarring, or heterotopic ossification
- The need for greater acetabular exposure
- Abductor laxity *with* an adequate trochanteric bed for fixation

Therefore based on these indications, the use of sliding TO is limited to complex primary THA and is rarely used in revision arthroplasty.

20.3.2 Technique

The description of the surgical technique summarizes methods from multiple authors [6, 8–10].

This procedure is primarily performed through a lateral or posterolateral approach. The fascia lata is incised in line with the skin incision. The gluteus maximus is identified proximal to the piriformis and it is developed with the underlying abductors. The fibers of gluteus maximus are bluntly split. Afterwards the anterior border of the gluteus medius and the interval between gluteus medius and minimus are identified. The interval between those muscles is developed from posteriorly to anteriorly. An incision of the vastus lateralis is performed beginning at the vastus ridge proximally and extended distally in line with the anterior border of the intermuscular septum. The vastus lateralis is elevated and retracted from the anterolateral aspect of the femoral shaft. The osteotomy is started proximally medial to the gluteus medius insertion into the greater trochanter with an oscillating saw, ensuring that the osteotomy remains lateral to the gluteus minimus. The osteotomy should extend distally beyond the vastus ridge. By its attachment to the joint capsule, the fragment should still be tethered to the proximal femur. Therefore, to avoid severe displacement from the trochanteric bed during external rotation of the hip, it is necessary to retract the posterior border of the fragment anterolaterally and the capsule tissue should be dissected from the anterior border of the fragment.

20.3.3 Fixation

There is considerable variation on fixation techniques compared to the extended trochanteric osteotomy (ETO). The following fixation methods can be used for this procedure:

- Cerclage wires [10–14]
- Cerclage wires/cable [8, 9]
- Cables/wires/cancellous screws [15]
- Trochanteric bolt/wires [16]
- Cortical screws [17]

- Wires/cortical screws [3]
- Locking plate/cerclage cables [18]
- Trochanteric bolt/washer [19]

20.3.4 Complications

In primary THA, nonunion rates range from 2.6 [12] to 16.7% [11]. The dislocation rate after sliding TO appears lower than that in the ETO with rates between 0 and 9.3% [8, 17]. Reasons for reoperations include aseptic loosening, neuropraxia, bursitis, trochanteric migration, heterotopic ossification, and abductor weakness. Despite these reasons for reoperation, not all complications require an additional revision surgery. When comparing the complication rates of different fixation methods, cerclage wires seem to outperform cortical screws, but data is insufficient to fully assess the performance among the various fixation methods.

For revision arthroplasty, nonunion rates range from 0 [15] to 31% [19], dislocation rate from 0 [16, 20] to 24.1% [19], and deep infection rate from 0 [10, 13, 15, 18, 20] to 34.5% [19]. There is a vast range in reoperation rates from 0 [9, 15] to 34.5% [19]. As indicated previously, comparing types of fixation and their outcome appears to be even more difficult due to the distinct variety in their study designs. However, cerclage wires seem to have a lower complication rate than bolts or locking plates, but cables seem to outperform wires with regard to union and prevention of subsidence [21].

20.4 Extended Trochanteric Osteotomy

20.4.1 Introduction

In 1989, Wagner was the first to describe a transfemoral approach to gain access to the proximal femur [22]. Through a posterolateral approach, the proximal femur was split longitudinally creating an osteotomized fragment comprising the greater trochanter and approximately half the circumference of the femoral shaft. The technique described by Wagner was later modified by Younger [23] and Paprosky [24], and is now known as the extended trochanteric osteotomy (ETO). The difference between the original transfemoral approach and modified method is that the osteotomy only involves approximately one-third of the femoral shaft circumference, while the vastus lateralis (divided in its midsubstance and retracted anteriorly and posteriorly) and glutei muscles still remain attached. Younger et al. [23] published this technique using a lateral approach as a modification to the anterolateral approach described by Wagner [22].

The ETO has gained wide acceptance as a suitable technique to facilitate the removal of well-fixed implants. Uncemented and cemented stem removals pose a challenge during revision THA and the ETO is a reliable method to create a controlled osteotomy of the proximal femur allowing access to the femoral canal [25]. The osteotomy created with this procedure can be of variable femoral diaphyseal length with the femoral fragment levered opened anterolaterally while retaining muscle and periosteal integrity.

The length of the osteotomy should be sufficient enough to access the bone-cement or bone-implant interface that will need to be removed during implant extraction. Care should be taken to also retain at least 4 cm of isthmic diaphyseal cortex for adequate fixation during reconstruction. The average length of the osteotomy has been reported to be between 12.5 cm and 14.1 cm, but the length is largely contingent on the implant in situ [26, 27].

The ETO remains a reliable technique to prevent further compromising of the bone stock when conducting a revision THA. As with all revision arthroplasties, preoperative templating, proper implant selection, and fixation techniques are crucial for good intraoperative and postoperative outcomes.

20.4.2 Indications

The ETO can serve as a useful supplement when conducting a revision THA due to aseptic loosening, failed hemiarthroplasties, periprosthetic fractures, or recurrent dislocations. The indications for this technique are the extraction of an osseointegrated stem, well-fixed cemented stem, and difficult-to-access cement mantle. Other indications are the need for improved access to acetabular component and varus remodeling of the proximal femur that can prohibit reaming of the distal cavity and fixation of the revision implant.

Aseptic loosening remains the most common indication requiring an ETO.

When Younger et al. first described the use of the ETO, 15 patients required the ETO for aseptic loosening (75%), 2 for recurrent dislocation (10%), 1 for femoral fracture (5%), and 1 for previous resection arthroplasty (5%) [23]. In a more recent and larger study, 119 patients had an ETO for aseptic loosening (75.8%), 11 for periprosthetic fracture (7.0%), 7 for periprosthetic infection (4.5%), 5 for implant breakage (3.2%), and 4 for hip fusion (2.5%) [28].

This technique has the advantage of providing wide exposure, distal visualization of the cement plug, safe circumferential cement removal, and excellent component fixation while providing high union rate [23]. In addition, the controlled osteotomy created by this technique should prevent further complications such as uncontrolled intraoperative fractures and canal perforations. The anatomy of the hip joint also allows significant abductor muscle tensioning without hindering reattachment stability. Proximal migration is prevented due to the presence of the gluteus medius, gluteus minimus, anterolateral muscle hinge, vastus lateralis, and periosteum. By retaining this soft-tissue envelope with the osteotomized bone, vascularity to the fragment is not compromised. This, coupled with the large surface area of the fragment, promotes healing of the osteotomy sites [23].

20.4.3 Technique

A standard posterolateral approach is used with an extension distal along the lateral border of the thigh (Fig. 20.1a). Use of as much previous incisions as possible is recommended. Subsequent dissection of the subcutaneous tissue down to the fascia is performed. The fascia is dissected in line with its fibers and the underlying fibers of the gluteus maximus. To release posterior tension, the femoral insertion of the gluteus maximus is identified and dissected. A posterior capsulotomy should be performed at the posterior border of the vastus lateralis and the gluteus medius along with the attachment of the external rotators to the posterior ridge of the greater trochanter and piriformis fossa.

After performing the posterolateral approach and dislocation of the hip in a controlled manner, the operated leg is placed in extension and internal rotation. For better exposure, an elevator is placed under the calcar. After placing the leg in flexion and internal rotation, the posterior border of the vastus lateralis is identified (Fig. 20.1b) and detached from the intermuscular septum. At this point, it is crucial to ligate or cauterize perforator vessels of the profunda femoris to reduce blood loss and gain better visualization. The vastus lateralis is retracted against the anterior femoral cortex (Fig. 20.1c, d). Care should be taken to ensure that the vastus lateralis attachment is maintained at the vastus ridge with the abductor muscle attachment.

To assure accurate length of the ETO, a ruler is used to mark the appropriate length of the osteotomy beginning at the tip of the greater trochanter. Prior to any osteotomy a prophylactic cable or wire is placed 1 cm distal to the planned transverse osteotomy site (Fig. 20.2). The osteotomy itself can be performed with a pencil burr on a high-speed drill and/or with an oscillating saw. The osteotomy should be flush with the implant surface or cement mantle. Extend the posterior limb of the osteotomy throughout the entire length of the ETO (Fig. 20.3a). To improve visualization during this step, the leg can be placed in extension and internal rotation. After performing the posterior cut of the ETO, the leg should be placed in external rotation to release the pseudocapsule at the anterior aspect of the greater trochanter. This step is crucial to gain adequate visualization to perform the anterior proximal cut of the osteotomy and to prevent from impeded

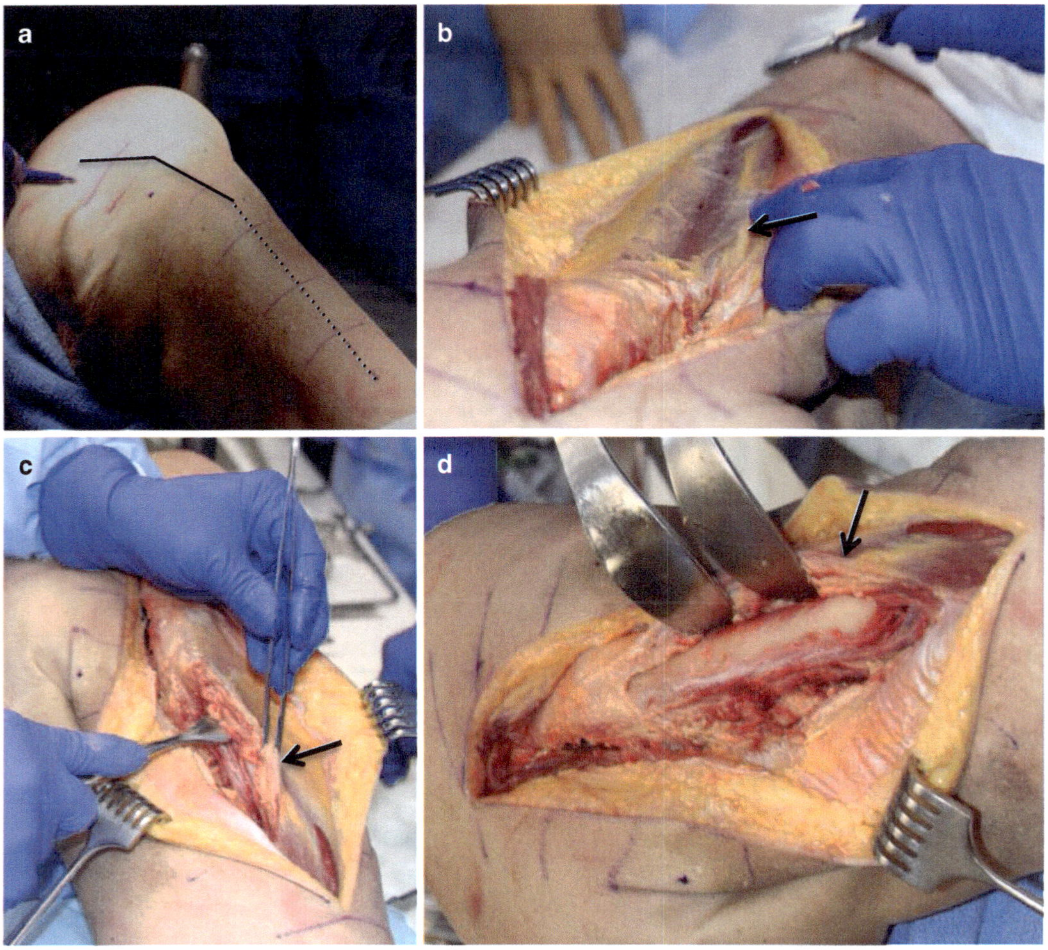

Fig. 20.1 (a–d) Exposure of the proximal femur with a skin incision using a standard posterolateral approach (continuous line) with distal extension along the lateral border of the thigh (dotted line) (**a**). The posterior border of the vastus lateralis (arrow) is identified (**b**). The fascia is split longitudinally and the vastus lateralis (arrow) is detached from the intermuscular septum (**c**). The vastus lateralis (arrow) is retracted against the anterior femoral cortex (**d**)

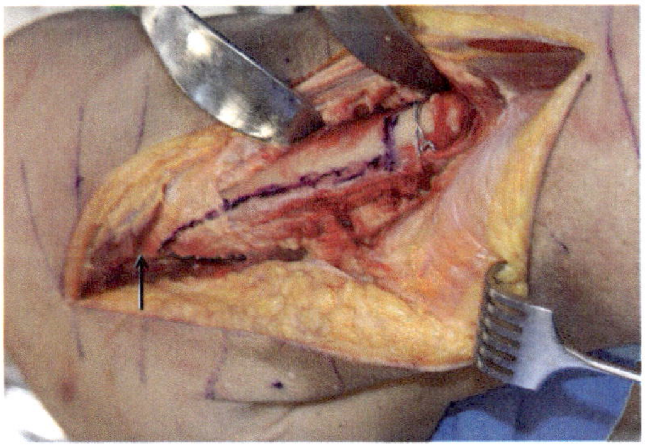

Fig. 20.2 The extent of the ETO is marked with a ruler using the greater trochanter as the starting point (arrow). Prior to the osteotomy, a prophylactic wire or cable is placed 1 cm distal to the transverse cut

reduction of the fragment due to tensile forces. Afterwards, the anterior osteotomy can be completed (Fig. 20.3b). The transverse cut of the osteotomy should extend approximately one-third of the femoral shaft circumference. Drill holes along the line of the transverse cut reduce the risk of uncontrolled fracture (Fig. 20.4).

After placing the leg in internal rotation, osteotomes are used to lift the osteotomized fragment from posteriorly to anteriorly (Figs. 20.5 and 20.6a). After performing all case-specific steps (e.g., removal of femoral implant; Fig. 20.6b), some authors suggest beginning with preparation and reaming of the femoral canal, although the senior author recommends beginning the femoral

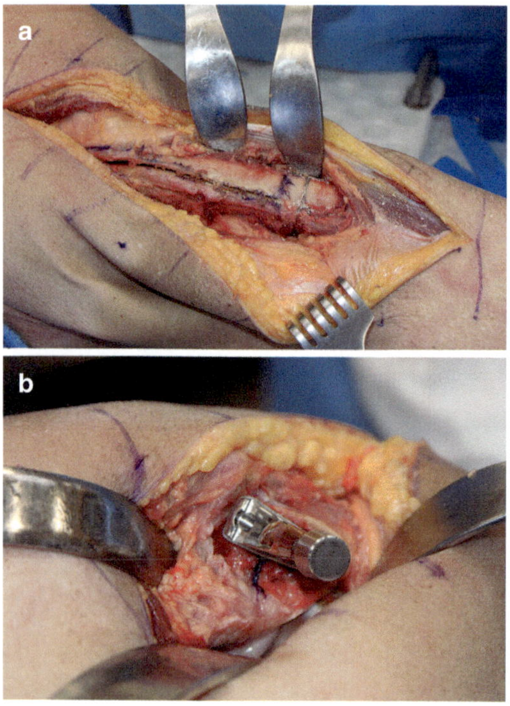

Fig. 20.3 (**a**, **b**) After performing the posterior cut of the ETO (**a**), the proximal anterior osteotomy is performed to prevent uncontrolled fracture in the trochanteric region (**b**)

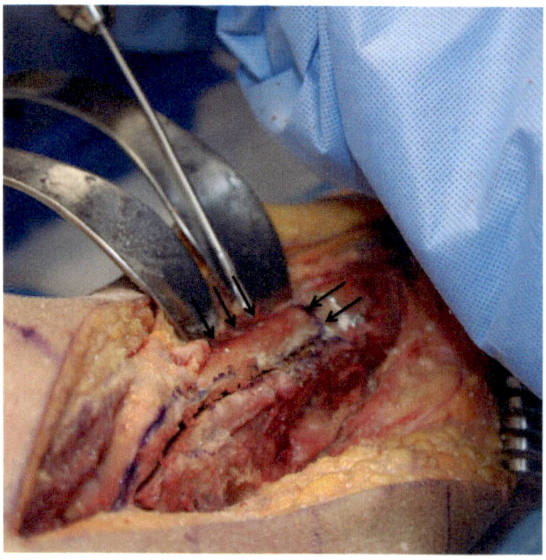

Fig. 20.4 Drill holes (arrows) along the anterior osteotomy site and along the transverse cut reduce uncontrolled fracture risk

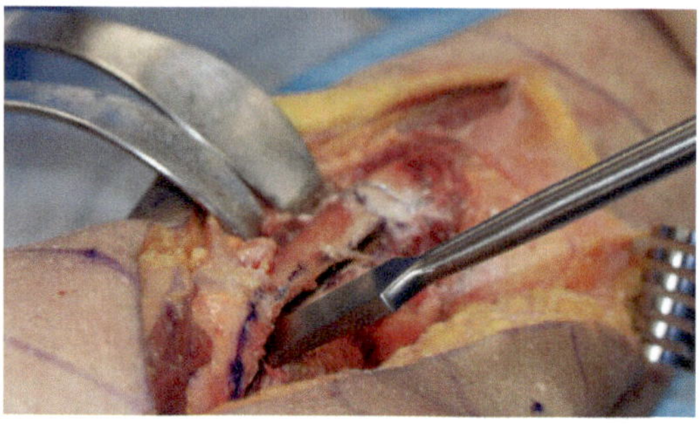

Fig. 20.5 Osteotomes are used to retract the osteotomized fragment from posterior to anterior

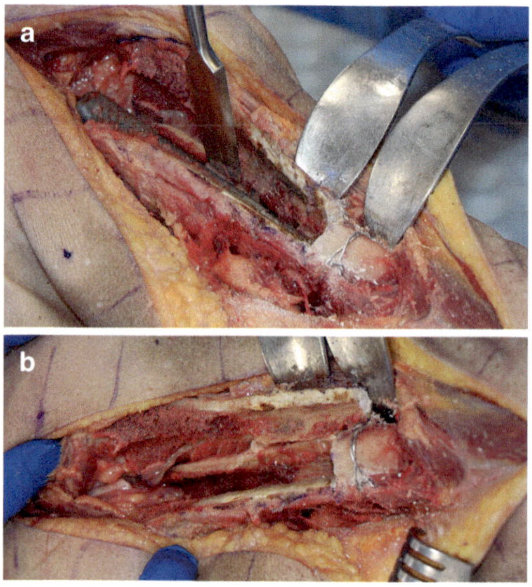

Fig. 20.6 (**a**, **b**) The osteotomy should be flush with the retained implant (**a**) in order to remove the implant with as little damage to the bone stock as possible (**b**)

reconstruction with the reduction and fixation of the osteotomized fragment. Two cables are usually sufficient for a stable fixation of the fragment (Fig. 20.7). Each cable should be passed deep between the femoral cortex and the vastus lateralis. A fracture reduction clamp can be helpful for this step. After satisfactory reduction of the fragment, femoral reconstruction can be performed (Figs. 20.8, 20.9, and 20.10).

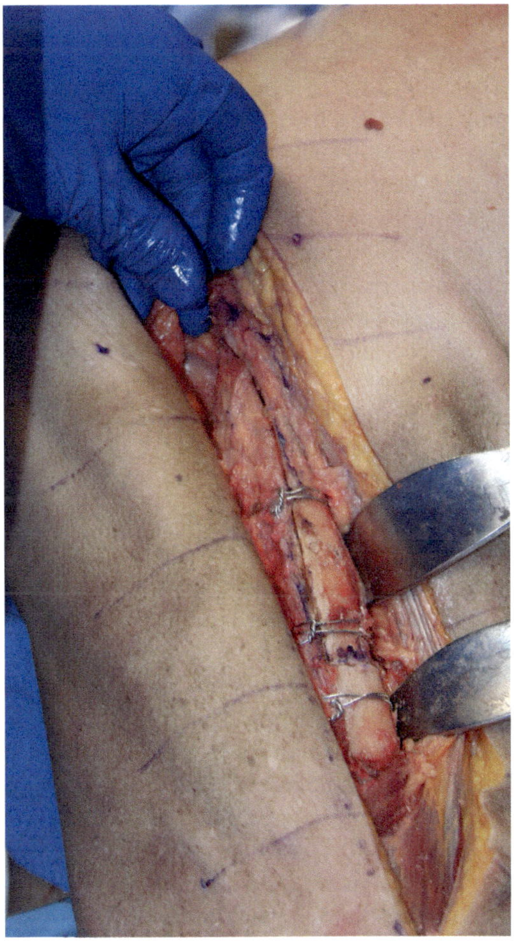

Fig. 20.7 After removal of the implant, the fragment is reduced and wires or cables are used for fixation. Usually, two wires are sufficient for stable fixation

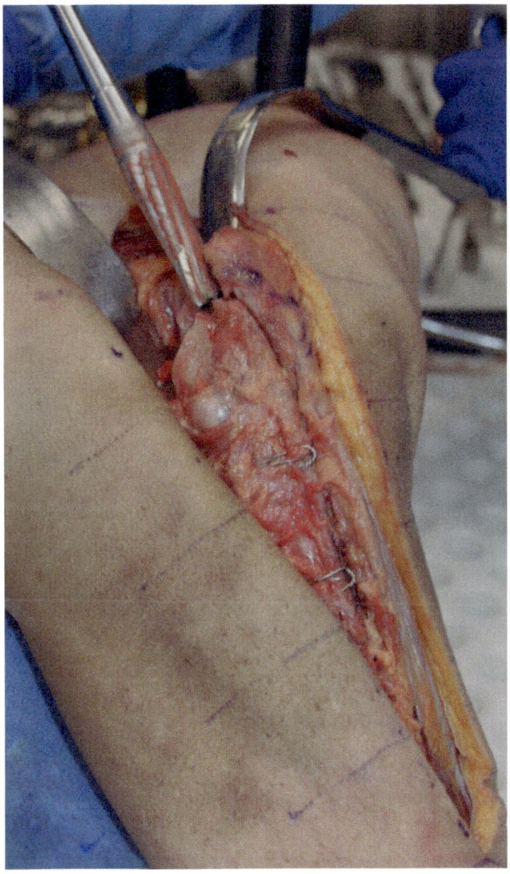

Fig. 20.8 Proximal femur preparation is initiated by reaming the femoral canal

20.4.4 Technical Considerations

20.4.4.1 Cemented Femoral Component

The difficulty of removing a cemented stem can vary depending on the type of implant and thickness of the cement mantle. Care should be taken to avoid fractures of the greater trochanter [29]. Overhanging bone and as much cement mantle as possible should be removed from the lateral aspect of the femur to reduce fracture risk.

If changing to a press-fit uncemented revision stem, the length of the ETO should allow 5–6 cm press fit distally if using a fully porous cylindrical stem. If a more contemporary tapered stem is used, only 1–2 cm of isthmus is necessary. After performing the ETO, the cement mantle can be removed in a piecemeal fashion with hand instruments or a high-speed burr. Once enough cement is removed around the implant, the implant should be extracted with an impactor. Special implant-specific extractors are often available as long as the specific implant details are known preoperatively. It is possible that a portion of cement is remaining distally to the prior extracted

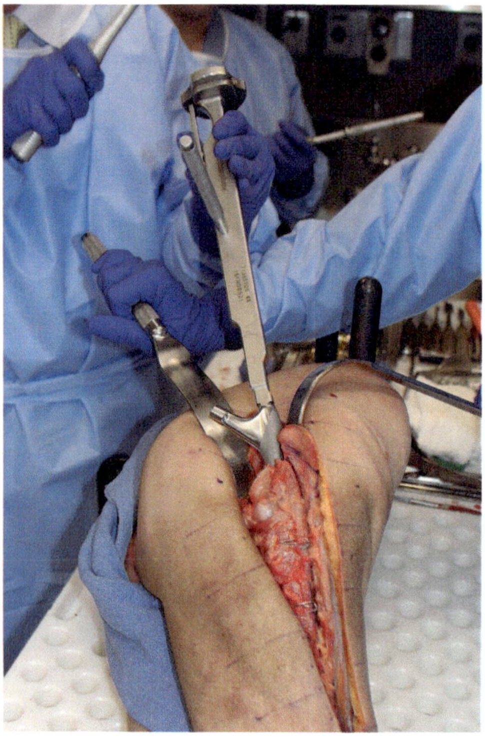

Fig. 20.9 After sizing with trial components, a press-fit uncemented revision stem can be implanted

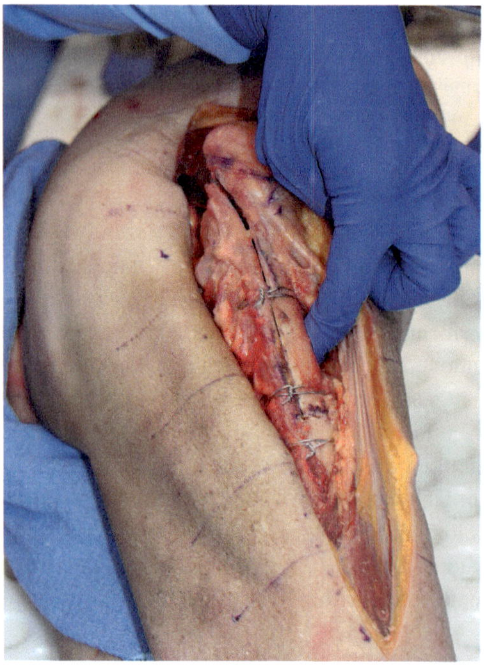

Fig. 20.10 Once the stem is implanted, it is assessed for stability and the osteotomized fragment is checked again for any dislocation or fracture signs

tip of the stem. Removal of the distal cement can be achieved with a drill and tap technique, where a hole is drilled through the center of the cement plug and a tap is inserted in the drilled hole, and backslapping. Another way to remove the distally fixed cement plug is the use of ultrasonic tools. These tools melt the cement mantle and small cement pieces can be removed. Advantage of these ultrasonic tools is the reduced fracture risk, but other complications such as thermal necrosis of the bone can occur [30].

20.4.4.2 Proximally or Extensively Coated Cementless Femoral Component

Proximally or extensively coated cementless femoral stems show the most unpredictability when they need to be removed. Therefore, it is vital to get the exact information about the type and model of the implant preoperatively. Bioreactive coatings, such as corundum-blasted surfaces, on the distal portion may provide such a strong fixation that an ETO is needed to remove the implant without causing a fracture [27]. After performing an ETO, a Gigli saw can be used to remove the medial portion of the stem for interface disruption. For the non-osteotomized part of the stem, a pencil burr can be helpful to interrupt the bone-stem interface. Removal of the implant should be performed with implant-specific instruments or slap hammers that rigidly attach to the implant.

20.4.4.3 Well-Fixed Tapered Fluted Stems

Removing a well-fixed, tapered fluted stem can be challenging due to the presence of a bow in the middle to distal portion. Therefore, using straight trephines is not possible in these cases. Secondly, the larger diameter in the more proximal part of the stem tapers to a smaller diameter. Hence, larger diameter trephines need to be used, increasing the risk of fracture at the distal portion of the stem. Additionally, these types of stems are usually used in cases where poor bone quality is already present at the time of implantation. As a result, a low threshold for performing an ETO is recommended in these cases.

20.4.4.4 Fixation Techniques

Proper fixation is essential to ensure sufficient healing of the femoral osteotomy fragment and this may be influenced by the hardware used during an ETO. Micromotion of the fragment coupled with the pull of the abductors can cause migration of the osteotomy and prevent bone growth.

The most common fixation techniques are of metallic wires or cables. A concern when using cables is the possibility that they fatigue. A cadaveric study quantitatively exploring the difference between cerclage wire and cable combinations found that the cable grip fixation was significantly more stable than the wire fixation [31]. In a retrospective review of 30 acute periprosthetic fractures requiring an ETO, there was no significant difference in time to union between Dall-Miles cable-plate fixation compared to cable-only fixation, although the cable-plate group showed significant improvements in modified Harris Hip Score with mean follow-up for cable-plate fixation and cable-only fixation of 32 months and 12 months, respectively [32].

20.4.4.5 Number of Cables Used for an ETO

The number of cables indicated is directly dependent on the length of the osteotomy [10]. To our knowledge no clinical study exists that compares the number of cables used for fixation of the osteotomized fragment. In a biomechanical study, Schwab et al. compared the efficacy of two versus three cables in nine paired cadaver legs [33]. They found no significant differences in peak force, stiffness, and axial, angular, and transverse displacement. No further data is available assessing the correlation between the number of cables used and postoperative complications. Additionally, the number of cables is also dependent on the length of the ETO [34]. The senior author of this chapter recommends using three cables in the setting of an ETO. The first cable is a prophylactic cable distally to the distal transverse osteotomy of the ETO to prevent further uncontrolled fracture and the other two cables are used for refixation of the osteotomized fragment.

20.4.5 Complications

One of the most common complications encountered in revision THA is intraoperative fractures. The Mayo Clinic joint registry reports an intraoperative fracture rate of 7.8% with revision THA [35]. The ETO should be used to mitigate the risk of intraoperative fractures while removing a femoral stem. Lerch et al. evaluated postoperative outcomes after an intraoperative fracture compared to an ETO and found significantly better clinical and radiographical outcomes in the ETO-treated patients further underscoring the utility of this procedure during revision THA [36].

20.4.6 Results

In a large series of 108 ETOs performed, 101 achieved fixation within 6 months, and although 7 did not heal, there was no displacement of the osteotomized fragment [37]. In 12 cases, a greater trochanter fracture was noted with proximal migration of 5–15 mm. One patient required trochanter reattachment. There was one failure of fixation due to infection and two due to stem subsidence and failure of osseointegration [37].

The ETO procedure also performs well with concomitant cemented impaction allografting for cases where there may be poor bone stock [38]. The direct lateral approach ETO has also shown reliable results with 89% union rates, low dislocation rates, but higher incidence of fracture and escape [39]. Selecting the appropriate implant for revision arthroplasties is essential for long-term stability and fixation. A modular stem can be used in patients with poor bone stock, although these designs have limitations. There is concern of fretting or fatigue fracture at the modular junction. In addition, 25% of patients fail to grow bony support at the modular junction 2 years postoperatively [40, 41].

20.5 Summary

Although trochanteric osteotomies are not commonly used, they offer greater exposure in complex primary and revision arthroplasty while providing a safe and reliable way to remove well-fixed implants or retained hardware. The techniques as described above should be in the repertoire of every adult joint reconstruction specialist but it should be noted that there is a substantial learning curve with these techniques. However with proper preoperative planning, appropriate implant, and hardware selection, the ETO remains a safe and useful approach to facilitate the extraction of femoral stem during revision arthroplasty surgery.

References

1. Charnley J. Arthroplasty of the hip. A new operation. Lancet (London, England). 1961;1(7187):1129–32.
2. Della Valle CJ, et al. Extended trochanteric osteotomy in complex primary total hip arthroplasty. A brief note. J Bone Joint Surg Am. 2003;85–A(12):2385–90.
3. Wieser K, Zingg P, Dora C. Trochanteric osteotomy in primary and revision total hip arthroplasty: risk factors for non-union. Arch Orthop Trauma Surg. 2012;132(5):711–7.
4. Laffosse J-M. Removal of well-fixed fixed femoral stems. Orthop Traumatol Surg Res. 2016;102:S177–87.
5. English TA. The trochanteric approach to the hip for prosthetic replacement. J Bone Joint Surg Am. 1975;57(8):1128–33.
6. Glassman AH, Engh CA, Bobyn JD. A technique of extensile exposure for total hip arthroplasty. J Arthroplast. 1987;2(1):11–21.
7. Archibeck MJ, et al. Trochanteric osteotomy and fixation during total hip arthroplasty. J Am Acad Orthop Surg. 2003;11(3):163–73.
8. Bal BS, et al. Anterior trochanteric slide osteotomy for primary total hip arthroplasty. Review of nonunion and complications. J Arthroplast. 2006;21(1):59–63.
9. Goodman S, et al. Modified sliding trochanteric osteotomy in revision total hip arthroplasty. J Arthroplast. 2004;19(8):1039–41.
10. Lakstein D, Backstein DJ, et al. Modified trochanteric slide for complex hip arthroplasty. J Arthroplast. 2010;25(3):363–8.
11. van der Grinten M, et al. Trochanteric osteotomy versus posterolateral approach: function the first year post surgery. A pilot study. BMC Musculoskelet Disord. 2011;12(1):138.
12. Hartofilakidis G, et al. Trochanteric osteotomy in total hip replacement for congenital hip disease. J Bone Joint Surg Br. 2011;93(5):601–7.
13. Lakstein D, Kosashvili Y, et al. Trochanteric slide osteotomy on previously osteotomized greater trochanters. Clin Orthop Relat Res. 2010;468(6):1630–4.
14. Nezry N, et al. Partial anterior trochanteric osteotomy in total hip arthroplasty: surgical technique and preliminary results of 127 cases. J Arthroplast. 2003;18(3):333–7.
15. Romero AC, Imrie S, Goodman SB. Sliding trochanteric osteotomy preserves favorable abductor biomechanics in revision total hip arthroplasty. J Arthroplast. 2001;16(1):55–64.
16. Emerson RH, Head WC, Higgins LL. A new method of trochanteric fixation after osteotomy in revision total hip arthroplasty with a calcar replacement femoral component. J Arthroplast. 2001;16(8 Suppl 1):76–80.
17. Beaulé PE, Shim P, Banga K. Clinical experience of Ganz surgical dislocation approach for metal-on-metal hip resurfacing. J Arthroplast. 2009;24(6):127–31.
18. Tetreault AK, McGrory BJ. Use of locking plates for fixation of the greater trochanter in patients with hip replacement. Arthroplast Today. 2016;2(4):187–92.
19. Chilvers M, et al. Trochanteric fixation in total hip arthroplasty using the S-ROM bolt and washer. J Arthroplast. 2002;17(6):740–6.
20. Langlais F, et al. Trochanteric slide osteotomy in revision total hip arthroplasty for loosening. J Bone Joint Surg Br. 2003;85(4):510–6.
21. Warren P, Thompson P, Fletcher M. Transfemoral implantation of the Wagner SL stem. Arch Orthop Trauma Surg. 2002;122(9):557–60.
22. Wagner H. [A revision prosthesis for the hip joint]. Der Orthopade. 1989;18(5):438–53. http://www.ncbi.nlm.nih.gov/pubmed/2812776. Accessed 27 Feb 2019.
23. Younger TI, et al. Extended proximal femoral osteotomy: a new technique for femoral revision arthroplasty. J Arthroplast. 1995;10(3):329–38.
24. Paprosky WG, Sporer SM. Controlled femoral fracture: easy in. J Arthroplast. 2003;18(3 Suppl 1):91–3.
25. Duncan C, Howell J, Masri B. Advanced reconstruction hip. In: Lieberman J, Berry D, editors. Advanced reconstruction hip. Rosemont: American Academy of Orthopaedic Surgeons; 2005. p. 299–310.
26. Chen WM, et al. Extended slide trochanteric osteotomy for revision total hip arthroplasty. J Bone Joint Surg Am. 2000;82(9):1215–9.
27. Miner TM, et al. The extended trochanteric osteotomy in revision hip arthroplasty: a critical review of 166 cases at mean 3-year, 9-month follow-up. J Arthroplast. 2001;16(8 Suppl 1):188–94.
28. Prudhon JL, Tardy N. Extended trochanteric osteotomy: comparison of 3 modes of fixation: metallic wires, cables, plate, about a series of 157 cases. SICOT J. 2018;4:21.
29. Paprosky WG, Weeden SH, Bowling JW. Component removal in revision total hip arthroplasty. Clin Orthop Relat Res. 2001;393:181–93.
30. Gardiner R, et al. Revision total hip arthroplasty using ultrasonically driven tools. A clinical evaluation. J Arthroplast. 1993;8(5):517–21. http://www.ncbi.nlm.nih.gov/pubmed/8245997. Accessed 1 Mar 2019.

31. Zhu Z, et al. An in-vitro biomechanical study of different fixation techniques for the extended trochanteric osteotomy in revision THA. J Orthop Surg Res. 2013;8(1):7.
32. Sheridan GA, et al. Extended trochanteric osteotomy (ETO) fixation for femoral stem revision in periprosthetic fractures: Dall–Miles plate versus cables. Eur J Orthop Surg Traumatol. 2018;28(3):471–6.
33. Schwab JH, et al. Optimal fixation for the extended trochanteric osteotomy. J Arthroplast. 2008;23(4):534–8.
34. Lakstein D, et al. The long modified extended sliding trochanteric osteotomy. Int Orthop. 2011;35(1):13–7.
35. Mardones R, et al. Extended femoral osteotomy for revision of hip arthroplasty: results and complications. J Arthroplast. 2005;20(1):79–83.
36. Lerch M, et al. Revision of total hip arthroplasty: clinical outcome of extended trochanteric osteotomy and intraoperative femoral fracture. Technol Health Care. 2008;16(4):293–300.
37. Wronka KS, Cnudde PHJ. Union rates and midterm results after Extended Trochanteric Osteotomy in Revision Hip Arthroplasty. Useful and safe technique. Acta Orthop Belg. 2017;83(1):53–6.
38. Charity J, et al. Extended trochanteric osteotomy followed by cemented impaction allografting in revision hip arthroplasty. J Arthroplast. 2013;28(1):154–60.
39. MacDonald SJ, et al. Extended trochanteric osteotomy via the direct lateral approach in revision hip arthroplasty. Clinl Orthop Relat Res. 2003;(417):210–6.
40. Cross MB, Paprosky WG. Managing femoral bone loss in revision total hip replacement: fluted tapered modular stems. Bone Joint J. 2013;95–B(11 Suppl A):95–7.
41. Ladurner A, Zdravkovic V, Grob K. Femoral bone restoration patterns in revision total hip arthroplasty using distally fixed modular tapered titanium stems and an extended trochanteric osteotomy approach. J Arthroplast. 2018;33(7):2210–7.

21 Acetabular Defects and Their Treatment

Emmanuel Gibon, Moussa Hamadouche, and Stuart B. Goodman

21.1 Indications for Acetabular Revision: Diagnosis and Symptoms

The demand for lower limb joint arthroplasty is rising at a staggering rate. Data from past studies [1, 2] and projection studies [3, 4] show that the number of revision total hip arthroplasties (THAs) will increase 137% over the next 25 years in the United States. Similar trends have been reported in the United Kingdom and Australia [5, 6]. Among revision THAs, Bozic et al. [7] have shown that acetabular component revision currently represents the third most common procedure (12.7%) following femoral component revision (13.2%) and all-component revision (41.1%). A more recent study by Gwam et al. [8] reported that acetabular component revision remained in third place (14.5%) but is now equal to head and liner revision.

The reasons for revision have changed somewhat over the last decade, as seen in Table 21.1. The difference in indication for surgery is the switch from "implant failure" in 2009 to "other mechanical problem" in 2017 for the third most common reason of acetabular component revision. This difference is likely due to the emergence of new bearing surfaces. Among these, ceramics and first- and second-generation highly cross-linked polyethylene (HXLPE) are increasingly used for primary THAs, markedly reducing wear and osteolysis [9–16]. However,

Table 21.1 Most common reasons for revisions of all components ("all revisions") and acetabular component revision in 2009 and 2017

	2009 [7]	2017 [8]
All revisions	Dislocation (22.5%) Mechanical loosening (19.7%) Infection (14.8%)	Dislocation (17.3%) Mechanical loosening (16.8%) Infection (12.8%)
Acetabular component revision	Dislocation (33.0%) Mechanical loosening (24.2%) Implant failure (10.8%)	Dislocation (24.7%) Mechanical loosening (21.7%) Other mechanical problem (18.1%)

E. Gibon (✉)
Division of Adult Reconstruction, Department of Orthopedics and Rehabilitation, University of Florida College of Medicine, University of Florida, Gainesville, FL, USA

M. Hamadouche
Clinical Orthopaedic Research Center, Centre Hospitalo-Universitaire Cochin-Port Royal, Paris, France
e-mail: moussa.hamadouche@aphp.fr

S. B. Goodman
Department of Orthopaedic Surgery, Stanford University, Stanford, CA, USA

Department of Bioengineering, Stanford University, Stanford, CA, USA
e-mail: goodbone@stanford.edu

W. R. Drescher et al. (eds.), *Advances in Specialist Hip Surgery*,
https://doi.org/10.1007/978-3-030-61830-8_21

despite dramatic reductions in implant failure, osteolysis accounts for up to 11% of revision THAs [7, 17].

Loose cemented acetabular components are generally not painful, as the loosening process is very slow; periprosthetic osteolysis results from cement fragmentation and loss of mechanical fixation, or polyethylene wear and centripetal osteolysis which undermines the cement-bone interface. The diagnosis of acetabular loosening of cemented cups is made in patients reporting a new onset of vague groin/buttock pain and limp; radiographs demonstrate progressive acetabular migration with a complete circumferential radiolucent line >2 mm in diameter. Cement fractures and conventional polyethylene (PE) wear with eccentricity of the femoral head and acetabular osteolysis may be noted.

Loose cementless acetabular components are virtually always painful, due to movement and abrasion of the stiff acetabular metallic shell directly on bone. Periprosthetic radiolucent lines, screw breakage, progressive cup migration, or entire displacement of the cup from the acetabular bone bed may be noted. These events are usually associated with sudden pain in the groin and buttock, often of a high intensity.

21.2 Preoperative Workup

An accurate, in-depth history and physical examination are critical steps in assessing the diagnosis of acetabular cup problems. Pain that is located in the groin or the buttock is usually indicative of acetabular cup issues, whereas thigh pain or referred knee pain is usually indicative of femoral component problems. The time of onset is also an important clue: unremitting pain since surgery with a noninfected cementless cup suggests that the cup has never osseointegrated. A history of delayed wound healing, large hematoma, wound drainage, unremitting fever, or chills implicates deep infection. Alternatively, periprosthetic osteolysis and wear are insidious and often not painful until catastrophic failure occurs such as with sudden cup migration, dislocation, PE liner dislodgement, or a fracture through an osteolytic area. The physical examination should start with an assessment of the patient's gait to look for a limp and to ask the location of painful areas. The skin around the wound should be carefully examined for redness, other signs of inflammation, a sinus, or drainage. The physical exam should be completed with a quick neurological examination, as lumbar spinal conditions can mimic pain emanating from the hip.

Subsequently, the surgeon obtains relevant imaging studies to assess the position of the cup and the surrounding bone structures. Plain radiographs should be ordered first as it gives the surgeon an overview of the pelvis and implant. The radiographs should include at least an anteroposterior (AP) view of the pelvis, a cross-table lateral view of the hip, and if indicated Judet oblique views [18]. Giori and Sidky [19] have also shown that lateral and high-angle oblique views of the pelvis can be useful to assess the posterior column. DeLee and Charnley created a system to report acetabular osteolysis by dividing the socket into three adjacent zones [20]. Two lines, one vertical and the other horizontal, cross at the center of the prosthetic femoral head. Zone I is designated superolateral, zone III is inferomedial, and zone II is in between. Chiang et al. [21] have shown that the pattern of osteolysis differs between cemented and cementless acetabular component. For cemented components, osteolysis predominantly occurs in DeLee zones III and I whereas osteolysis is mostly observed in DeLee zones II and III for cementless components. More advanced imaging modalities are also useful. CT scanning can be used to visualize osteolysis and bone defects around the acetabular component. However, in the presence of a metal-back prosthesis, a special acquisition called MARS (Metal Artifact Reduction Software) should be used to mitigate the brightness of the metal. MRI (as opposed to CT) is more helpful when analyzing soft-tissue masses and deficiencies; however MARS MRI is preferred when a metal-back acetabular component is present. Robinson et al. [22] have shown that CT is superior to MRI to evaluate osteolysis whereas MRI is more effective to characterize soft-tissue anomalies such as pseudotumors.

In order to help rule out an infection, a blood sample with a complete blood count, an erythrocyte sedimentation rate (ESR), and C-reactive protein (CRP) should be ordered [23]. The International Consensus Meeting (ICM) definition of Prosthetic Joint Infection (PJI) added a new scoring system in 2018 with a sensitivity of 97.7% and a specificity of 99.5% [24, 25]. This scoring system is a combination of major and minor criteria using established diagnostic tests both in the synovial fluid (white blood cell counts and neutrophil percentage) and in the blood (ESR, CRP, or D-dimer) and also new tests in the synovial fluid (alpha-defensin and leukocyte esterase). Two positive cultures with the same bacteria from the synovial fluid aspirate are considered to be diagnostic for PJI. Emerging diagnostic tests are interleukin-6 and the use of molecular technologies such as next-generation sequencing (NGS). In general, radionuclide imaging has not proven to be useful diagnostically, and therefore is not taken into account in the new PJI scoring system.

Joint fluid and saline aspirate should be cultured on enriched media for a minimum of 10 but ideally 14 days. This increases the probability of isolating and identifying slow-growing pathogens such as *Corynebacterium acnes*. In immunocompromised patients, fungal and mycobacterial cultures should also be sent. Close and frequent communication with the microbiology laboratory optimizes the diagnosis.

21.3 Classification of Acetabular Bone Loss After THR

The severity of the osteolysis can be categorized using different classifications (Table 21.2).

A useful classification should be highly descriptive, should be progressive in terms of bone loss, and should help the surgeon in the decision-making process for reconstruction. Given these goals, the Paprosky classification fulfills these requirements and is the most widely used one at present.

Table 21.2 Current classifications for acetabular defects

Classification	Assessment
Engh et al. [26]	Is based on the integrity of the rim and the bed
Gustilo and Pasternak [27]	Is based on the integrity of the acetabular walls
D'Antonio et al. [28] (a.k.a. AAOS)	Is based on acetabular segmental and cavitary deficiencies
Gross et al. [29]	Is based on contained/uncontained bone loss including the percentage of bone defect of the acetabulum
Saleh et al. [30]	Is based on bone defects after removal of the acetabular implant
Paprosky et al. [31]	Is based on the presence or absence of key supporting structures of the acetabulum • **Type I:** has the least bone loss; the acetabulum has a supportive rim and demonstrates no significant osteolysis of the teardrop or ischium • **Type II:** acetabular bone loss is more extensive; there is loss of bone superiorly in the dome, and moderate bone loss in the ischium and inferior teardrop. The acetabular rim is still capable of providing support for a metallic shell. The subtypes denote how the previous cup has migrated: superomedially (IIa), superolaterally (IIb), or directly medially (IIc) • **Type III:** defects are the most extensive. Bone loss has destroyed the dome superiorly such that cup migration is greater than 2 cm; furthermore, the bone loss superiorly and in the ischium inferiorly are to such a degree that the rim alone cannot support an acetabular shell (IIIa). The IIIb defects are even more extensive such that both rim deficiency and bone ingrowth will not be supported • **Type IV:** pelvic discontinuity

21.4 Basic Tenets to Guide the Reconstruction

Reconstruction of the acetabulum in the setting of revision THA should be carefully prepared with a clear preoperative plan. The radiographs should be current and scaled appropriately (100%) for templating, and the appropriate implants and other hardware should be available and compatible with existing retained implants (e.g., femoral head and Morse taper need to be compatible). As some cases can be challenging, multiple assistants are usually warranted. As the course of surgery can suddenly change due to an intraoperative complication, it is recommended to have a backup plan and appropriate instrumentation and hardware. The extent of the intraoperative bone loss is often worse than the size predicted from the preoperative X-rays, especially behind the acetabulum [32]. Moreover, an unexpected fracture or pelvic discontinuity can be discovered or created while performing the revision, requiring changing the plan during surgery.

Given the fact that reconstructive procedures are usually long, patients often undergo general anesthesia together with spinal anesthesia in order to be comfortably positioned and limit blood loss by decreasing systemic blood pressure and peripheral vascular resistance. The estimated blood loss for isolated acetabular revision is approximately 650 mL and for both acetabular and femoral revision around 1100 mL [33]. These authors also showed that the use of intravenous tranexamic acid significantly decreased the drop in hemoglobin for isolated acetabular component revision (as well as for major revisions). Other studies have also demonstrated the efficiency of intraoperative red blood cell-retrieval devices to mitigate blood loss [34, 35].

It is recommended to use a surgical approach that allows for a large and extensile exposure for both the acetabular and the femoral implants. A posterior approach is preferred, allowing for a wide exposure and a clear view of the upper third and medullary canal of the femur. This approach also allows for distal extension if a femoral osteotomy is needed. A trochanteric osteotomy is performed when there is nonunion of a previous trochanteric osteotomy, or when even wider exposure is necessary.

The surgeon should remove any existing sinus tracks, all the way to the implant or joint space. If the surgical approach is through old nonvascular scar tissue, it should be excised. The surgeon then excises all necrotic and inflammatory soft tissue until reaching normal healthy tissue. The synovectomy should be circumferential, during and after implant removal. If present, the surgeon should excise existing bone sequestra, perforating bone fistulas and impediments such as heterotopic ossifications should be excised. It is important to take five joint fluid and tissue samples for bacterial analysis.

For a cementless acetabular cup, an algorithm based on different criteria [36, 37] has been elaborated in order to help the surgeon in the decision-making process as to whether or not to retain the cup and only change the liner, or revise the entire cup (Table 21.3).

Naudie and Engh reported that liner exchange is indicated when there is approximately 1.5 mm of liner thickness remaining [38]. Recently, Narkbunnam et al. [39] showed that liner exchange and cementing a new liner provided satisfactory outcomes. For cementing a liner into an existing acceptable shell Callaghan et al. reported that liners should be chosen to allow for a 2–4 mm cement mantle between the outer liner and inner surface of the cementless shell [40]. If the liner is smooth, it should be scored to allow cement to penetrate into ridges for added fixation.

Table 21.3 Decision-making algorithm for cementless acetabular cups [36, 37]

Cup stable		Cup unstable
Answer the following: (a) Is the cup position acceptable? (b) Is the cup survivorship acceptable? (c) Is the cup modular? (d) Is the cup without damage? (e) Is the locking mechanism intact? (f) Can a liner of sufficient thickness be inserted?		↓
YES to all above	NO to at least 1 above	
= Type 1	= Type 2	= Type 3
Retain cup Modular liner exchange Debride lesions Bone grafting if possible	Cup revision Debride nonviable tissue and osteolytic lesions Bone grafting	

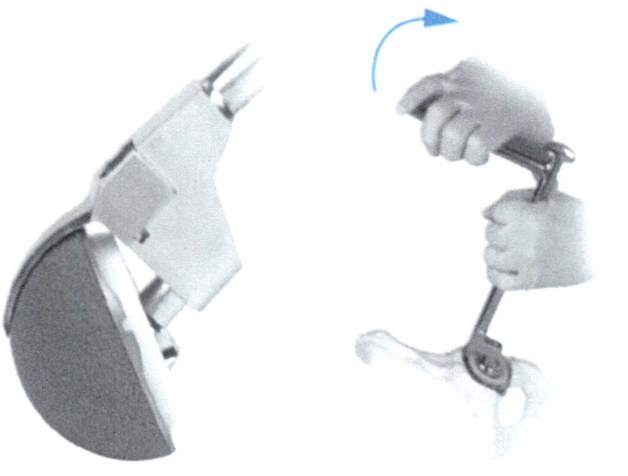

Fig. 21.1 The explant acetabular cup removal system (used with permission from Zimmer Biomet, Warsaw, IN, USA)

When a full acetabular revision is indicated, one starts by freeing the edges of the implant with a curved chisel. Then a device such as the Explant Acetabular Cup Removal System (Zimmer Biomet, Warsaw, IN, USA) (Fig. 21.1) or similar device, or a series of chisels for the acetabulum, can be used. Adelani et al. have shown that the explant system allowed less bone loss when removing well-fixed acetabular components than Aufranc gouges [41]. Then, after implant removal, inter-positional fibrous membranes should be removed using a curette and the acetabulum prepared with reamers in order to expose healthy, bleeding bone. At this time the Paprosky classification can be used to assess the extent of the defects.

For a cemented acetabular cup, the cup is removed with chisels. It is mandatory to remove all cement and foreign material (screws, bone-graft substitutes, old infected graft), being mindful of any endopelvic cement. A preoperative CT angiography might be necessary to assess the localization of blood vessels with regard to any endopelvic hardware or cement.

The reconstruction then proceeds according to the following principles:

1. The acetabular reconstruction must be focused on obtaining initial robust mechanical stability.
2. If possible, the goal is to restore the normal hip center of rotation to facilitate satisfactory long-term outcomes [42].
3. Contained loss of bone stock (cavitary defects) can be successfully treated by impaction grafting with morselized allograft bone [43]. The host bone must be viable for this technique to be successful; Paprosky type I and II cases are ideal indications.
4. An entirely circumferential rim fit is not mandatory but preferable. When contact between viable bleeding host bone and a porous coated acetabular component is greater than 50% and mechanical stability can be achieved, then osseointegration is expected [44–48]. Moreover, numerous screws or pegs are highly desirable, as bone ingrowth is most extensive around these devices.
5. When 50% contact cannot be obtained between host bone and acetabular component, the surgeon has several options including the use of an acetabular reinforcement ring [49–51] or acetabular augments and screws [52, 53]. This is usually the case for Paprosky type IIb and IIIa.
6. Type IIIb defects are extremely demanding. Rarely, some cases are performed in two stages, first restoring bone stock and second the final reconstruction. Supplemental support is always necessary such as acetabular rings, cup-cage constructs, custom-made implants, or even massive tumor surgery implants (Fig. 21.2).
7. Pelvic discontinuity is perhaps one of the most challenging cases to manage (Fig. 21.3). To address this challenge, two techniques are usually performed involving (A) stabilization or effective bypass of the discontinuity and using the reconstruction techniques mentioned above [54, 55] or (B) using the acetabular distraction technique (Fig. 21.4) to wedge a large porous metallic cup (jumbo cup) [56, 57].
8. To ensure extra stability, large femoral heads (32 mm or more) should be used according to the size of the socket to allow sufficient polyethylene thickness. Haw et al. [58] showed that with a 3.9 mm cross-linked polyethylene (XLPE) thin liner, wear rate of 36 mm femoral head does not increase significantly. However, most surgeons prefer polyethylene thickness

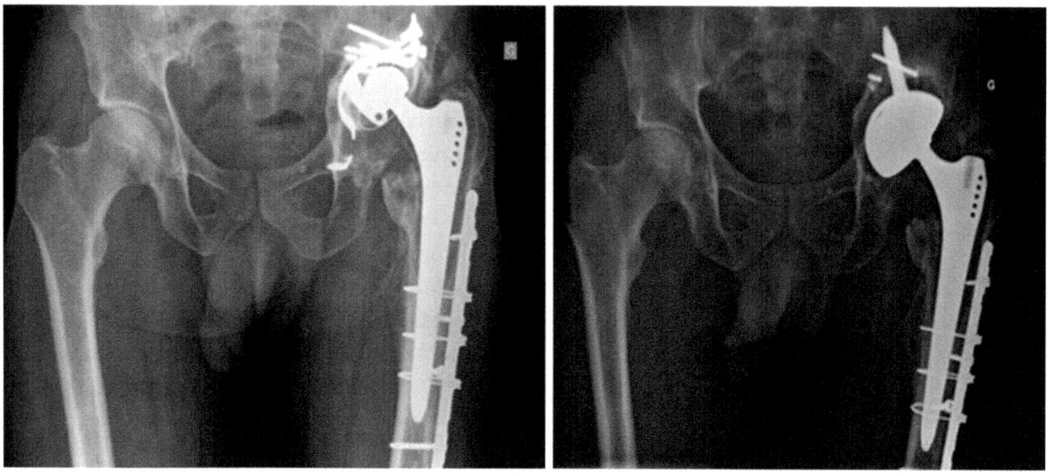

Fig. 21.2 Example of a Paprosky type IIIb acetabular defect of the left hip. The revision was performed using a tumor surgery implant: a coned acetabular ("ice-cream cone") prosthesis

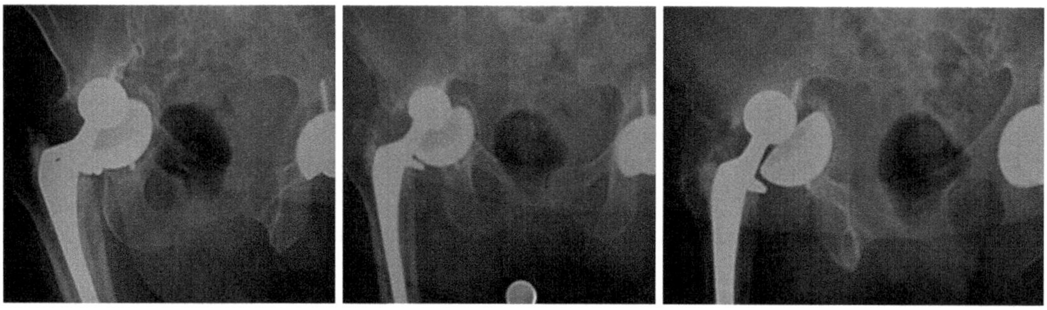

Fig. 21.3 Example of a Paprosky type IV acetabular defect (pelvic discontinuity) at the right hip

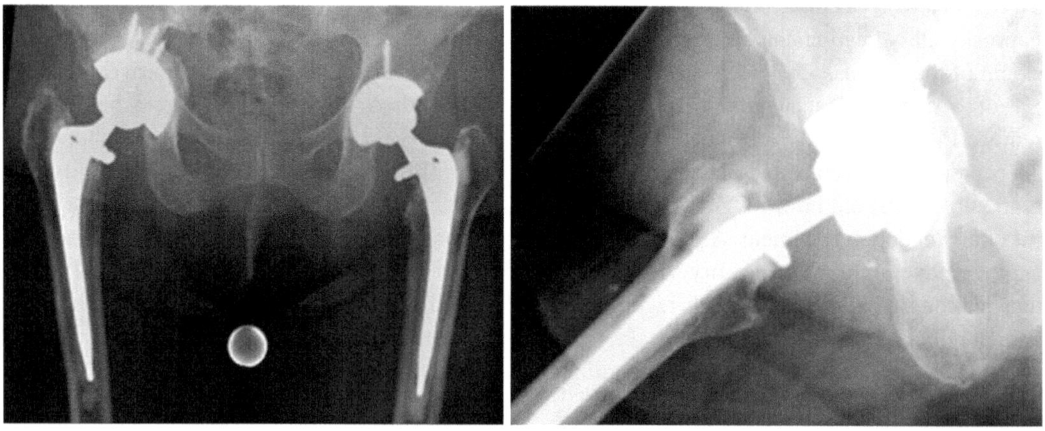

Fig. 21.4 The distraction technique with impaction grafting used to revise the case presented in Fig. 21.3

to be greater than 4 mm. If instability is still worrisome, implants such as constrained liners, dual mobility, or tripolar constructs can be used.

9. Postoperative bracing is controversial. Bracing theoretically limits the range of motion (thereby protecting the newly reconstructed hip from dislocation) and facilitates soft-tissue healing.

21.5 Options for Restoring Lost Bone

1. Bone autograft represents the best material as it is osteoconductive, osteoinductive, and osteogenic. As a living material, autograft also provides osteogenic cells and growth factors. The drawback is that the supply is limited either to remote harvesting sites (e.g., iliac crest or proximal tibia) or from local tissues harvested while performing the revision (e.g., acetabular reaming). However, harvesting bone from remote sites is associated with up to 8.6% major complications [59]. Therefore, to avoid this issue, a new technique of bone marrow aspiration has been developed. Bone marrow cells are aspirated from the iliac crest and then concentrated using a centrifuge [60–62]. Hernigou et al. have shown that bone marrow aspiration is associated with ten times less complication than the usual open technique [63]. Once the cells have been concentrated they can be added to a scaffold (e.g., demineralized bone matrix or allograft croutons), which will subsequently fill out the defect. This technique can be applied to an isolated liner exchange in a well-fixed cup with a threatening small area of osteolysis when the latter is treated with bone grafting [64].
2. An alternative to autologous bone graft is freeze-dried allograft cancellous bone croutons. These are obtained from cadavers, then prepared and shaped by companies, and sold as small rectangular pieces of bone. These croutons can be mixed with harvested bone marrow cells or acetabular reaming, then placed in the acetabular defect, and compacted with a "reverse reaming" technique. Etienne et al. [65] reported that this technique provided a stable reconstruction in 98% of cases at a mean of 7-year follow-up.
3. Structural allografts represent another option for acetabular reconstruction. "Structural" means that a larger bulk piece of bone is used. The major concern is the fate of the allograft with subsequent risk of failure due to resorption and collapse leading to implant loosening. Structural allografts are provided by a bone bank and can be a femoral head [66, 67] or part of the distal femur [68], or even an acetabulum. Jasty and Harris [69] reported a failure rate of 32% at 6 years with a mean time to failure of 5.4 years. Failure was attributed to marked resorption of the graft in all but one of the failed cases. Garbuz et al. [42] reported a series of 38 hips that showed successful results at a mean of 7.5 years when an acetabular reinforcement device (cage) supported the structural allograft; most of the reconstructions without a device failed. Therefore, these authors advocated the use of an acetabular reinforcement ring in association with a structural allograft. Presently, structural porous metallic augments fixed with screws (Fig. 21.5) have fulfilled most of the previous indications for structural allografts, except in younger patients when long-term bone restoration is important.
4. The last option to restore the lost bone is the use of bone substitutes such as calcium sulfate, calcium phosphate/carbonates, or hydroxyapatite (HA) products. They have weak mechanical properties and therefore are usually not used alone for acetabular reconstruction. Tanaka and colleagues [70, 71] used HA granules mixed with autologous bone graft and showed satisfactory clinical and radiologic results at 12.8 years when used with a Kerboull acetabular reinforcement device.

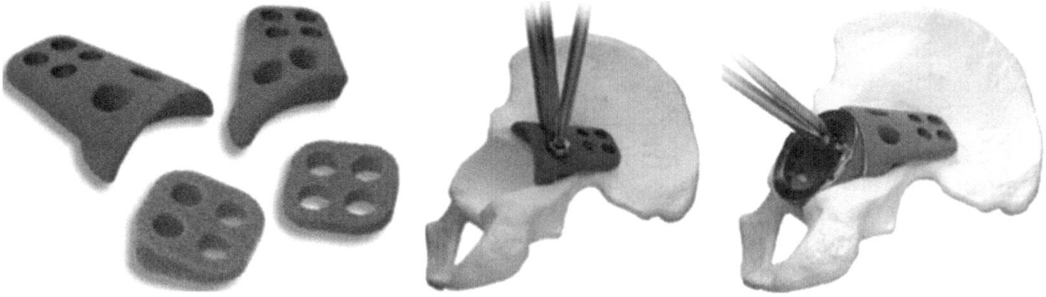

Fig. 21.5 Trabecular metal augments (used with permission from Zimmer Biomet, Warsaw, IN, USA)

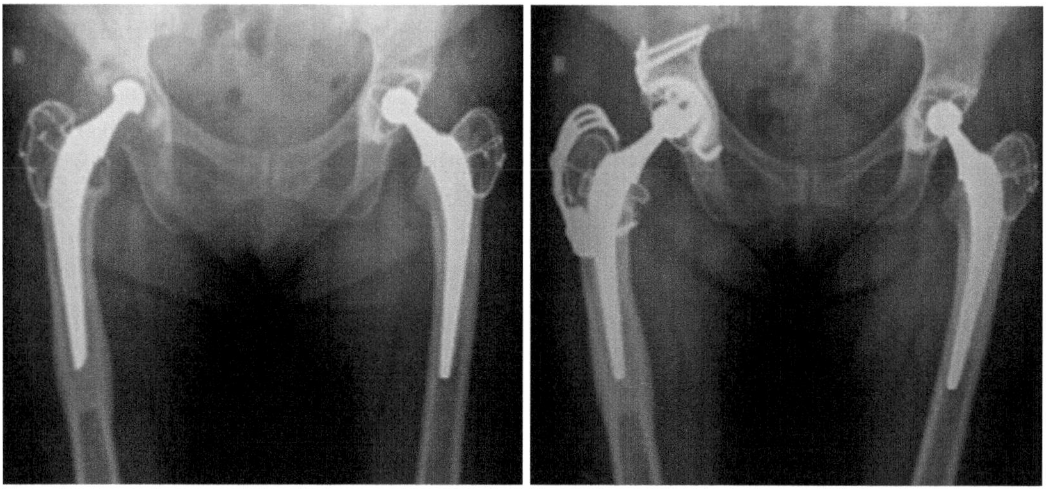

Fig. 21.6 Example of a Paprosky type IIIa acetabular defect at the right hip. The reconstruction was performed using structural bone allograft and the Kerboull acetabular reinforcement ring

21.6 Options for Implants

To manage acetabular defects, various techniques using different implants have been reported. The use of tantalum porous metal implants [53, 72–75], Burch-Schneider cage [76–79], Müller ring [80], Ganz ring [81], Kerboull ring [82] (Fig. 21.6), morselized bone graft and metal mesh technique developed by Sloof et al. [83], and recently customized cages [84] has been reported. However, cementless cups and screws associated with impaction grafting are the mainstay of reconstruction.

To ensure robust and reliable osseointegration, newer implants are made of metallic shells with porous coatings mimicking cancellous bone and are associated with numerous holes for screw fixation. These implants provide a friction fit and immediate strong mechanical stability. Batuyong et al. [74] showed 92% osseointegration at 37 months for Paprosky type III acetabular defects using porous tantalum implants.

In line with this philosophy of immediate robust mechanical stability using cementless implants, acetabular augments are now increasingly used. They can be made of porous tantalum, titanium, or other metals [85]. These devices avoid using structural allografts, and provide mechanical structural support like bone graft. A large number of publications have substantiated their efficacy and safety for acetabular reconstruction [53, 75, 86]. The cup-cage technique (Fig. 21.7)

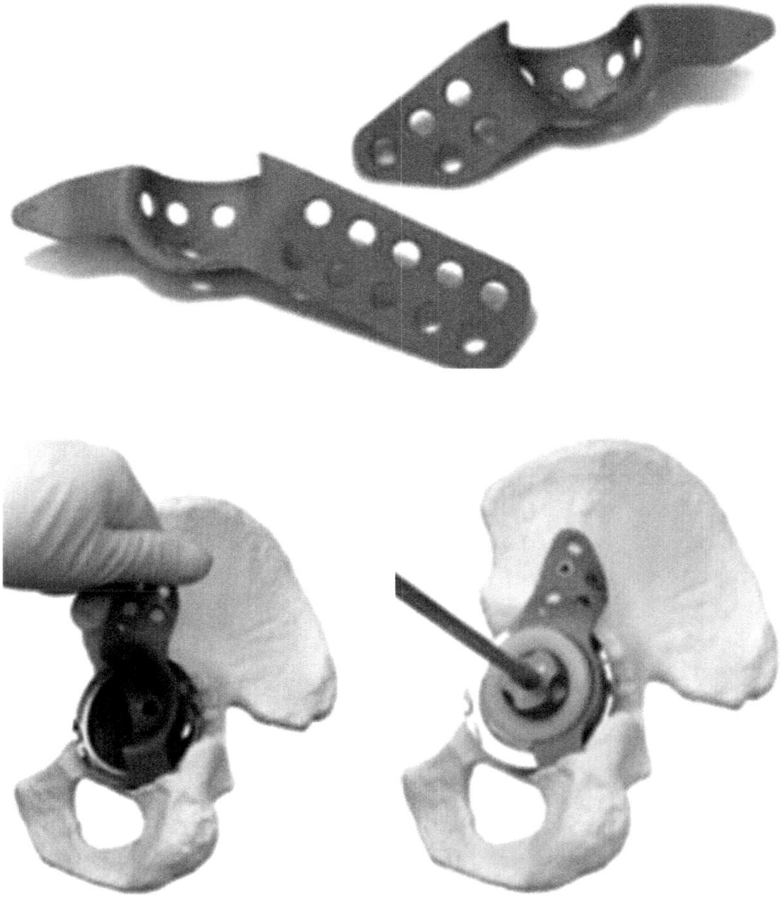

Fig. 21.7 The cup-cage construct (used with permission from Zimmer Biomet, Warsaw, IN, USA)

is also based on obtaining initial mechanical stability provided by a porous acetabular shell [87]. The technique consists of a trabecular metal (TM) acetabular shell and an ilioischial antiprotrusio cage placed over the cup (full cup-cage construct). The desired outcome of this construct was based on the fact that no bone ingrowth could be obtained into the cage whereas a TM acetabular shell enables and promotes bone ingrowth when placed first. Kosashvili et al. [88] reported on a series of 26 cases of acetabular revision including 24 patients with pelvic discontinuity and severe acetabular bone defects (a mean of 15.8% contact with bleeding host bone). After filling the defects with morselized bone graft, the cup and the cage were placed. A polyethylene liner was then cemented into the cage. At a mean of 3.7-year follow-up, the authors reported 3 (11.5%) cases of construct migration. Later on, the same group presented an extended follow-up study of the initial series and compared it with a group of cases with pelvic discontinuity reconstructed with a conventional cage (without trabecular metal) [89]. The cup-cage group had a survivorship of 87.2% whereas the conventional cage group had a survivorship of 49.9% at 5.8 years and 6.8 years, respectively. Similar outcomes were reported by Amenabar et al. [90] who treated Gross type IV (uncontained loss of bone stock involving >50% of the acetabulum and affecting both columns) and Gross type V (pelvic discontinuity) acetabular deficiencies. The authors showed a 10-year survival rate of 85%.

These constructs have replaced traditional stainless steel roof rings [91] and cages that often failed later due to lack of osseointegration.

21.7 Summary

An acetabular revision surgery should be carefully planned and all instrument, prosthetic, and biologic needs anticipated preoperatively. After ruling out infection, the potential reconstruction is assessed preoperatively and confirmed intraoperatively using the Paprosky classification. Minor defects can be treated with impaction grafting with a cementless cup and screws, which provide satisfactory stability. For larger major defects, the use of porous metal implants (augments and shells) and occasionally cup-cage or custom implants is indicated. On very rare occasions, with massive bone loss, reconstruction can be staged.

References

1. Kurtz SM, Ong KL, Schmier J, Zhao K, Mowat F, Lau E. Primary and revision arthroplasty surgery caseloads in the United States from 1990 to 2004. J Arthroplast. 2009;24(2):195–203. https://doi.org/10.1016/j.arth.2007.11.015.
2. Kurtz S, Mowat F, Ong K, Chan N, Lau E, Halpern M. Prevalence of primary and revision total hip and knee arthroplasty in the United States from 1990 through 2002. J Bone Joint Surg Am. 2005;87(7):1487–97. https://doi.org/10.2106/JBJS.D.02441.
3. Kurtz SM, Ong KL, Lau E, Bozic KJ. Impact of the economic downturn on total joint replacement demand in the United States: updated projections to 2021. J Bone Joint Surg Am. 2014;96(8):624–30. https://doi.org/10.2106/JBJS.M.00285.
4. Kurtz S, Ong K, Lau E, Mowat F, Halpern M. Projections of primary and revision hip and knee arthroplasty in the United States from 2005 to 2030. J Bone Joint Surg Am. 2007;89(4):780–5. https://doi.org/10.2106/JBJS.F.00222.
5. Inacio MCS, Graves SE, Pratt NL, Roughead EE, Nemes S. Increase in total joint arthroplasty projected from 2014 to 2046 in Australia: a conservative local model with international implications. Clin Orthop Relat Res. 2017;475(8):2130–7. https://doi.org/10.1007/s11999-017-5377-7.
6. Patel A, Pavlou G, Mújica-Mota RE, Toms AD. The epidemiology of revision total knee and hip arthroplasty in England and Wales: a comparative analysis with projections for the United States. A study using the National Joint Registry dataset. Bone Joint J. 2015;97-B(8):1076–81. https://doi.org/10.1302/0301-620X.97B8.35170.
7. Bozic KJ, Kurtz SM, Lau E, Ong K, Vail TP, Berry DJ. The epidemiology of revision total hip arthroplasty in the United States. J Bone Joint Surg Am. 2009;91(1):128–33. https://doi.org/10.2106/JBJS.H.00155.
8. Gwam CU, Mistry JB, Mohamed NS, Thomas M, Bigart KC, Mont MA, et al. Current epidemiology of revision total hip arthroplasty in the United States: National Inpatient Sample 2009 to 2013. J Arthroplast. 2017;32(7):2088–92. https://doi.org/10.1016/j.arth.2017.02.046.
9. Hanna SA, Somerville L, McCalden RW, Naudie DD, MacDonald SJ. Highly cross-linked polyethylene decreases the rate of revision of total hip arthroplasty compared with conventional polyethylene at 13 years' follow-up. Bone Joint J. 2016;98-B(1):28–32. https://doi.org/10.1302/0301-620X.98B1.36527.
10. Shen C, Tang ZH, Hu JZ, Zou GY, Xiao RC, Yan DX. Does cross-linked polyethylene decrease the revision rate of total hip arthroplasty compared with conventional polyethylene? A meta-analysis. Orthop Traumatol Surg Res. 2014;100(7):745–50. https://doi.org/10.1016/j.otsr.2014.07.015.
11. Bitsch RG, Loidolt T, Heisel C, Ball S, Schmalzried TP. Reduction of osteolysis with use of Marathon cross-linked polyethylene. A concise follow-up, at a minimum of five years, of a previous report. J Bone Joint Surg Am. 2008;90(7):1487–91. https://doi.org/10.2106/JBJS.F.00991.
12. Epinette J-A, Jolles-Haeberli BM. Comparative results from a national joint registry hip data set of a new cross-linked annealed polyethylene vs. both conventional polyethylene and ceramic bearings. J Arthroplast. 2016;31(7):1483–91. https://doi.org/10.1016/j.arth.2015.12.041.
13. Scemama C, Anract P, Dumaine V, Babinet A, Courpied JP, Hamadouche M. Does vitamin E-blended polyethylene reduce wear in primary total hip arthroplasty: a blinded randomised clinical trial. Int Orthop. 2017;41(6):1113–8. https://doi.org/10.1007/s00264-016-3320-2.
14. Scemama C, Dora C, Langlois J, Hamadouche M. Minimum five-year wear rate of metal-on-highly cross-linked polyethylene in primary total hip arthroplasty. Int Orthop. 2015;39(6):1051–5. https://doi.org/10.1007/s00264-014-2609-2.
15. Mu Z, Tian J, Wu T, Yang J, Pei F. A systematic review of radiological outcomes of highly cross-linked polyethylene versus conventional polyethylene in total hip arthroplasty. Int Orthop. 2009;33(3):599–604. https://doi.org/10.1007/s00264-008-0716-7.
16. Oral E, Muratoglu OK. Vitamin E diffused, highly crosslinked UHMWPE: a review. Int Orthop. 2011;35(2):215–23. https://doi.org/10.1007/s00264-010-1161-y.
17. Delaunay C, Hamadouche M, Girard J, Duhamel A, So FG. What are the causes for failures of primary hip arthroplasties in France? Clin Orthop Relat Res. 2013;471(12):3863–9. https://doi.org/10.1007/s11999-013-2935-5.
18. Thomas A, Epstein NJ, Stevens K, Goodman SB. Utility of Judet oblique X-rays in preoperative

assessment of acetabular periprosthetic osteolysis: a preliminary study. Am J Orthop. 2007;36(7):E107–10.
19. Giori NJ, Sidky AO. Lateral and high-angle oblique radiographs of the pelvis aid in diagnosing pelvic discontinuity after total hip arthroplasty. J Arthroplast. 2011;26(1):110–2. https://doi.org/10.1016/j.arth.2009.12.006.
20. DeLee JG, Charnley J. Radiological demarcation of cemented sockets in total hip replacement. Clin Orthop Relat Res. 1976;(121):20–32.
21. Chiang PP, Burke DW, Freiberg AA, Rubash HE. Osteolysis of the pelvis: evaluation and treatment. Clin Orthop Relat Res. 2003;417:164–74. https://doi.org/10.1097/01.blo.0000096816.78689.e5.
22. Robinson E, Henckel J, Sabah S, Satchithananda K, Skinner J, Hart A. Cross-sectional imaging of metal-on-metal hip arthroplasties. Can we substitute MARS MRI with CT? Acta Orthop. 2014;85(6):577–84. https://doi.org/10.3109/17453674.2014.964618.
23. Lee K-J, Goodman SB. Identification of periprosthetic joint infection after total hip arthroplasty. J Orthop Transl. 2015;3(1):21–5. https://doi.org/10.1016/j.jot.2014.10.001.
24. Goswami K, Parvizi J, Maxwell Courtney P. Current recommendations for the diagnosis of acute and chronic PJI for hip and knee-cell counts, alpha-defensin, leukocyte esterase, next-generation sequencing. Curr Rev Musculoskelet Med. 2018;11(3):428–38. https://doi.org/10.1007/s12178-018-9513-0.
25. Parvizi J, Tan TL, Goswami K, Higuera C, Della Valle C, Chen AF, et al. The 2018 definition of periprosthetic hip and knee infection: an evidence-based and validated criteria. J Arthroplast. 2018;33(5):1309–14.e2. https://doi.org/10.1016/j.arth.2018.02.078.
26. Engh CA, Glassman AH, Griffin WL, Mayer JG. Results of cementless revision for failed cemented total hip arthroplasty. Clin Orthop Relat Res. 1988;(235):91–110.
27. Gustilo RB, Pasternak HS. Revision total hip arthroplasty with titanium ingrowth prosthesis and bone grafting for failed cemented femoral component loosening. Clin Orthop Relat Res. 1988;(235):111–9.
28. D'Antonio JA, Capello WN, Borden LS, Bargar WL, Bierbaum BF, Boettcher WG, et al. Classification and management of acetabular abnormalities in total hip arthroplasty. Clin Orthop Relat Res. 1989;(243):126–37.
29. Gross AE, Allan DG, Catre M, Garbuz DS, Stockley I. Bone grafts in hip replacement surgery. The pelvic side. Orthop Clin North Am. 1993;24(4):679–95.
30. Saleh KJ, Holtzman J, Gafni Asaleh L, Jaroszynski G, Wong P, Woodgate I, et al. Development, test reliability and validation of a classification for revision hip arthroplasty. J Orthop Res. 2001;19(1):50–6. https://doi.org/10.1016/S0736-0266(00)00021-8.
31. Paprosky WG, Perona PG, Lawrence JM. Acetabular defect classification and surgical reconstruction in revision arthroplasty. A 6-year follow-up evaluation. J Arthroplast. 1994;9(1):33–44.
32. Dumbleton JH, Manley MT, Edidin AA. A literature review of the association between wear rate and osteolysis in total hip arthroplasty. J Arthroplast. 2002;17(5):649–61.
33. Peck J, Kepecs DM, Mei B, Safir OA, Backstein D, Gross AE, et al. The effect of preoperative administration of intravenous tranexamic acid during revision hip arthroplasty: a retrospective study. J Bone Joint Surg Am. 2018;100(17):1509–16. https://doi.org/10.2106/JBJS.17.01212.
34. Greenky M, Shaner J, Rasouli MR, Han S-B, Parvizi J, Hozack WJ. Intraoperative blood salvage in revision total hip arthroplasty: who benefits most? J Arthroplast. 2014;29(6):1298–300. https://doi.org/10.1016/j.arth.2013.12.009.
35. Zarin J, Grosvenor D, Schurman D, Goodman S. Efficacy of intraoperative blood collection and reinfusion in revision total hip arthroplasty. J Bone Joint Surg Am. 2003;85-A(11):2147–51.
36. Maloney WJ, Paprosky W, Engh CA, Rubash H. Surgical treatment of pelvic osteolysis. Clin Orthop Relat Res. 2001;393:78–84.
37. Rubash HE, Sinha RK, Paprosky W, Engh CA, Maloney WJ. A new classification system for the management of acetabular osteolysis after total hip arthroplasty. Instr Course Lect. 1999;48:37–42.
38. Naudie DDR, Engh CA. Surgical management of polyethylene wear and pelvic osteolysis with modular uncemented acetabular components. J Arthroplast. 2004;19(4 Suppl 1):124–9.
39. Narkbunnam R, Amanatullah DF, Electricwala AJ, Huddleston JI, Maloney WJ, Goodman SB. Outcome of 4 surgical treatments for wear and osteolysis of cementless acetabular components. J Arthroplast. 2017;32(9):2799–805. https://doi.org/10.1016/j.arth.2017.04.028.
40. Callaghan JJ, Hennessy DW, Liu SS, Goetz KE, Heiner AD. Cementing acetabular liners into secure cementless shells for polyethylene wear provides durable mid-term fixation. Clin Orthop Relat Res. 2012;470(11):3142–7. https://doi.org/10.1007/s11999-012-2380-x.
41. Adelani MA, Goodman SB, Maloney WJ, Huddleston JI. Removal of well-fixed cementless acetabular components in revision total hip arthroplasty. Orthopedics. 2016;39(2):e280–4. https://doi.org/10.3928/01477447-20160129-04.
42. Garbuz D, Morsi E, Gross AE. Revision of the acetabular component of a total hip arthroplasty with a massive structural allograft. Study with a minimum five-year follow-up. J Bone Joint Surg Am. 1996;78(5):693–7.
43. Busch VJJF, Gardeniers JWM, Verdonschot N, Slooff TJJH, Schreurs BW. Acetabular reconstruction with impaction bone-grafting and a cemented cup in patients younger than fifty years old: a concise follow-up, at twenty to twenty-eight years, of a previous report. J Bone Joint Surg Am. 2011;93(4):367–71. https://doi.org/10.2106/JBJS.I.01532.

44. Della Valle CJ, Berger RA, Rosenberg AG, Galante JO. Cementless acetabular reconstruction in revision total hip arthroplasty. Clin Orthop Relat Res. 2004;(420):96–100.
45. Hallstrom BR, Golladay GJ, Vittetoe DA, Harris WH. Cementless acetabular revision with the Harris-Galante porous prosthesis. Results after a minimum of ten years of follow-up. J Bone Joint Surg Am. 2004;86-A(5):1007–11.
46. Park DK, Della Valle CJ, Quigley L, Moric M, Rosenberg AG, Galante JO. Revision of the acetabular component without cement. A concise follow-up, at twenty to twenty-four years, of a previous report. J Bone Joint Surg Am. 2009;91(2):350–5. https://doi.org/10.2106/JBJS.H.00302.
47. Templeton JE, Callaghan JJ, Goetz DD, Sullivan PM, Johnston RC. Revision of a cemented acetabular component to a cementless acetabular component. A ten to fourteen-year follow-up study. J Bone Joint Surg Am. 2001;83-A(11):1706–11.
48. Trumm BN, Callaghan JJ, Liu SS, Goetz DD, Johnston RC. Revision with cementless acetabular components: a concise follow-up, at a minimum of twenty years, of previous reports. J Bone Joint Surg Am. 2012;94(21):2001–4. https://doi.org/10.2106/JBJS.L.00058.
49. Boscainos PJ, Kellett CF, Maury AC, Backstein D, Gross AE. Management of periacetabular bone loss in revision hip arthroplasty. Clin Orthop Relat Res. 2007;465:159–65. https://doi.org/10.1097/BLO.0b013e3181560c6c.
50. Garcia-Cimbrelo E. Porous-coated cementless acetabular cups in revision surgery: a 6- to 11-year follow-up study. J Arthroplast. 1999;14(4):397–406.
51. Goodman S, Saastamoinen H, Shasha N, Gross A. Complications of ilioischial reconstruction rings in revision total hip arthroplasty. J Arthroplast. 2004;19(4):436–46.
52. Jenkins DR, Odland AN, Sierra RJ, Hanssen AD, Lewallen DG. Minimum five-year outcomes with porous tantalum acetabular cup and augment construct in complex revision total hip arthroplasty. J Bone Joint Surg Am. 2017;99(10):e49. https://doi.org/10.2106/JBJS.16.00125.
53. Grappiolo G, Loppini M, Longo UG, Traverso F, Mazziotta G, Denaro V. Trabecular metal augments for the management of Paprosky Type III defects without pelvic discontinuity. J Arthroplast. 2015;30(6):1024–9. https://doi.org/10.1016/j.arth.2015.01.001.
54. Schwarzkopf R, Ihn HE, Ries MD. Pelvic discontinuity: modern techniques and outcomes for treating pelvic disassociation. Hip Int. 2015;25(4):368–74. https://doi.org/10.5301/hipint.5000270.
55. Abdelnasser MK, Klenke FM, Whitlock P, Khalil AM, Khalifa YE, Ali HM, et al. Management of pelvic discontinuity in revision total hip arthroplasty: a review of the literature. Hip Int. 2015;25(2):120–6. https://doi.org/10.5301/hipint.5000201.
56. Sheth NP, Melnic CM, Paprosky WG. Acetabular distraction: an alternative for severe acetabular bone loss and chronic pelvic discontinuity. Bone Joint J. 2014;96-B(11 Suppl A):36–42. https://doi.org/10.1302/0301-620X.96B11.34455.
57. Brown NM, Hellman M, Haughom BH, Shah RP, Sporer SM, Paprosky WG. Acetabular distraction: an alternative approach to pelvic discontinuity in failed total hip replacement. Bone Joint J. 2014;96-B(11 Suppl A):73–7. https://doi.org/10.1302/0301-620X.96B11.34316.
58. Haw JG, Battenberg AK, Huang D-CT, Schmalzried TP. Wear rates of larger-diameter cross-linked polyethylene at 5 to 13 years: does liner thickness or component position matter? J Arthroplast. 2017;32(4):1381–6. https://doi.org/10.1016/j.arth.2016.11.022.
59. Younger EM, Chapman MW. Morbidity at bone graft donor sites. J Orthop Trauma. 1989;3(3):192–5.
60. Hernigou J, Picard L, Alves A, Silvera J, Homma Y, Hernigou P. Understanding bone safety zones during bone marrow aspiration from the iliac crest: the sector rule. Int Orthop. 2014;38(11):2377–84. https://doi.org/10.1007/s00264-014-2343-9.
61. Hernigou J, Alves A, Homma Y, Guissou I, Hernigou P. Anatomy of the ilium for bone marrow aspiration: map of sectors and implication for safe trocar placement. Int Orthop. 2014;38(12):2585–90. https://doi.org/10.1007/s00264-014-2353-7.
62. Jäger M, Herten M, Fochtmann U, Fischer J, Hernigou P, Zilkens C, et al. Bridging the gap: bone marrow aspiration concentrate reduces autologous bone grafting in osseous defects. J Orthop Res. 2011;29(2):173–80. https://doi.org/10.1002/jor.21230.
63. Hernigou P, Desroches A, Queinnec S, Flouzat Lachaniette CH, Poignard A, Allain J, et al. Morbidity of graft harvesting versus bone marrow aspiration in cell regenerative therapy. Int Orthop. 2014;38(9):1855–60. https://doi.org/10.1007/s00264-014-2318-x.
64. Maloney WJ, Herzwurm P, Paprosky W, Rubash HE, Engh CA. Treatment of pelvic osteolysis associated with a stable acetabular component inserted without cement as part of a total hip replacement. J Bone Joint Surg Am. 1997;79(11):1628–34.
65. Etienne G, Bezwada HP, Hungerford DS, Mont MA. The incorporation of morselized bone grafts in cementless acetabular revisions. Clin Orthop Relat Res. 2004;(428):241–6.
66. Harris WH. Allografting in total hip arthroplasty: in adults with severe acetabular deficiency including a surgical technique for bolting the graft to the ilium. Clin Orthop Relat Res. 1982;(162):150–64.
67. Harris WH, Crothers O, Oh I. Total hip replacement and femoral-head bone-grafting for severe acetabular deficiency in adults. J Bone Joint Surg Am. 1977;59(6):752–9.
68. Sporer SM, O'Rourke M, Chong P, Paprosky WG. The use of structural distal femoral allografts for acetabular reconstruction. Surgical technique. J Bone Joint Surg Am. 2006;88(Suppl 1 Pt 1):92–9. https://doi.org/10.2106/JBJS.E.00903.

69. Jasty M, Harris WH. Salvage total hip reconstruction in patients with major acetabular bone deficiency using structural femoral head allografts. J Bone Joint Surg Br. 1990;72(1):63–7.
70. Kim Y, Tanaka C, Kanoe H. Long-term outcome of acetabular reconstruction using a Kerboull-type acetabular reinforcement device with hydroxyapatite granule and structural autograft for AAOS type II and III acetabular defects. J Arthroplast. 2015;30(10):1810–4. https://doi.org/10.1016/j.arth.2015.04.034.
71. Tanaka C, Shikata J, Ikenaga M, Takahashi M. Acetabular reconstruction using a Kerboull-type acetabular reinforcement device and hydroxyapatite granules: a 3- to 8-year follow-up study. J Arthroplast. 2003;18(6):719–25.
72. Weeden SH, Schmidt RH. The use of tantalum porous metal implants for Paprosky 3A and 3B defects. J Arthroplast. 2007;22(6 Suppl 2):151–5. https://doi.org/10.1016/j.arth.2007.04.024.
73. Del Gaizo DJ, Kancherla V, Sporer SM, Paprosky WG. Tantalum augments for Paprosky IIIA defects remain stable at midterm follow-up. Clin Orthop Relat Res. 2012;470(2):395–401. https://doi.org/10.1007/s11999-011-2170-x.
74. Batuyong ED, Brock HS, Thiruvengadam N, Maloney WJ, Goodman SB, Huddleston JI. Outcome of porous tantalum acetabular components for Paprosky type 3 and 4 acetabular defects. J Arthroplast. 2014;29(6):1318–22. https://doi.org/10.1016/j.arth.2013.12.002.
75. Clement RGE, Ray AG, MacDonald DJ, Wade FA, Burnett R, Moran M. Trabecular metal use in Paprosky type 2 and 3 acetabular defects: 5-year follow-up. J Arthroplast. 2016;31(4):863–7. https://doi.org/10.1016/j.arth.2015.10.033.
76. Ilyas I, Alrumaih HA, Kashif S, Rabbani SA, Faqihi AH. Revision of type III and type IVB acetabular defects with Burch-Schneider anti-protrusio cages. J Arthroplast. 2015;30(2):259–64. https://doi.org/10.1016/j.arth.2014.08.014.
77. Hsu C-C, Hsu C-H, Yen S-H, Wang J-W. Use of the Burch-Schneider cage and structural allografts in complex acetabular deficiency: 3- to 10-year follow up. Kaohsiung J Med Sci. 2015;31(10):540–7. https://doi.org/10.1016/j.kjms.2015.08.001.
78. Jones L, Grammatopoulos G, Singer G. The Burch-Schneider cage: 9-year survival in Paprosky type 3 acetabular defects. Clinical and radiological follow-up. Hip Int. 2012;22(1):28–34. https://doi.org/10.5301/HIP.2012.9078.
79. Berry DJ, Müller ME. Revision arthroplasty using an anti-protrusio cage for massive acetabular bone deficiency. J Bone Joint Surg Br. 1992;74(5):711–5.
80. Kösters C, Schliemann B, Decking D, Simon U, Zurstegge M, Decking J. The Müller acetabular reinforcement ring—still an option in acetabular revision of Paprosky 2 defects? Long-term results after 10 years. Acta Orthop Belg. 2015;81(2):257–63.
81. Gerber A, Pisan M, Zurakowski D, Isler B. Ganz reinforcement ring for reconstruction of acetabular defects in revision total hip arthroplasty. J Bone Joint Surg Am. 2003;85-A(12):2358–64.
82. Gibon E, Barut N, Courpied J-P, Hamadouche M. Revision total hip arthroplasty using the Kerboull acetabular reinforcement device for Paprosky type III defects involving the inferior margin of the acetabulum: a minimum five-year follow-up study. Bone Joint J. 2018;100-B(6):725–32.
83. Slooff TJ, Huiskes R, van Horn J, Lemmens AJ. Bone grafting in total hip replacement for acetabular protrusion. Acta Orthop Scand. 1984;55(6):593–6.
84. Mao Y, Xu C, Xu J, Li H, Liu F, Yu D, et al. The use of customized cages in revision total hip arthroplasty for Paprosky type III acetabular bone defects. Int Orthop. 2015;39(10):2023–30. https://doi.org/10.1007/s00264-015-2965-6.
85. Abolghasemian M, Tangsataporn S, Sternheim A, Backstein D, Safir O, Gross AE. Combined trabecular metal acetabular shell and augment for acetabular revision with substantial bone loss: a mid-term review. Bone Joint J. 2013;95-B(2):166–72. https://doi.org/10.1302/0301-620X.95B2.30608.
86. Whitehouse MR, Masri BA, Duncan CP, Garbuz DS. Continued good results with modular trabecular metal augments for acetabular defects in hip arthroplasty at 7 to 11 years. Clin Orthop Relat Res. 2015;473(2):521–7. https://doi.org/10.1007/s11999-014-3861-x.
87. Hanssen AD, Lewallen DG. Modular acetabular augments: composite void fillers. Orthopedics. 2005;28(9):971–2.
88. Kosashvili Y, Backstein D, Safir O, Lakstein D, Gross AE. Acetabular revision using an anti-protrusion (ilio-ischial) cage and trabecular metal acetabular component for severe acetabular bone loss associated with pelvic discontinuity. J Bone Joint Surg Br. 2009;91(7):870–6. https://doi.org/10.1302/0301-620X.91B7.22181.
89. Abolghasemian M, Tangsaraporn S, Drexler M, Barbuto R, Backstein D, Safir O, et al. The challenge of pelvic discontinuity: cup-cage reconstruction does better than conventional cages in mid-term. Bone Joint J. 2014;96-B(2):195–200. https://doi.org/10.1302/0301-620X.96B2.31907.
90. Amenabar T, Rahman WA, Hetaimish BM, Kuzyk PR, Safir OA, Gross AE. Promising mid-term results with a cup-cage construct for large acetabular defects and pelvic discontinuity. Clin Orthop Relat Res. 2016;474(2):408–14. https://doi.org/10.1007/s11999-015-4210-4.
91. Gibon E, Kerboull L, Courpied J-P, Hamadouche M. Acetabular reinforcement rings associated with allograft for severe acetabular defects. Int Orthop. 2019;43(3):561–71. https://doi.org/10.1007/s00264-018-4142-1.

22 Surgical Management of Femoral Bone Loss

Anton Khlopas, Linsen T. Samuel, and Atul F. Kamath

22.1 Indications for Femoral Revision

Total hip arthroplasty (THA) has been shown to be one of the most successful and cost-effective surgical interventions, and the incidence of this procedure is increasing [1, 2]. Current population-based estimates conclude that the number of revision THA cases is projected to increase substantially over the next 25 years in the United States [2–5]. Based on respective national joint registries, the projections are similar for other countries [6, 7]. In an epidemiological study of revision THA, femoral component revision is the second most common procedure (13.2%), following both-component revision (41.1%) [8]. The most common reasons for revision THA reported in this study were instability/dislocation (22.5%), mechanical loosening (19.7%), and infection (14.8%) [8]. Specifically, mechanical loosening was the most common reason for isolated femoral component revision (24.7%) [8]. In another study of the National Inpatient Sample, Gwam et al. found that dislocation was the main indication for revision THA (17.3%), followed by mechanical loosening (16.8%) [9]. In the same study, the authors concluded that the mean total charge for revision THA was $77,851.24. It is important to understand the epidemiology of revision THA in the next decade and beyond, given the emergence of new bearing surfaces such as ceramics and highly cross-linked polyethylene, which have reduced osteolysis as a cause of 11% of revisions (head and liner exchange) [10–13].

22.2 Preoperative Workup

Every patient with a painful THA should have a thorough history taken and physical examination performed. Patients with femoral component issues usually complain of groin, thigh pain, start-up pain, and often ipsilateral referred knee pain. If the patient does complain of pain, it is important to clarify several issues: when it started (immediately after the surgery vs. several weeks or months after), the timeframe of onset (gradually increasing pain vs. sudden onset of severe pain), any associated trauma or injury, compliance with postoperative instructions, progression of pain, and any signs of infection (fever/chills, delayed wound healing, drainage, hematoma). These signs, in addition to appropriate imaging, will help distinguish between periprosthetic fracture (sudden), subsidence and periprosthetic osteolysis or loosening (progressive until potential catastrophic failure), and infection (acute versus chronic).

A. Khlopas · L. T. Samuel · A. F. Kamath (✉)
Department of Orthopaedic Surgery, Cleveland Clinic Foundation, Cleveland, OH, USA
e-mail: khlopaa@ccf.org; kamatha@ccf.org

W. R. Drescher et al. (eds.), *Advances in Specialist Hip Surgery*,
https://doi.org/10.1007/978-3-030-61830-8_22

Every physical examination should begin with evaluation of the patient's gait, followed by close inspection of the skin around the incision and throughout the lower extremity. Any erythema, wound dehiscence, drainage/sinus tract, swelling, or warmth should be noted. A history of early wound-healing problems may inform occult infection. This should be followed by range-of-motion evaluation when appropriate. A careful evaluation of the ipsilateral knee and lumbar spine should be performed to rule out referred pain from other locations, or overlapping pain syndromes.

Radiographic evaluation should always start with calibrated anteroposterior (AP) view of the pelvis, AP view of the hip, and a lateral view of the hip. Commonly, an AP and lateral view of the femur is necessary to rule out any associated pathology. Most fractures, subsidence, osteolysis, or loosening can be observed on plain radiographs, especially when serial radiographs are viewed. However, in some cases a computed tomography (CT) scan may be used to identify subtle fractures and versional abnormalities (stems often fail into varus and retroversion). A modern multidetector CT imaging protocol is preferred to reduce metal artifacts [14]. In addition, it can be used to further assess or evaluate fracture morphology, implant stability, periarticular masses, fluid collections, soft-tissue ossifications, and bone stock which may be helpful for preoperative planning. In addition, 3-dimensional (3D) reconstruction may be used to better understand fracture morphology. Additional radiation exposure risk should be evaluated on a case-by-case basis.

Magnetic resonance imaging (MRI) has become an increasingly useful diagnostic tool for evaluation of THA implants with development of metal artifact reduction techniques for improved depiction of bone, implant-tissue interfaces, and periprosthetic soft tissues [15]. Some of the pathologies that can be identified with MRI include osseous stress reactions, nondisplaced fractures, bone resorption, aseptic loosening, infection, heterotopic ossification, local tissue reactions to metal products (e.g., adverse metal reactions/metallosis), and neoplasms.

If infection is suspected, workup should begin with a complete blood count (CBC), erythrocyte sedimentation rate (ESR), and C-reactive protein (CRP) [16]. The Musculoskeletal Infection Society (MSIS) criteria for periprosthetic joint infection were introduced in 2011 and have been modified in 2018, demonstrating a sensitivity of 97.7% and specificity of 99.5% [17]. These diagnostic criteria use various laboratory (in addition to key clinical) findings for diagnosis of periprosthetic joint infection (PJI), including synovial fluid white blood cell (WBC) count and neutrophil percentage, blood ESR, CRP or D-dimer, synovial fluid alpha defensin, and leukocyte esterase. Synovial fluid should be sent for aerobic, anaerobic, and, in immunocompromised patients, fungal and mycobacterial cultures.

22.3 Classification of Femoral Bone Loss

Femoral component loosening, osteolysis, stress shielding, multiple revisions, periprosthetic fracture, and infection often result in progressive bone loss of the proximal femur. In addition, intraoperative techniques of removing the failed femoral stem and, if present, cement often result in further defects in the bone stock. A reproducible way of classifying femoral bone loss can be helpful for preoperative planning. Several classification systems have been developed, including the American Academy of Orthopaedic Surgeons (AAOS) classification system, and perhaps the more commonly used Paprosky classification system [18–20]. The AAOS system divides defects into segmental (loss of supporting cortical bone) and cavitary (loss of cancellous medullary bone) deficiencies (Fig. 22.1) [18]; the Paprosky system divides defects on the basis of metaphyseal and diaphyseal bone loss (Fig. 22.2) [19, 20]; and the Vancouver classification system can be used in cases of periprosthetic femur fracture (Fig. 22.3) [21].

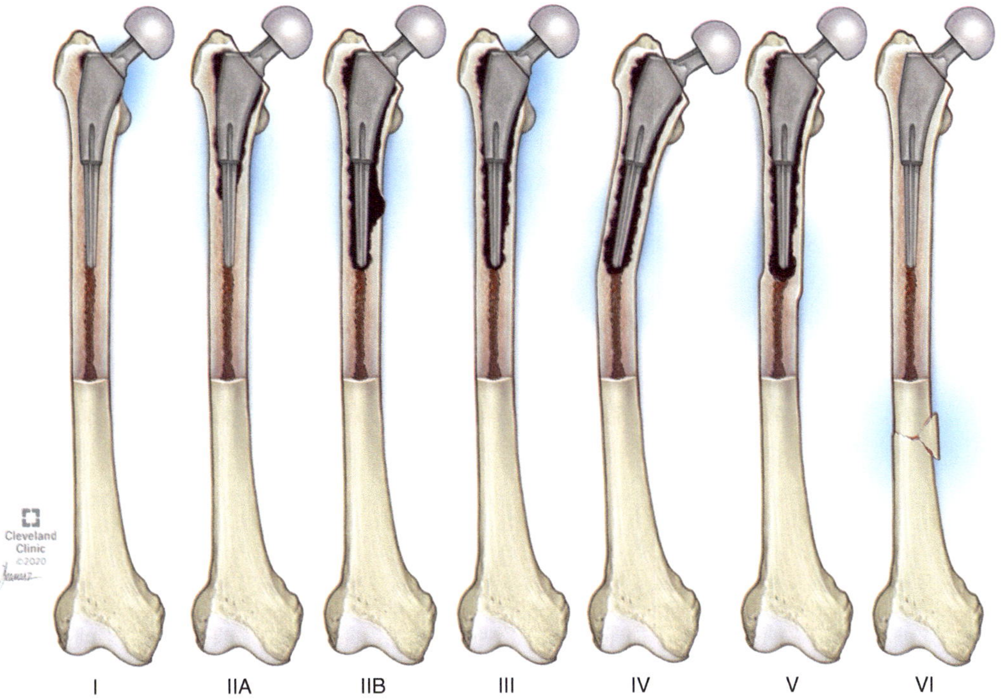

Fig. 22.1 American Academy of Orthopaedic Surgeons (AAOS) classification of femoral bone loss. Type I (segmental): Loss of bone off the supporting shell of the femur; type II (cavitary): loss of endosteal bone with an intact cortical shell; type III (combined): combination of a type I (segmental) and type II (cavitary) deficiency; type IV (malalignment): loss of the normal femoral geometry due to prior surgery, trauma, or disease; type V (stenosis): obliteration of the canal due to trauma, fixation devices, or bony hypertrophy; type VI (femoral discontinuity): loss of femoral integrity from fracture of nonunion (reprinted with permission, Cleveland Clinic Center for Medical Art & Photography © 2020. All Rights Reserved)

Fig. 22.2 Paprosky classification of femoral bone loss. Type I: Minimal metaphyseal cancellous bone loss and intact diaphysis; type II: loss of the whole metaphysis to the level of the lesser trochanter distally; type IIIA: extensive bone defect in proximal femur, but adequate diaphyseal bone (>4 cm of intact diaphyseal bone); type IIIB: intact diaphyseal bone <4 cm; type IV: inadequate diaphysis with no support for cementless fixation (reprinted with permission, Cleveland Clinic Center for Medical Art & Photography © 2020. All Rights Reserved)

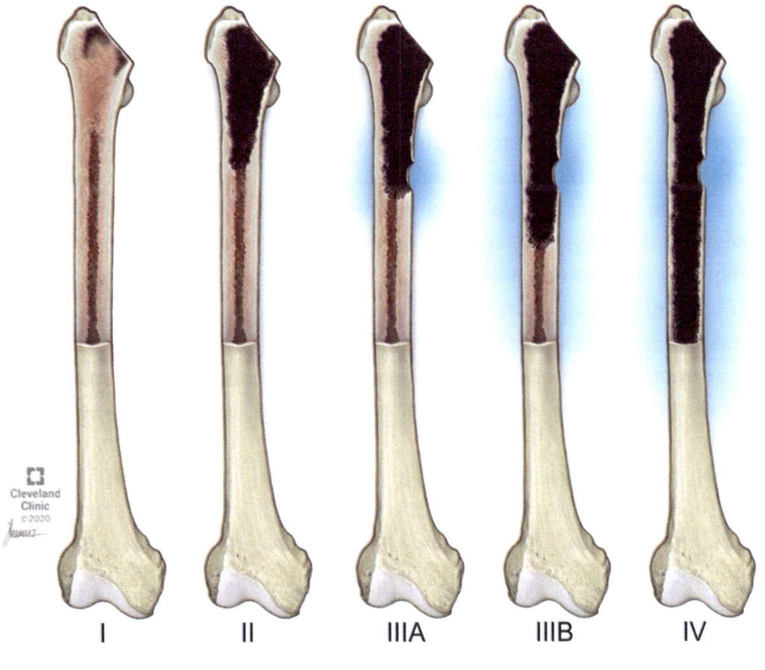

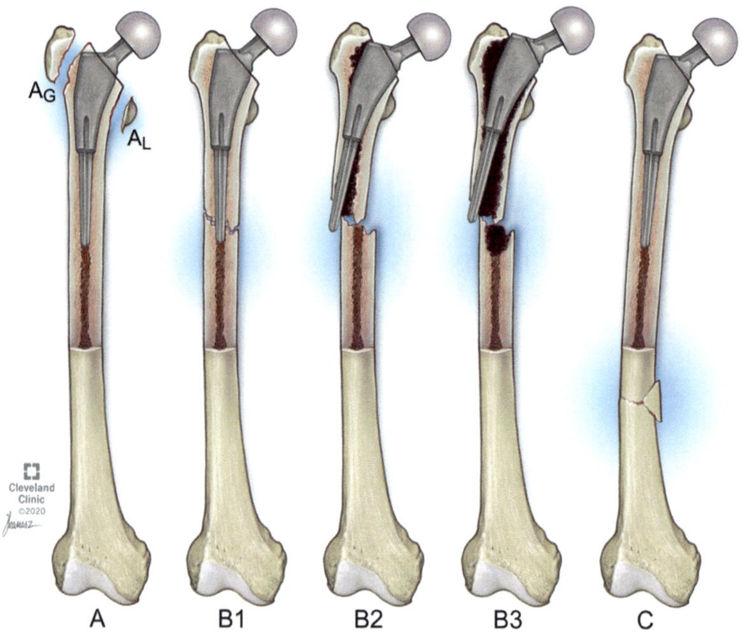

Fig. 22.3 Vancouver classification of femoral periprosthetic fractures. Type A: Fracture in the trochanteric region (A_G: fracture of the greater trochanter; A_L: fracture of the lesser trochanter); type B: fracture around the proximal femoral stem (B1: well-fixed femoral stem; B2: loose femoral stem with good-quality proximal bone stock; B3: loose stem with poor-quality proximal bone stock); type C: fracture occurring well below the distal tip of the femoral stem (reprinted with permission, Cleveland Clinic Center for Medical Art & Photography © 2020. All Rights Reserved)

22.4 Tenets of Reconstruction

1. Femoral reconstruction must be focused on obtaining mechanical axial and rotational stability of the stem.
2. If possible, limb length should be restored.
3. For cavitary defects, consider impaction grafting with morselized allograft bone.
4. As circumferential stem fit is desired, large segmental defects may reduce the stability of the stem and should be addressed.
5. If instability is present, large femoral heads, dual mobility or tripolar constructs, and constrained liners should be considered. Constraint may be preferred in the setting of complete abductor deficiency.
6. Appropriate load transmission to the femur for both axial and rotational stress should be obtained. High torsional loads may occur during common activities of daily living, including ascending stairs and getting out of chair.
7. It is important to assess the integrity and stability of the abductor musculature and other muscles surrounding the hip; if trochanteric osteotomy is performed, secure re-fixation is important; consider muscle transfer (e.g., Whiteside transfer [22]) for abductor deficiency management in conjunction with bony/prosthetic reconstruction techniques.

22.5 Surgical Options

In revision THA, it is important to preserve as much bone as possible during exposure and explantation to maintain bone stock for reconstruction. Several options for restoring lost bone and/or defects are currently available, including impaction bone grafting, strut allograft, cemented or cementless metal implants, and combination of all of the above. To select the appropriate reconstruction option, the surgeon

Table 22.1 Paprosky classification of femoral bone loss and recommended reconstruction options

Type	Definition	Reconstruction options (author preference)
I	Minimal metaphyseal bone loss	Cementless fixation, proximally fitting, collared, or extensively porous coated stem; cemented fixation
II	Moderate-to-severe metaphyseal bone loss	Cementless extensively porous coated stem; cemented fixation
IIIA	Severe metaphyseal bone loss with >4 cm of isthmus intact	Extensively porous coated stem (if <19 mm in diameter) versus modular fluted tapered stem (preferentially used in cases where >19 mm in diameter stem is required); impaction grafting plus cemented stem
IIIB	Severe metaphyseal bone loss with <4 cm of isthmus intact	Modular fluted tapered stem
IV	Complete loss of metaphyseal and diaphyseal bone	Allograft prosthetic composite (in young), cemented stem/impaction grafting plus cemented stem, modular fluted tapered stem, femoral replacement/ megaprosthesis

should rely on his or her training and experience. The authors' preferred reconstructive options based on the degree of bone loss are provided in Table 22.1.

22.6 Available Implants

22.6.1 Extensively Porous Coated Stems

Extensively porous coated femoral stems have been commonly used with good outcomes in the primary and revision setting. Engh et al. reviewed 25 patients who underwent revision THA with extensively porous coated components at a minimum of 10-year follow-up [23]. The 10-year survivorship of the femoral component was 89% [23]. In a similar study, Hamilton et al. reviewed 905 femoral revisions utilizing extensively porous coated stems and demonstrated 97.5% survivorship at 5 years and 95.9% survivorship at 10 years [24]. Similarly, Chung et al. performed a retrospective review of 96 femoral revisions utilizing extensively porous coated stems in Paprosky type III defects. At a mean follow-up of 65.7 months, one patient developed a periprosthetic fracture which was treated with fixation, three patients developed intraoperative perforations treated with structural bone grafts and cable fixation, and no patients required revision of the femoral component [25]. Overall, extensively porous coated femoral stems remain a viable option in the armamentarium. However, in a more recent study of 51 patients treated with 10-in. or 9-in. calcar extensively porous coated stem, Sporer and Paprosky demonstrated a failure rate of 0% in type IIIB defects with femoral canal measuring less than 19 mm in diameter, and 18% in patients with femoral canal greater than 19 mm in diameter at 4.2 years of follow-up [26]. In addition, patients with type IV defects had a failure rate of 37.5% with porous coated stem use [26]. The authors of this chapter will routinely place a fully coated stem in the revision setting if removal of the failed femoral stem can be done without an extended trochanteric osteotomy with no significant proximal femoral bone remodeling (Fig. 22.4).

22.6.2 Cemented vs. Cementless Modular and Monoblock Fluted Tapered Stems

There is a general lack of studies comparing the survivorship and outcomes of cemented versus newer generation cementless femoral stems [27–30]. In a study of 2296 revision THAs, Tyson et al. demonstrated that 10-year survival was similar in cementless (85% (95% CI 83–87)) and cemented stems (88% (95% CI 86–90)) [29]. Cementless stems were more often re-revised for infection and dislocation, while cemented stems were more likely re-revised for aseptic loosening. Cemented stems may have lower re-revision for

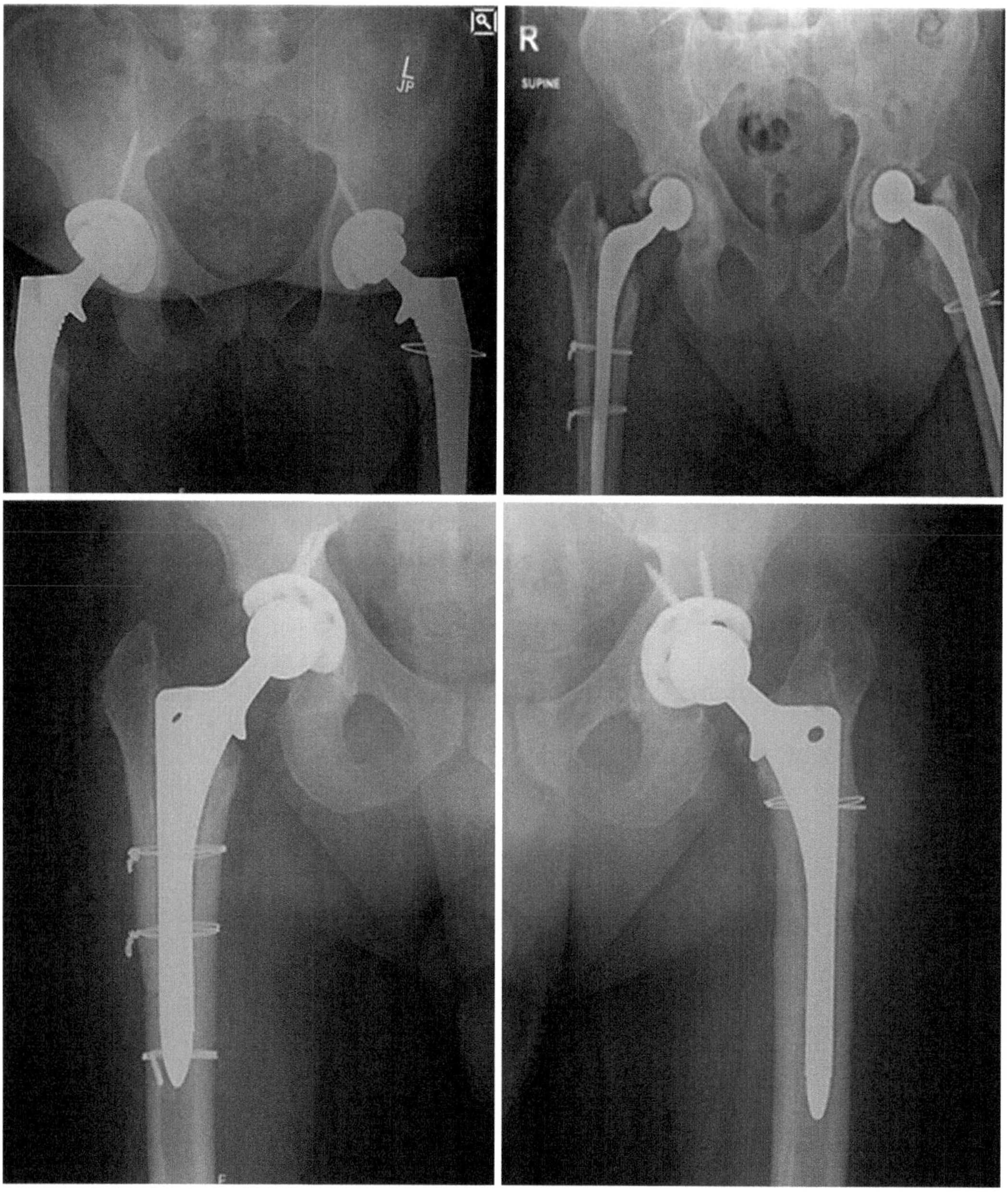

Fig. 22.4 Patient with bilateral periprosthetic hip infections treated with sequential, two-stage revisions with explantation through extended trochanteric osteotomies. Extensively coated femoral stems were used at the time of second-stage reimplantation

infection because of the use of antibiotic cement. Cementless femoral stems may be superior because the proximal part of the stem may be exchanged or repositioned in dislocation and instability cases, which cannot be accomplished in the same fashion with cemented non-modular stems (limited ability with cement-in-cement revision). Many factors may influence the choice between cemented and cementless stems including bone defect size, varus remodeling, patient age, comorbidities, and surgeon training and skills.

Several studies have demonstrated higher survival rate after revision of the femoral component with cemented when compared to a cementless stem. In a study utilizing the Swedish Hip Arthroplasty Register, Weiss et al. identified 812 consecutive revision THAs treated with a modular cementless stem (mean follow-up 3.4 years) and 1073 cemented long stems (mean follow-up 4.2 years) [30]. The authors demonstrated an increased risk of reoperation (HR 1.7, 95% CI: 1.3–2.4) and revision (HR 1.9, 95% CI: 1.2–3.1) in the cementless cohort [30]. Hernigou et al. performed a comparison study of 85 cementless distal locked stems and 124 extensively long cemented stems in patients with previous revision and severe bone loss [28]. The authors demonstrated an increased risk of pain, periprosthetic fracture, and revision in cementless stems (21%) when compared to the cemented stem (0%) cohort [28].

All of the abovementioned studies compared cemented stems to older generation cementless designs. The newer modular fluted tapered stems have demonstrated improved survivorship, decreased risk of subsidence, and improved restoration of limb length and femoral offset in short- and midterm follow-up to date (Fig. 22.5). In a study of 129 patients with Paprosky type 3 and 4 femoral defects treated with modular tapered fluted stems, Otero et al. demonstrated aseptic survivorship of 98.4% and overall survivorship of 95% at a mean of 3.75-year follow-up [31]. In a similar study of 519 modular fluted tapered stems used in aseptic femoral revision, Abdel et al. demonstrated 96% overall survivorship at 10 years and improved Harris Hip Score at 2 years and at final follow-up ($p < 0.001$) [32]. In a level II prospective comparative study of patients with Paprosky type 1 and 2 femoral bone loss during revision, Iorio et al. compared 43 cementless modular stems with 43 cemented stems and demonstrated that, at 8-year mean follow-up, there were no differences in functional outcomes or revision rates (2.3 vs. 4.6%, $p = 0.557$) [27].

Although modular tapered fluted cementless stems are increasingly used in complex revision cases, non-modular (monolithic) stems can still be an excellent option. In a study of 160 consecutive modular and 129 consecutive non-modular fluted tapered stems, Huang et al. demonstrated no significant difference in functional outcome and 8-year survival rate (94.43% and 96.69%, $p = 0.99$) between the two groups [33]. However, less subsidence ($p = 0.001$) and more intraoperative fractures (16.9% vs. 7.0%, $p = 0.01$) occurred in the modular group [33].

22.6.3 Proximal Femoral Replacement

Proximal femoral replacement is an option for patients with large proximal bony defects [34]. This treatment modality is in large reserved for those patients with unreconstructable deficiencies of the proximal femur, often including significant damage to the greater trochanter/abductor mechanism. One of the important drawbacks to this method is challenges associated with abductor mechanism connection to the metallic proximal femur. Attempts at ameliorating this by creating special attachment points for abductor repair on the prosthesis have been somewhat successful, but adductor deficiency remains a major complication of this procedure.

In a retrospective review, Parvizi et al. identified 48 patients with a mean age of 74 years who underwent a proximal femoral replacement (modular megaprosthesis) with or without bone grafting [35]. At a mean of 36.5-month follow-up, there was a significant improvement in Harris Hip Score ($p < 0.05$). In addition, the overall survivorship of the implant was 87% at 1 year and 73% at 5 years [35]. In a similar study, Viste et al. retrospectively reviewed the outcomes of 44 patients who underwent revision THA to proximal femoral replacement, with a mean age of 79 years [36]. The overall implant survivorship was 86% at 5 years and 66% at 10 years, and the mean Harris Hip Score improved from 42.8 to 68.5 ($p = 0.0009$) [36]. Grammatopoulos et al. reviewed 79 patients who underwent 80 proximal femur replacements for non-tumor indications and demonstrated 5-year survival of 87% [37]. Therefore, proximal femur replacement is a viable procedure in a specific salvage patient population. However it is associated with lower overall survivorship,

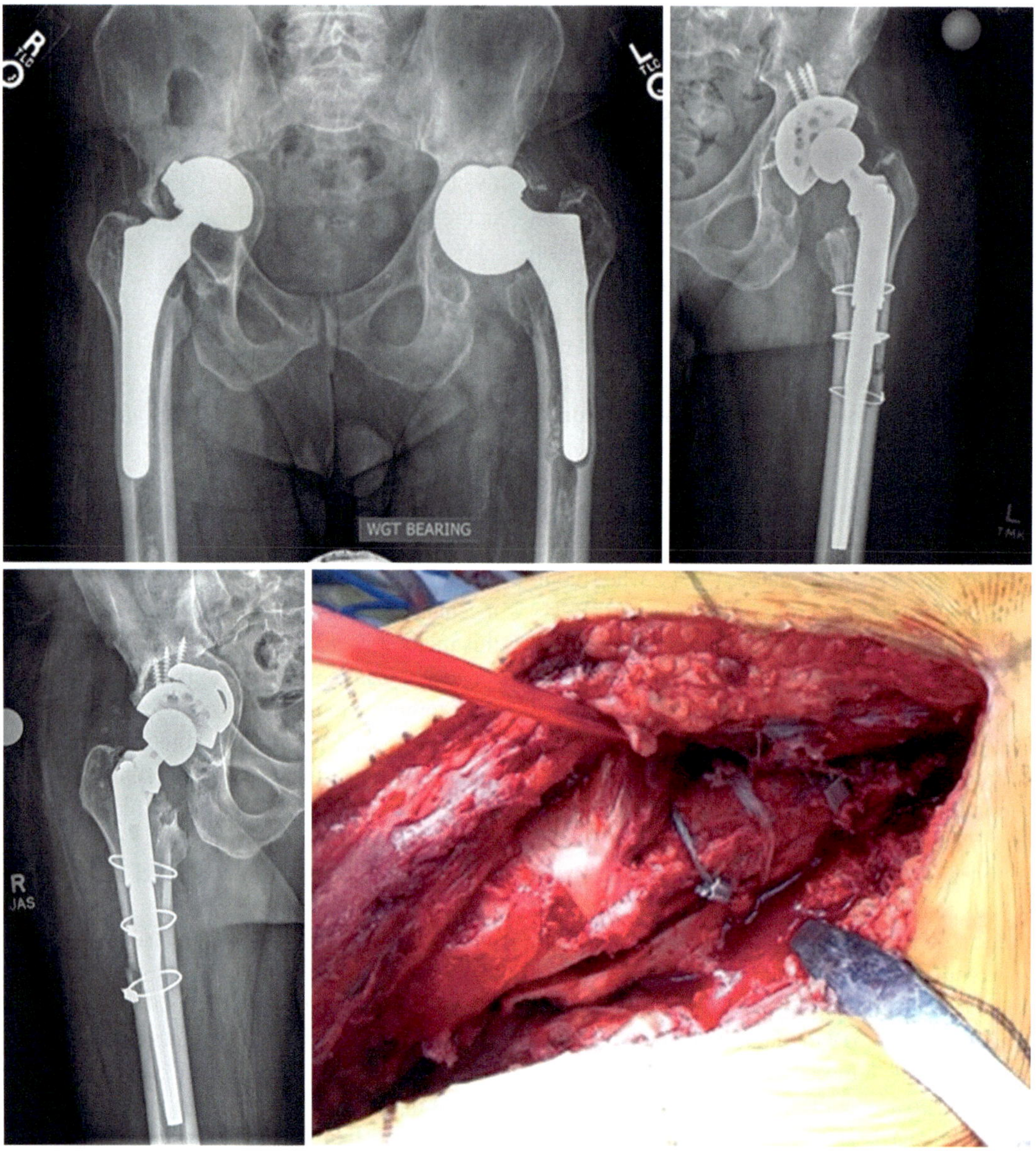

Fig. 22.5 Patient with aseptic loosening of bilateral femoral stems, with varus remodeling, treated with modular fluted tapered stems through an extended trochanteric osteotomy. Intraoperative image demonstrating repair of the greater trochanteric osteotomy segment

increased dislocation risk, and increased risk of infection [38] (Figs. 22.6 and 22.7).

22.6.4 Allograft Prosthetic Composite

The allograft prosthetic composite utilizes a cemented long stem and an allograft of the proximal femur attached to the host bone distally [39, 40]. This fixation option may be advantageous in the younger patient where prosthetic replacement may be preferentially avoided. This technique requires a sized allograft to be cut at an appropriate level to match the host bone. This allograft is subsequently reamed and broached, and a long stem is cemented. This is followed by implantation of the composite into the host, which is usually per-

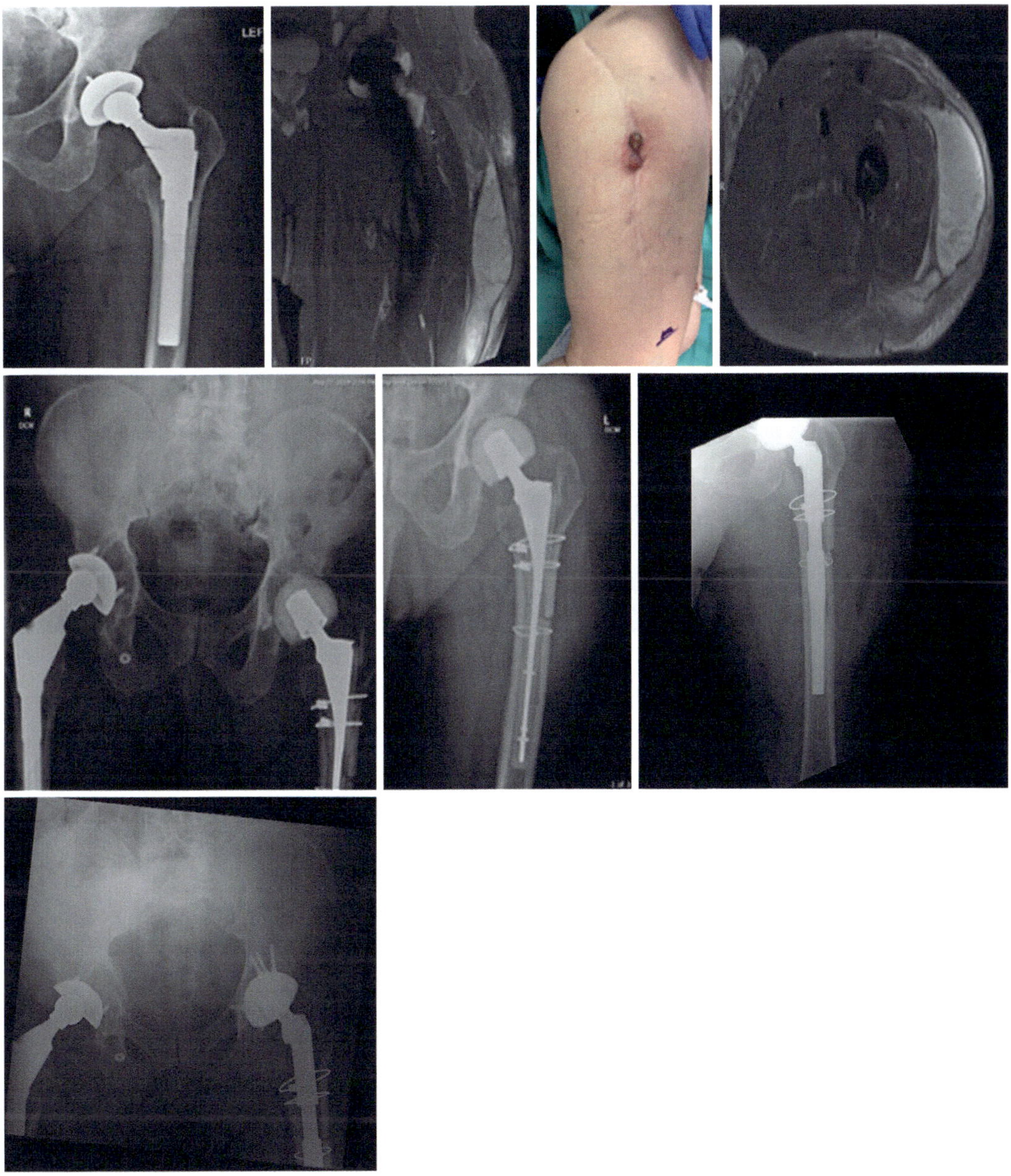

Fig. 22.6 Patient with infected left total hip arthroplasty and large pseudotumor collection in the anterolateral thigh with draining sinus, treated with two-stage revision and modular fluted tapered stem through an extended trochanteric osteotomy

formed with cement, although press-fit reconstruction is a reasonable alternative. This may be accomplished with or without an interlocking step-cut at the composite junction. Although commonly performed at some specialized centers, these procedures are associated with a high number of complications, including infection, graft resorption, failure of graft incorporation, nonunion, theoretical disease transmission, aseptic loosening, and periprosthetic fracture [41].

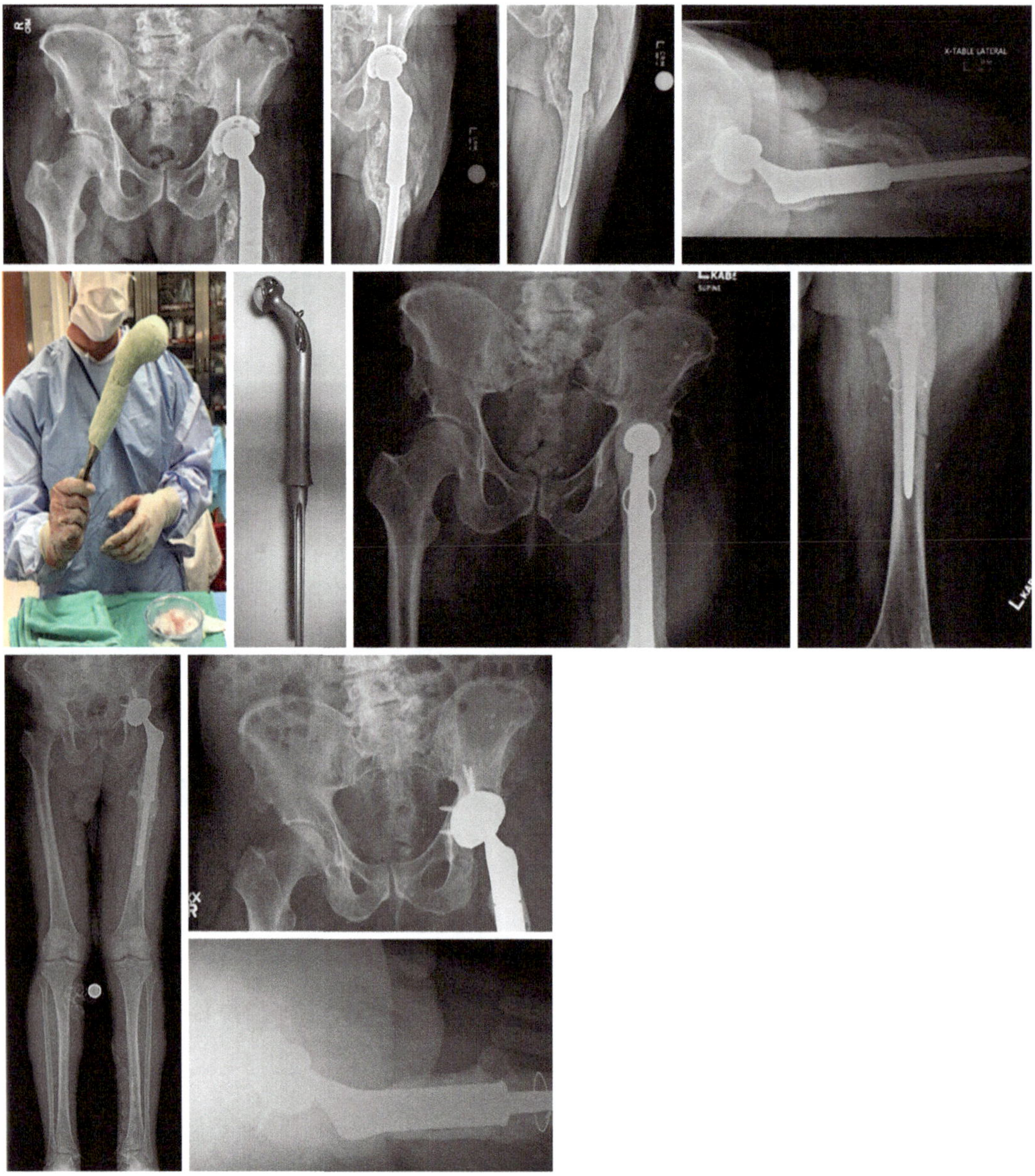

Fig. 22.7 Infected proximal femoral replacement and massive heterotopic ossification treated with a two-stage revision utilizing a monoblock stem as a temporary proximal femoral replacement spacer

22.6.5 Impaction Bone Grafting

Impaction bone grafting has been extensively used to treat severe femoral bone loss during revision THA in centers worldwide [42–44]. In this technique it is imperative to contain the impacted bone within the medullary cavity, which may be supplemented with a metal mesh [45]. Impaction bone grafting is usually used to treat segmental defects; however, several authors have extended the indication of this procedure to complete circumferential proximal cortical bone loss [45]. This technique is usually used in combination with a cemented femoral stem. In a study of 540 revision THAs utilizing femoral impaction grafting and cemented femoral stem, Laberton et al. demonstrated 10-year aseptic survival rate of the implant of 98% and 10-year overall survival rate of 84.2% [46]. In a similar study, Wilson et al. demonstrated a 20-year aseptic survivorship of 98.8% and overall 20-year survivorship of 87.7% in the largest series to date of femoral impaction grafting (705 revisions) [47]. However, impaction bone grafting is not performed uniformly across all orthopedic centers; requires extensive training in technique, specialized instrumentation, and large amount of allograft; and is time consuming. Some studies have demonstrated that impaction bone grafting is associated with higher infection rates, and higher overall complication rates when compared to uncemented distally fixed tapered stems [48].

22.6.6 Other Options

Total femoral replacement may be used in cases where there is severe proximal bone loss and distal bone stock is compromised by failed total hip/knee arthroplasty or periprosthetic fracture, or if there is insufficient bone stock in the distal femur to support a proximal reconstruction [49]. Resection arthroplasty may be a salvage option for the treatment of failed THA or limb-threatening issue or massive uncontrolled infection. This may be used after multiple failed revision procedures in low-demand/medically infirm patient [50]. In addition, this may be a temporary option for patients with severe sepsis and inability to eradicate periprosthetic joint infection, with a goal of reconstruction in the future. This procedure may provide eradication of infection and pain relief; however, limited function is expected [50] and multiple temporary limb-spanning spacer options have been proposed.

22.7 Summary

In summary, patients with femoral bone defects should be carefully evaluated, beginning with a detailed physical exam, appropriate imaging studies, and infection workup. Preoperative and intraoperative assessment of the degree of bone loss should be performed utilizing available classification systems in order to establish a preoperative plan and to have the required instrumentation and implants available in the operating room. Many factors contribute to the selection of the most appropriate reconstructive technique, including patient comorbidities, anatomy, degree of bone loss, and surgeon experience and training.

References

1. Elmallah RK, Chughtai M, Adib F, Bozic KJ, Kurtz SM, Mont MA. Determining health-related quality-of-life outcomes using the SF-6D following total hip arthroplasty. J Bone Joint Surg. 2017;99(6):494–8. https://doi.org/10.2106/JBJS.15.01351.
2. Kurtz S, Ong K, Lau E, Mowat F, Halpern M. Projections of primary and revision hip and knee arthroplasty in the United States from 2005 to 2030. J Bone Joint Surg Am. 2007;89(4):780–5. https://doi.org/10.2106/JBJS.F.00222.
3. Kurtz SM, Ong KL, Lau E, Bozic KJ. Impact of the economic downturn on total joint replacement demand in the United States: updated projections to 2021. J Bone Joint Surg Am. 2014;96(8):624–30. https://doi.org/10.2106/JBJS.M.00285.
4. Kurtz SM, Ong KL, Schmier J, Zhao K, Mowat F, Lau E. Primary and revision arthroplasty surgery caseloads in the United States from 1990 to 2004. J Arthroplast. 2009;24(2):195–203. https://doi.org/10.1016/j.arth.2007.11.015.
5. Kurtz S, Mowat F, Ong K, Chan N, Lau E, Halpern M. Prevalence of primary and revision total hip and knee arthroplasty in the United States from 1990 through 2002. J Bone Joint Surg Am. 2005;87(7):1487. https://doi.org/10.2106/JBJS.D.02441.
6. Inacio MCS, Graves SE, Pratt NL, Roughead EE, Nemes S. Increase in total joint arthroplasty projected from 2014 to 2046 in Australia: a conservative local model with international implications. Clin Orthop Relat Res. 2017;475(8):2130–7. https://doi.org/10.1007/s11999-017-5377-7.
7. Patel A, Pavlou G, Mújica-Mota RE, Toms AD. The epidemiology of revision total knee and hip arthroplasty in England and Wales: a comparative analysis with projections for the United States. A study using the National Joint Registry dataset. Bone Joint J. 2015;97-B(8):1076–81. https://doi.org/10.1302/0301-620X.97B8.35170.
8. Bozic KJ, Kurtz SM, Lau E, Ong K, Chiu V, Vail TP, Rubash HE, Berry DJ. The epidemiology of revision total knee arthroplasty in the United States. Clin Orthop Relat Res. 2010;468(1):45–51. https://doi.org/10.1007/s11999-009-0945-0.
9. Gwam CU, Mistry JB, Mohamed NS, Thomas M, Bigart KC, Mont MA, Delanois RE. Current epidemiology of revision total hip arthroplasty in the

United States: National Inpatient Sample 2009 to 2013. J Arthroplast. 2017;32(7):2088–92. https://doi.org/10.1016/j.arth.2017.02.046.
10. Bozic KJ, Kurtz SM, Lau E, Ong K, Vail TP, Berry DJ. The epidemiology of revision total hip arthroplasty in the United States. J Bone Joint Surg Am. 2009;91(1):128–33. https://doi.org/10.2106/JBJS.H.00155.
11. Delaunay C, Hamadouche M, Girard J, Duhamel A, SoFCOT Group. What are the causes for failures of primary hip arthroplasties in France? Clin Orthop Relat Res. 2013;471(12):3863–9. https://doi.org/10.1007/s11999-013-2935-5.
12. Hanna SA, Somerville L, McCalden RW, Naudie DD, MacDonald SJ. Highly cross-linked polyethylene decreases the rate of revision of total hip arthroplasty compared with conventional polyethylene at 13 years' follow-up. Bone Joint J. 2016;98-B(1):28–32. https://doi.org/10.1302/0301-620X.98B1.36527.
13. Shen C, Tang Z-H, Hu J-Z, Zou G-Y, Xiao R-C, Yan D-X. Does cross-linked polyethylene decrease the revision rate of total hip arthroplasty compared with conventional polyethylene? A meta-analysis. Orthop Traumatol Surg Res. 2014;100(7):745–50. https://doi.org/10.1016/j.otsr.2014.07.015.
14. Roth TD, Maertz NA, Parr JA, Buckwalter KA, Choplin RH. CT of the hip prosthesis: appearance of components, fixation, and complications. Radiographics. 2012;32(4):1089–107. https://doi.org/10.1148/rg.324115183.
15. Fritz J, Lurie B, Miller TT, Potter HG. MR imaging of hip arthroplasty implants. Radiographics. 2014;34(4):E106–32. https://doi.org/10.1148/rg.344140010.
16. Springer BD. The diagnosis of periprosthetic joint infection. J Arthroplast. 2015;30(6):908–11. https://doi.org/10.1016/j.arth.2015.03.042.
17. Parvizi J, Tan TL, Goswami K, Higuera C, Della Valle C, Chen AF, Shohat N. The 2018 definition of periprosthetic hip and knee infection: an evidence-based and validated criteria. J Arthroplasty. 2018;33(5):1309–1314.e2. https://doi.org/10.1016/j.arth.2018.02.078.
18. D'Antonio J, McCarthy JC, Bargar WL, Borden LS, Cappelo WN, Collis DK, Steinberg ME, Wedge JH. Classification of femoral abnormalities in total hip arthroplasty. Clin Orthop Relat Res. 1993;296:133–9.
19. Della Valle CJ, Paprosky WG. The femur in revision total hip arthroplasty evaluation and classification. Clin Orthop Relat Res. 2004;420:55–62. https://doi.org/10.1097/00003086-200403000-00009.
20. Valle C, Della J, Paprosky WG. Classification and an algorithmic approach to the reconstruction of femoral deficiency in revision total hip arthroplasty. J Bone Joint Surg Am. 2003;85-A(Suppl):1–6. https://doi.org/10.2106/00004623-200300004-00001.
21. Brady OH, Garbuz DS, Masri BA, Duncan CP. The reliability and validity of the Vancouver classification of femoral fractures after hip replacement. J Arthroplast. 2000;15(1):59–62. https://doi.org/10.1016/s0883-5403(00)91181-1.
22. Whiteside LA. Surgical technique: transfer of the anterior portion of the gluteus maximus muscle for abductor deficiency of the hip. Clin Orthop Relat Res. 2012;470(2):503–10. https://doi.org/10.1007/s11999-011-1975-y.
23. Engh CA, Ellis TJ, Koralewicz LM, McAuley JP, Engh CA. Extensively porous-coated femoral revision for severe femoral bone loss: minimum 10-year follow-up. J Arthroplast. 2002;17(8):955–60. https://doi.org/10.1054/arth.2002.35794.
24. Hamilton WG, Cashen DV, Ho H, Hopper RH, Engh CA. Extensively porous-coated stems for femoral revision. A choice for all seasons. J Arthroplasty. 2007;22(4 Suppl):106–10. https://doi.org/10.1016/j.arth.2007.01.002.
25. Chung LH, Wu PK, Chen CF, Chen WM, Chen TH, Liu CL. Extensively porous-coated stems for femoral revision: reliable choice for stem revision in Paprosky femoral type III defects. Orthopedics. 2012;35(7):e1017–21. https://doi.org/10.3928/01477447-20120621-13.
26. Sporer SM, Paprosky WG. Revision total hip arthroplasty: the limits of fully coated stems. Clin Orthop Relat Res. 2003;417:203–9. https://doi.org/10.1097/01.blo.0000096803.78689.0c.
27. Iorio R, Healy WL, Presutti AH. A prospective outcomes analysis of femoral component fixation in revision total hip arthroplasty. J Arthroplasty. 2008;23(5):662–9. https://doi.org/10.1016/j.arth.2007.06.009.
28. Philippe H, Nicolas D, Jerome D, Isaac G, Alexandre P, Jerome A, Flouzat Lachaniette CH. Long, titanium, cemented stems decreased late periprosthetic fractures and revisions in patients with severe bone loss and previous revision. Int Orthop. 2015;39(4):639–44. https://doi.org/10.1007/s00264-014-2528-2.
29. Tyson Y, Rolfson O, Kärrholm J, Hailer NP, Mohaddes M. Uncemented or cemented revision stems? Analysis of 2,296 first-time hip revision arthroplasties performed due to aseptic loosening, reported to the Swedish Hip Arthroplasty Register. Acta Orthop. 2019;90(5):421–6. https://doi.org/10.1080/17453674.2019.1624336.
30. Weiss RJ, Stark A, Kärrholm J. A modular cementless stem vs. cemented long-stem prostheses in revision surgery of the hip: a population-based study from the Swedish Hip Arthroplasty Register. Acta Orthop. 2011;82(2):136–42. https://doi.org/10.3109/17453674.2011.566145.
31. Otero JE, Martin JR, Rowe TM, Odum SM, Mason JB. Radiographic and clinical outcomes of modular tapered fluted stems for femoral revision for Paprosky III and IV femoral defects or Vancouver B2 and B3 femoral fractures. J Arthroplasty. 2020;35(4):1069–73. https://doi.org/10.1016/j.arth.2019.11.039.
32. Abdel MP, Cottino U, Larson DR, Hanssen AD, Lewallen DG, Berry DJ. Modular fluted tapered stems in aseptic revision total hip arthroplasty. J Bone

Joint Surg Am. 2017;99(10):873–81. https://doi.org/10.2106/JBJS.16.00423. Lippincott Williams and Wilkins.

33. Huang Y, Zhou Y, Shao H, Gu J, Tang H, Tang Q. What is the difference between modular and non-modular tapered fluted titanium stems in revision total hip arthroplasty. J Arthroplasty. 2017;32(10):3108–13. https://doi.org/10.1016/j.arth.2017.05.021.
34. Malkani AL, Paiso JM, Sim FH. Proximal femoral replacement with megaprosthesis. Instr Course Lect. 2000;49:141–6.
35. Parvizi J, Tarity TD, Slenker N, Wade F, Trappler R, Hozack WJ, Sim FH. Proximal femoral replacement in patients with non-neoplastic conditions. J Bone Joint Surg Am. 2007;89(5):1036–43. https://doi.org/10.2106/JBJS.F.00241.
36. Viste A, Perry KI, Taunton MJ, Hanssen AD, Abdel MP. Proximal femoral replacement in contemporary revision total hip arthroplasty for severe femoral bone loss: a review of outcomes. Bone Joint J. 2017;99-B(3):325–9. https://doi.org/10.1302/0301-620X.99B3.BJJ-2016-0822.R1.
37. Grammatopoulos G, Alvand A, Martin H, Whitwell D, Taylor A, Gibbons CLMH. Five-year outcome of proximal femoral endoprosthetic arthroplasty for non-tumour indications. Bone Joint J. 2016;98-B(11):1463–70. https://doi.org/10.1302/0301-620X.98B11.BJJ-2016-0244.R1.
38. Parvizi J, Sim FH. Proximal femoral replacements with megaprostheses. Clin Orthop Relat Res. 2004;420:169–75. https://doi.org/10.1097/00003086-200403000-00023.
39. Lee SH, Ahn YJ, Chung SJ, Kim BK, Hwang JH. The use of allograft prosthesis composite for extensive proximal femoral bone deficiencies: a 2- to 9.8-year follow-up study. J Arthroplast. 2009;24(8):1241–8. https://doi.org/10.1016/j.arth.2009.06.006.
40. Sakellariou VI, Babis GC. Management bone loss of the proximal femur in revision hip arthroplasty: update on reconstructive options. World J Orthop. 2014;5(5):614–22. https://doi.org/10.5312/wjo.v5.i5.614.
41. Rogers BA, Sternheim A, De Iorio M, Backstein D, Safir O, Gross AE. Proximal femoral allograft in revision hip surgery with severe femoral bone loss: a systematic review and meta-analysis. J Arthroplast. 2012;27(6):829–36.e1. https://doi.org/10.1016/j.arth.2011.10.014.
42. Fetzer GB, Callaghan JJ, Templeton JE, Goetz DD, Sullivan PM, Johnston RC. Impaction allografting with cement for extensive femoral bone loss in revision hip surgery: a 4- to 8-year follow-up study. J Arthroplast. 2001;16(8 Suppl 1):195–202. https://doi.org/10.1054/arth.2001.29136.
43. Gie GA, Linder L, Ling RS, Simon JP, Slooff TJ, Timperley AJ. Impacted cancellous allografts and cement for revision total hip arthroplasty. J Bone Joint Surg Br. 1993;75(1):14–21.
44. Leone WA, Naughton M, Gratto-Cox G, Luland CM, Kilgore JE, Hill GE. The effect of preoperative planning and impaction grafting surgical technique on intraoperative and postoperative complication rate for femoral revision patients with moderate to severe bone loss. J Arthroplast. 2008;23(3):383–94. https://doi.org/10.1016/j.arth.2007.02.017.
45. Buttaro MA, Comba F, Piccaluga F. Proximal femoral reconstructions with bone impaction grafting and metal mesh. Clin Orthop Relat Res. 2009;467(9):2325–34. https://doi.org/10.1007/s11999-009-0777-y.
46. Lamberton TD, Kenny PJ, Whitehouse SL, Timperley AJ, Gie GA. Femoral impaction grafting in revision total hip arthroplasty. J Arthroplast. 2011;26(8):1154–60. https://doi.org/10.1016/j.arth.2011.03.028.
47. Wilson MJ, Hook S, Whitehouse SL, Timperley AJ, Gie GA. Femoral impaction bone grafting in revision hip arthroplasty 705 cases from the originating centre. Bone Joint J. 2016;98-B(12):1611–9. https://doi.org/10.1302/0301-620X.98B12.37414.
48. Diaz-Dilernia F, Slullitel PA, Oñativia JI, Comba FM, Piccaluga F, Buttaro MA. Impaction bone grafting or uncemented modular stems for the treatment of type B3 periprosthetic femoral fractures? A complication rate analysis. J Arthroplast. 2019;34(9):2051–7. https://doi.org/10.1016/j.arth.2019.04.047.
49. Friesecke C, Plutat J, Block A. Revision arthroplasty with use of a total femur prosthesis. J Bone Joint Surg Am. 2005;87(12):2693–701. https://doi.org/10.2106/JBJS.D.02770.
50. Grauer JD, Amstutz HC, O'Carroll PF, Dorey FJ. Resection arthroplasty of the hip. J Bone Joint Surg Am. 1989;71(5):669–78.

GPSR Compliance

The European Union's (EU) General Product Safety Regulation (GPSR) is a set of rules that requires consumer products to be safe and our obligations to ensure this.

If you have any concerns about our products, you can contact us on ProductSafety@springernature.com

In case Publisher is established outside the EU, the EU authorized representative is:

Springer Nature Customer Service Center GmbH
Europaplatz 3
69115 Heidelberg, Germany

Batch number: 10731385

Printed by Printforce, the Netherlands